The Hands-on Guide to Surgical Training

The Hands-on Guide to Surgical Training

MATTHEW STEPHENSON
SURGICAL REGISTRAR
South East Thames Rotation

WILEY-BLACKWELL
A John Wiley & Sons, Ltd., Publication

Wiley-Blackwell is an imprint of John Wiley & Sons, formed by the merger of Wiley's global Scientific, Technical and Medical business with Blackwell Publishing.

Registered office: John Wiley & Sons, Ltd, The Atrium, Southern Gate, Chichester, West Sussex, PO19 8SQ, UK

Editorial offices: 9600 Garsington Road, Oxford, OX4 2DQ, UK
The Atrium, Southern Gate, Chichester, West Sussex, PO19 8SQ, UK
111 River Street, Hoboken, NJ 07030-5774, USA

For details of our global editorial offices, for customer services and for information about how to apply for permission to reuse the copyright material in this book please see our website at www.wiley.com/wiley-blackwell.

Library of Congress Cataloging-in-Publication Data
Stephenson, Matthew.
The hands-on guide to surgical training / Matthew Stephenson.
p. ; cm.
Includes bibliographical references and index.
ISBN 978-0-470-67261-7 (pbk. : alk. paper)
I. Title.
[DNLM: 1. Specialties, Surgical. 2. Surgical Procedures, Operative.
3. Vocational Guidance. WO 100]

617′.9076–dc23

2011034251

A catalogue record for this book is available from the British Library.

Set in 8/10 pt Humanist by Toppan Best-set Premedia Limited
Printed and bound in Malaysia by Vivar Printing Sdn Bhd

1 2012

Contents

Preface vi
Introduction vii
Contributors ix
So you want to be a surgeon? xi
Abbreviations xvii

Clinical

1 Theatres 1
- Surgical instruments 1
- Sutures 10
- Theatre etiquette 12
- Patient safety and the WHO surgical checklist 17
- How to write the operation note 22
- Introduction to operative sections 26
- Appendicectomy 26
- Inguinal hernia repair 31
- Dynamic hip screw 37

2 Wards 45
3 Clinics 71
4 On Call 78

Non-clinical

Generic stage

5 The Foundation Years 89
6 The Core Training Years 100
7 The Specialty Training Years 122

Surgical specialties

8 General Surgery 140
9 Urology 148
10 Cardiothoracic Surgery 156
11 Oral and maxillofacial surgery 160
12 Ear, nose and throat surgery (Otorhinolaryngology – head and neck surgery) 166
13 Paediatric surgery 171
14 Neurosurgery 179
15 Orthopaedics 186
16 Plastic Surgery 193

Other issues

17 Applying for Jobs 201
18 Flexible Training and Women in Surgery 219
19 Academic Surgery 225
20 Other Issues in Surgical Training 233
21 Fellowships 250
22 Approaching Consultancy 256

Appendix 1: Preoperative assessment 264
Appendix 2: Consent 286
Appendix 3: Local Anaesthetics 292

Index 295

Preface

It is a most gratifying sign of the rapid progress of our time that our best textbooks become antiquated so quickly.
Theodor Billroth (one of the founding fathers of abdominal surgery, 1829–1894)

There has been a need for a coherent resource for surgical trainees along the whole pathway of training for many years now, to offer some career advice and practical advice. The problem with writing such a book is in striking the balance between generic advice and specific advice. The former can make the book too vague and unhelpful, the latter means that by the time of publication the book is already long out of date, and this is particularly true in these changeable times post-MMC. Hopefully this book has struck a reasonable balance, but necessarily a book like this can only be historical, future-proofing the contents is impossible.

There are also of course variations in terms of location – some things are done differently between the regions of the UK. Where it's relevant, for instance in matters of recruitment, since the majority of trainees work in England this has generally been discussed primarily; however, where there are regional differences these have all been described.

Never more so is an author setting himself up for becoming out of date almost immediately than when publishing current prices. There would be an argument not to have included money talk at all, but the most recent figures have been included as a rough guide to give the reader an idea of the financial impact surgical training can have. It would be nice to see one set of these financial figures, our salary, become out of date as soon after publication of this book as possible; however, at the time of going to print, the government has frozen doctors' salaries for two years so it's likely, unfortunately, that these will be roughly accurate for longer than we would like.

This is a 'mixed ability' book. There will be bits that may seem irrelevant and too junior for you, or the other way around. Just ignore the bits that aren't helpful to you. The aim of this book is to be useful to a whole range of surgical and would-be surgical trainees. If you're a man, for instance, you probably won't find the Women in surgery section in Chapter 18 very helpful. There is also a need for overseas doctors coming to work in the UK to understand the system, which explains why sometimes the absolute basics are explored.

Finally, whichever career path you decide to follow, be it surgical or non-surgical, hepatopancreaticobiliary or otorhinolaryngology – I wish you the very best of luck.

Introduction

The life so short, the craft so long to learn.
Hippocrates (c. 460 BC–370 BC)

Surgical training has come a long way, for better or for worse. Until the mid-19th century you didn't need to go to university to become a surgeon. If you had the inclination for cutting people open with little or no anaesthetic, you would attach yourself to an already established surgeon. Much like becoming a tradesman's apprentice. Meanwhile our wealthier medical forebears would be living it up at university gaining a doctorate. They'd become 'Dr So and So', while we'd still be Mr (and no one's changed that system since, in most of the UK). We would at least have had to take an examination at the end of our apprenticeship and in London this was conducted by the Surgeons' Company, formed in 1745 as a break-away group from the Worshipful Company of Barbers. This illustriously named group was formed in 1308.

Back in those days a religious monk would be your GP, attending to all your medical and surgical needs. However, under papal decree they weren't allowed to spill blood, and given that practically all treatments back then involved spilling blood, this was an obstacle to them doing a good day's work. So they would work with the barbers who would not only give you a short back and sides and a wet shave, but chop off your leg, too.

Over the centuries surgery gradually became more advanced, hence the split in 1745 following power struggles between the barbers and the barber surgeons. In 1800, the Surgeons' Company became the Royal College of Surgeons of England. The Royal College of Surgeons of Edinburgh, however, claims a longer independent history, being formed in 1505 but with a not that dissimilar background of barber origins, too.

What on earth has all this got to do with you getting an ST3 job? Well not much actually. The more recent history of surgical training, however, will have an impact (see Chapter 20). It must be basic human nature that every generation believes themselves to be in the middle of the greatest change in history, be it in 1745, 1800 or 2012. Nevertheless, it can't be disputed that Modernising Medical Careers, the New Deal, the European Working Time Directive, public disclosure of outcome figures and even the fallout from Harold Shipman, have rocked our modern world of surgery. They have resulted in reduced working times, altered career progression and changes in how we prove our competence and probity. However, whatever changes politicians, managers or even senior doctors make, the core fundamentals of learning how to be a surgeon remain the same as they were during the time of the Worshipful Company of Barbers: study the theory of surgery and practise the art.

As a surgical trainee you'll spend your working day between four specific clinical categories: theatre, wards, clinic and on call. So that's how the clinical chapters have been arranged. The aim is not to repeat the basic science of surgery – that's been covered extensively elsewhere – it's to help with the practical aspects of working as a surgical trainee. For example, what are all those surgical instruments called? How do you effectively lead a surgical ward round? How long postop do you take out a T-tube and why? A complex discussion about aetiopathogenesis it is not. Furthermore, the clinical section is weighted towards general surgery. This is because general surgical jobs are far commoner than paediatric or cardiothoracic surgical attachments and to go into the minutiae of clinical management in each of the surgical disciplines would make this into a very different book.

The other main section of the book is related not to clinical work, but to all other non-clinical areas, much of it to assist in career guidance. There are three chapters relating to the three stages of training: foundation, core and specialty, which cover the generic aspects of those years. Each is divided into sections such as the aims of that stage, recruitment processes and competition, courses to attend and exams to take.

Following this there is a detailed look at each of the nine surgical specialties written by a senior trainee or consultant working in each of them, giving you an inside look at the specialty: how that specialty recruits, what it's like at core training level, specialty training level and consultant level, along with recommended courses to attend.

Finally we look at the process of getting jobs, women in surgery, flexible training, research and clinical governance, political issues affecting surgery and the end game of training: consultancy.

Contributors

Mr Sam Andrews MA, MS, FRCS (Gen.Surg)
Consultant Vascular Surgeon
Medway NHS Foundation Trust

Mr Sion P Barnard MSc, FRCS (C-Th)
Consultant Thoracic Surgeon
Freeman Hospital, Newcastle

Miss Ginny Bowbrick FRCS (Gen.Surg)
Consultant Vascular Surgeon
Medway NHS Foundation Trust

Mr Richard Burnham MFDS, MRCS
Specialty Registrar Oral and Maxillofacial Surgery
West Midlands Deanery

Mr Christopher M Butler MS, FRCS
Consultant General Surgeon
Medway Maritime Hospital

Miss Clare Byrne FRCS
Consultant General and Colorectal Surgeon
Lewisham Healthcare NHS Trust

Miss Sophie J Camp MA (Oxon), MRCS, PhD
Neurosurgery Specialty Registrar
Charing Cross Hospital, London

Ms Tamzin Cuming FRCS (Gen.Surg)
Colorectal Specialty Registrar
North East Thames Rotation

Miss Helen Dent MSc, MRCS
Surgical Trainee
Medway Maritime Hospital

Mr George HC Evans MA, MChir, FRCS
Consultant General and Vascular Surgeon
East Sussex Hospitals NHS Trust

Mr Iain Findlay MRCS
Trauma and Orthopaedics Specialty Registrar
King's College Hospital, London

Mrs Cheryl Funnell RGN
Lead Practitioner, General and Emergency Team and Registered Nurse
East Sussex Hospitals NHS Trust

Dr Shelly Griffiths MB, BS, MA (Cantab)
Core Surgical Trainee
South West Peninsula Deanery

Mr Amyn Haji MA, MSc, FRCS (Gen. Surg)
Consultant Colorectal Surgeon
King's College Hospital, London

Mrs Lisa Leonard BA, MSc, FRCS (Tr and Orth)
Consultant Orthopaedic Surgeon
Brighton and Sussex University Hospitals

Mr Wasim Mahmalji MSc, MRCS
Urology Specialty Registrar
South Thames Rotation

Miss Petra Marsh BSc, MRCS
Surgical Specialty Registrar
South East Thames Rotation

Mr James E Mitchell MRCS
ENT Specialty Registrar
St George's Hospital, London

Mr Max Pachl MRCS
Paediatric Surgery Specialty Registrar
Birmingham Children's Hospital

Mr Sofiane Rimouche BMedSci, MRCS
Plastic Surgery Specialty Registrar
North Western Rotation

Mr Matt Stephenson MSc, MRCS
General Surgical Specialty Registrar
South East Thames Rotation

Stephen Whitehead MChir, FRCS
Consultant General Surgeon
East Sussex Hospitals NHS Trust

So you want to be a surgeon?

You must always be students, learning and unlearning till your life's end, and if, gentlemen, you are not prepared to follow your profession in this spirit, I implore you to leave its ranks and betake yourself to some third-class trade.
Joseph Lister (British surgeon, 1827–1912)

Few careers could possibly offer as much opportunity for witnessing human suffering and being able to cure it, or for acquiring such a vast scientific knowledge and applying it to something so tangible. Not to mention the job security, the earning potential, the global portability and even the social status.

There are many great things about being a surgeon but there are also some drawbacks, some big drawbacks. Few careers could possibly offer as much opportunity for witnessing human suffering and making it even worse, or take so long and so much effort to acquire the vast scientific knowledge and experience required. Not to mention the unsociable hours, the career dead ends, the burdensome responsibility or the low pay compared with equivalent positions in the city.

Despite all this, surgical training remains highly competitive. It's not worth bothering unless you're sure that the pros outweigh the cons for you. The problem there is how could you possibly know until you've tried it? And not just as a foundation doctor or core trainee. Until you've felt the pain of an operation you've performed go badly wrong, or the gut wrenching ache of a major decision you've made lead to a serious adverse outcome, or had your finger up an nonagenarian's backside at 3am on a Saturday night because you're still doing nights well into your thirties, can you really see past the glamour of life as a surgeon.

In the not too distant past, trainees had, to all intents and purposes, as much time as they liked to try out different surgical jobs in the form of senior house officer posts – gaining experience, preparing for exams and confirming or refuting in their minds whether surgery was right for them. Modernising Medical Careers changed all that and you are now expected to commit at an earlier stage and choose a specialty much sooner. Neurosurgery, for instance, currently recruits nationally from FY2 to run-through training to consultant level. Because of the European Working Time Directive you'll also have less time at work to get the experience you need to make up your mind.

All of that said, you need to decide carefully – very carefully – and after taking as much advice from people as you can, that surgery is right for you. Many people don't, won't or can't see beyond the glossy side. If you're in it, at worst for the money and social status or at best because you like the idea of cutting things out of people and making them better, think again. There are other jobs that pay far better and for all the patients for whom you have the satisfaction of a clean, complication-free operation, there are many more you'll have to treat for chronic conditions, non-operative conditions or conditions serious enough that they're in ITU for months. Not everything in surgery will give you such quick gratification.

People often have misleading notions about who makes a good surgeon and you need to be cautious when interpreting their advice to you and establish **why** they think you'll be a good surgeon. For instance, you will not be better suited to surgery just because you are: (a) a rugby player; (b) dislike medicine; (c) like making snappy decisions; (d) have a type A personality; and (e) are male.

Forget the stereotype. Gregarious male rugby players who dislike the slower pace of medicine and like making snappy decisions do not make better surgeons than anyone else. Being a good surgeon requires a distinct skill set unrelated to sporting prowess.

1 You must be **intelligent**, at least as intelligent as a medic. You need to grasp in full detail, complex anatomy, physiological principles and the pathology that affects them.

2 You must be able to **make a decision**. Not a snappy one, you need a mind that can quickly and efficiently process information, weigh it, come to a conclusion and deliver your decision. And it must be with the acceptance that it might be wrong but you will learn from it. To be excessively scared of making difficult decisions quickly for fear of getting it wrong is a contraindication to surgery as a career.

3 You must be able to **cope under pressure** and **retain your judgement**.

4 You must be reasonably **dextrous**, with **good hand–eye coordination** and **spatial awareness**.

5 Whatever any moderniser says, you must accept a **work–life balance heavily weighted towards work**. Not only may you still be doing nights 10 years after qualifying when your family is at home, but to get the necessary experience you'll have to accept coming in on days off and staying late where necessary.

6 You must be **tough skinned** enough to **cope with your own failure**, with suffering, with covert bullying, with not getting jobs and with the hours, but not so much that you don't lose your humanity.

7 You must be **prepared to jump through hoops**: audit, exams, courses, interviews, publications, etc., and be patient enough to still be competing with others for career development and doing exams even though your contemporaries may have already reached the heights of their careers.

8 You must be a **good communicator**, like any other doctor.

9 You must like **working in a team**, taking both team participant and team leader roles readily.

10 You must like **problem solving**, although this is by no means specific to surgery.

Despite all the challenges and drawbacks of choosing to train in surgery you will be rewarded with some indescribably wonderful experiences in life if you do. It's difficult to compare the satisfaction from saving life or limb, in a way that no other specialty does. Learning the craft of surgery – the feel of putting knife to skin, dissecting out a tumour, identifying and preserving structures that you become familiar with like old friends, fixing broken bones, decompressing suffocating neural tissue, taking out old worn-out and putting in new – brings a kind of pleasure to your work that's impossible to explain to one who's never experienced it. Once you've had a taste, you'll know if it's for you.

I'm a medical student, what should I do now?

So if you've given it the requisite thought and decided yes, I am going to ruin my life and become a surgeon, what should you do now to increase the chances of success. Actually there's quite a lot, and it all relates to showing your early commitment to surgery.

1 Most importantly, start developing your **portfolio** (see Chapter 7). Obviously to begin with there won't be much to put in it, but every little bit helps.

2 Join, or if there isn't one already set up, a **local surgical society** at your medical school. The Royal College of Surgeons has information on its website to help form these. For bonus points you could sit on the Medical Student Liaison Committee (MSLC).

3 Take an **elective** with a surgical attachment.

4 Attend a free **surgical careers afternoon** at the Royal College of Surgeons (run twice a year) – you'll get a free certificate to kick your portfolio off.

5 Become an **affiliate member** of the Royal College of Surgeons (£15 per annum).

6 Get involved in a surgical **audit** – best done during a surgical attachment – someone's bound to be doing one, so get involved.

7 Do an **intercalated BSc** – it doesn't have to be, but ideally would be surgically related. Whatever it is, work hard and aim to get a publication out of it. Even just one publication will stand you in good stead for years to come.

8 Unrelated to a BSc, ask around at your nearest surgical academic department and offer to do anything to get involved in **research** that might lead to a paper.

9 **Work hard** academically – winning **prizes** in medical school will provide more points on future application forms than you realise. There's often a section for prizes and most people have to leave it empty.

10 **Prizes prizes prizes**. Apply for the Professor Harold Ellis Medical Student Prize for Surgery run through the RCS; the Hunterian Society offers a prize, as do many other local surgical societies – keep your ear to the ground.

11 Go on the **Systematic Training in Acute Illness Recognition and Treatment for Surgery** (START Surgery) course run by the Royal College of Surgeons for final year medical students and foundation doctors.

12 Join ASIT (Association of Surgeons in Training). This is now possible for medical student and costs £30 per annum. It will keep you abreast of current issues in surgical training.

13 If you're a woman, join **Women in Surgery** (see Chapter 18).

What kind of surgery?

Obviously it isn't enough just to say you want to be a surgeon, eventually (but not for a good while if you're still a medical student or foundation doctor) you'll have to decide which area of surgery interests you most. There are nine specialties within surgery:

- cardiothoracic surgery
- general surgery
- neurosurgery
- oral and maxillofacial surgery
- otorhinolaryngology (ENT)
- paediatric surgery
- plastic surgery
- trauma and orthopaedic surgery
- urology.

In addition to this, there is the field of academic surgery, which is heavily weighted towards research. Furthermore, by around 2013, it's likely that vascular surgery will have split off from general surgery altogether to have formed its own independent tenth specialty. There are more detailed exposés of these specialties in Chapters 8–16, but the following is a brief idea. Besides each specialty is the number of ST3 posts that were available in that specialty nationally in 2008 and the ratio of applications to posts the same year (for a more thorough look at competition ratios, see Chapter 8).

Cardiothoracic surgery (2008, 5 posts; ratio 1 : 23)

Heart, lungs, oesophagus and other chest disorders. You would eventually choose either cardiac or thoracic, not both usually. It also includes transplantation surgery. Common cardiac operations are coronary artery bypass grafting and valve operations, while thoracic ones are lobectomies and pneumonectomies, now more often thoracoscopic rather than open. Much of the work over the past decade has been extracted by cardiologists, as endovascular techniques have gained in popularity. It's a very intensive career choice with often complex patients.

General surgery (2008, 80 posts; ratio 1 : 19)

A very large specialty now in practice split into many smaller subspecialties. It's no longer possible to become a 'true' general surgeon and be able to cover the whole range unfortunately. The main subspecialties are:

- upper gastrointestinal
- lower gastrointestinal
- hepatopancreaticobiliary
- breast
- transplant
- vascular
- endocrine

Generally, you would subspecialise in one of these but would continue to do a general workload so that there are enough consultants to cover the on-call commitments but your elective work will be more limited to your subspecialty. Often now, however, new breast consultants will specialise only in breast, and vascular consultants only in vascular. This trend will almost certainly continue.

Neurosurgery (2008, 5 posts (ST1); ratio 1 : 5)

Brain, spinal cord and peripheral nerves. For a small specialty it's also quite subspecialised with areas including paediatric, neuro-oncology, functional neurosurgery, skull-base surgery and spinal surgery (the largest). The patients are often very high dependency and a strong grasp of neurology is essential. Neurosurgery is unique in that there is run-through recruitment at ST1 level, not ST3. Applicants frequently are very well qualified, often with postgraduate degrees.

Oral and maxillofacial surgery (OMFS) (2008, 17 posts; ratio 1 : 13)

Facial bones, face and neck. You have to hold both a medical and dental degree, so the training pathway is slightly longer, but not as much as you might think (see Chapter 11). On-call commitments are low. The unique thing about OMFS is the opportunity to combine operating on both bone and soft tissue in good measure.

Otorhinolaryngology (ENT) (2008, 19 posts; ratio 1 : 14)

Head and neck, skull base and facial plastics. There is a heavy preponderance of day case work – much time is spent on diagnosis and outpatient treatment. On-call commitments are quite low.

Paediatric surgery (2008, 1 post; ratio 1 : 40)

From the fetal period to the teenage years (usually 16 is the cut-off). The vast majority of surgery on children is performed by non-specialist paediatric surgeons; however, some conditions require specialist input, especially in the very young or in oncology. Day case surgery is particularly common. You will be limited to the geographical location you can work; this specialty is small.

Plastic surgery (2008, 9 posts; ratio 1 : 23)

Essentially surgery on the soft tissues, mainly reconstructive. Common elective cases are breast reconstruction, cleft lip and palate, and other facial deformities. Emergency work includes hand trauma and burns. On-call commitment is quite high, especially with burns, and severe facial and hand injuries. There is also the option of training in cosmetic surgery.

Trauma and orthopaedic surgery (2008, 50 posts; ratio 1 : 15)

Bones, joints and associated soft tissues. Also quite subspecialised to regional areas, e.g. knee, hip, foot and ankle, etc., although for emergency work you will continue to cover the whole range. There is quite a demanding on-call component.

Urology (2008, 14 posts; ratio 1 : 15)

The urogenital system. Common pathology you'd deal with includes renal stones, cancer (especially of the prostate, bladder, testis and kidney), incontinence, erectile dysfunction and prostate disorders. Much of urology can be done on a day case or even outpatient basis.

Career structure overview

As things stand, after qualifying as a doctor you will undertake two years as a foundation doctor. During this time you will want to undertake as many surgical jobs as possible, as well as an A&E post. You then apply for a core surgical training rotation, which lasts two years and generally comprises six-month jobs (or apply directly to ST1 run-through neurosurgery). It's during this time you will be expected to get your Membership of the Royal College of Surgeons (MRCS) exams, and in the case of ENT trainees, your Diploma in Otolaryngology – Head and Neck Surgery (DOHNS) diploma. The pathway for OMFS trainees is entirely different (see Chapter 11). This is the time to get your final preparation in order for competition into higher surgical training.

Once you've completed your core training posts and obtained MRCS you would apply for ST3 in your chosen specialty – this is essentially a first-year registrar job. If you don't have MRCS yet, or for various other reasons, you might do a CT3 year, which is essentially a grace year – you won't be able to proceed to ST3 without MRCS. From ST3 you rotate through your region in six-month jobs covering various areas of your specialty, and you usually have to choose your subspecialty. All the specialties go up to ST8 except urology, which runs to ST7.

Once you've successfully completed your registrar years, and have passed the exit exam in your chosen specialty you can apply for a Certificate of Completion of Training (CCT), which entitles you to enter your name on the specialist register and apply for a consultant job.

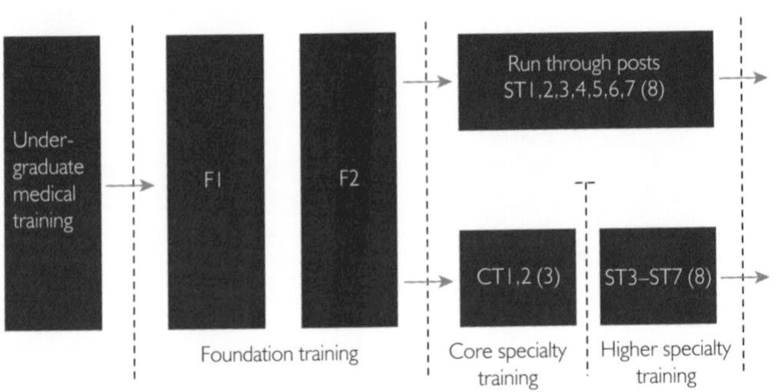

(Diagram adapted from image by David Rice, KSS Deanary, 2008)

Abbreviations

ABPI	ankle-brachial pressure index
ACCS	acute common care stem
ACF	Academic Clinical Fellowship
AES	assigned educational supervisor
ALS	Advanced Life Support
AP	anteroposterior
APLS	Advanced Paediatric Life Support
ARCP	Annual Review of Competence Progression
ARR	absolute risk reduction
ASA	American Association of Anesthesiologists
ASGBI	Association of Surgeons of Great Britain & Northern Ireland
ASIS	anterior superior iliac spine
ASIT	Association of Surgeons in Training
ATLS	Advanced Trauma Life Support
AUA	American Urological Association
AUGIS	Association of Upper Gastrointestinal Surgeons
BAAPS	British Association of Aesthetic Surgeons
BBA	British Burns Association
BAETS	British Association of Endocrine & Thyroid Surgeons
BAOMS	British Association of Oral and Maxillofacial Surgeons
BAPES	British Association of Paediatric Endoscopic Surgeons
BAPRAS	British Association of Plastic Reconstructive and Aesthetic Surgery
BAPS	British Association of Paediatric Surgeons
BAPU	British Association of Paediatric Urologists
BAUS	British Association of Urological Surgeons
BOTA	British Orthopaedic Trainee's Association
BSS	Basic Surgical Skills
BSSH	British Society for Surgery of the Hand
CABG	coronary artery bypass graft
CBD	case-based discussion
CCAM	congenital cystic adenomatous malformation
CCBST	Certificate of Completion of Basic Surgical Training
CCLG	Childrens Cancer and Leukaemia Group
CCrISP	Care of the Critically Ill Surgical Patient
CCT	Certificate of Completion of Training
CEPOD	Confidential Enquiry into Peri Operative Deaths
CEX	clinical evaluation exercise
CfWI	Centre for Workforce Intelligence
CI	confidence interval

CNS central nervous system

CONSORT Consolidated Standards of Reporting Trials

COPD chronic obstructive pulmonary disease

CPR cardiopulmonary resuscitation

CRP C-reactive protein

CSDH chronic subdural haematoma

CSF cerebrospinal fluid

CT computed tomography; core training

CTA computed tomography angiography

CTPA computed tomography pulmonary angiogram

CV curriculum vitae

CVP central venous pressure

DP dorsalis pedis

CH Department of Health

DHS dynamic hip screw

DNAR do not attempt resuscitation

DNUK Doctors.net.uk

DOHNS Diploma in Otolaryngology – Head and Neck Surgery

DOPS direct observation of procedural skills

DRE digital rectal examination

DSA digital subtraction angiography

DVT deep vein thrombosis

EAU European Association of Urology

ECG electrocardiogram

ECMO extracorporeal membrane oxygenation

EEA European Economic Area

eLPRAS e-learning plastic surgery resource

EMI extended matching item

ERCP endoscopic retrograde cholangiopancreatography

ESPU European Society for Paediatric Urologists

EUA examination under anaesthetic

EUPSA European Association of Paediatric Surgeons

EVAR endovascular aneurysm repair

EVD external ventricular drain

EWDT European Working Time Directive

FACD Foundation Achievement of Competency Document

FAST focused assessment sonography in trauma

FNA fine needle aspiration

FRCS Fellowship of the Royal College of Surgeons

FS Foundation School

FTSTA fixed-term specialty training appointment

FY foundation year

GA general anaesthetic

GB gall bladder

GCS Glasgow Coma Scale

GI gastrointestinal

GMC General Medical Council

GTN glyceryl trinitrate

HCG human chorionic gonadotropin

HIDA hepatobiliary iminodiacetic acid

HPB hepatopancreaticobiliary

HST higher surgical training

ICH intracerebral haematoma

ICP intracranial pressure

IF impact factor

IMCA Independent Mental Capacity Advocate

IPEG	International Paediatric Endosurgery Group
ISCP	Intercollegiate Surgical Curriculum Programme
IV	intravenous
IVC	inferior vena cava
JCST	Joint Committee on Surgical Training
LAS	locum appointment for service
LAT	locum appointment for training
LCP	Liverpool Care Pathway
LDH	lactate dehydrogenase
LTFT	Less Than Full Time Training
MBOS	Maximum Surgical Blood Ordering Schedule
MCA	Mental Capacity Act
MCQ	multiple-choice question
MDT	multidisciplinary team
MMC	Modernising Medical Careers
MPET	Multi Professional Education and Training
MRA	magnetic resonance angiography
MRCS	Membership of the Royal College of Surgeons
MRI	magnetic resonance imaging
MSF	multi-source feedback
MSLC	Medical Student Liaison Committee
MSU	mid-stream urine
MTAS	Medical Training Application Service
NCEPOD	National Confidential Enquiry into Patient Outcome and Death
NEC	necrotising enterocolitis
NES	NHS Education for Scotland
NG	nasogastric
NHSLA	NHS Litigation Authority
NICU	neonatal critical care
NNT	number needed to treat
NPSA	National Patient Safety Agency
NSAID	non-steroidal anti-inflammatory drug
NTN	national training number
OCAP	Orthopaedic Curriculum and Assessment Project
OGD	oesophagogastroduodenoscopy
OMFS	oral and maxillofacial surgery
OOP	Out of Programme
OOPC	Out of Programme for Career Breaks
OOPE	Out of Programme for Clinical Experience
OOPR	Out of Programme for Research
OOPT	Out of Programme for Approved Clinical Training
OSATS	Objective Structured Assessments of Technical Skills
OSCE	Objective Structured Clinical Examination
PACS	picture archiving and communications system
PALS	Paediatric Advanced Life Support
PAT	peer assessment tools
PBA	procedure-based assessment
PD	programme director
PE	pulmonary embolus
PEG	percutaneous endoscopic gastrostomy
PICU	paediatric critical care

PLASTA	Plastic Surgery Trainees Association
PMETB	Postgraduate Medical Education and Training Board
PPV	patent process vaginalis
PRHO	pre-registration house officer
PT	posterior tibial
RCS	Royal College of Surgeons
RITA	Record of In-Training Assessment
RR	relative risk
RSM	Royal Society of Medicine
SDOPS	direct observation of procedural skills in surgery
SHO	senior house officer
SpR	specialist registrar
ST	specialty training
STA	Specialist Training Authority
START	Systematic Training in Acute Illness Recognition and Treatment
STEP	Surgeons in Training Education Programme
StR	specialty registrar
STROBE	Strengthening the Reporting of Observational Studies in Epidemiology
TAB	team assessment of behaviour
TEDS	thromboembolic deterrent stockings
TMJ	temporomandibular joint
TOF	tracheo-oesophageal fistula
TPD	training programme director
TTO	to take out
TURBT	transurethral resection of bladder tumour
TURP	transurethral resections of prostate
USMLE	United States Medical Licensing Examination
USS	ultrasound scans
VAC	vacuum-assisted closure
VAD	ventricular assist device
VATS	video-assisted thoracic surgery
VP	ventriculoperitoneal
VTS	vocational training scheme
WBA	workplace-based assessment
WHO	World Health Organization
WOFAPS	World Federation of Associations of Paediatric Surgeons

Chapter 1
THEATRES

Surgical instruments, 1
Sutures, 10
Theatre etiquette, 12
Patient safety and the WHO surgical checklist, 17
How to write the operation note, 22
Introduction to operative sections, 26
Appendicectomy, 26
Inguinal hernia repair, 31
Dynamic hip screw, 37

Surgical instruments

Matt Stephenson and Cheryl Funnell

Introduction

So many things in surgery are never actually taught; you will just be expected to pick them up by osmosis during your time in theatre. Learning the names of surgical instruments is one of those things. There is no secret course or lecture you've missed, it simply doesn't get taught to trainee surgeons. Yet it sounds so much more professional to ask for Gillies Forceps rather than 'some tweezers'.

One of the big problems with learning the names of instruments is that some hospitals call certain instruments one thing while others call them something else; this is usually the case at least with scissors and forceps. There is little continuity between units, sometimes even day surgery will call an instrument one thing and the main theatres another – all in the same hospital. However, you can turn this to your advantage; you can quite easily make up any name you like, who are they to say you're wrong? OK perhaps not.

Some have eponymous names, others simply are called what they are. Even if you don't learn the eponymous names (if there is one), learn how to describe the instrument, e.g. long dissecting scissors versus stitch cutting scissors. We have used some of the more commonly used names here, but in your own hospital they may very well be different.

There is such a vast array of instruments they cannot all be covered here. The best way to learn each of their names and what their special powers are, is to spend some time with an experienced scrub person.

The Hands-on Guide to Surgical Training, First Edition. Matthew Stephenson.

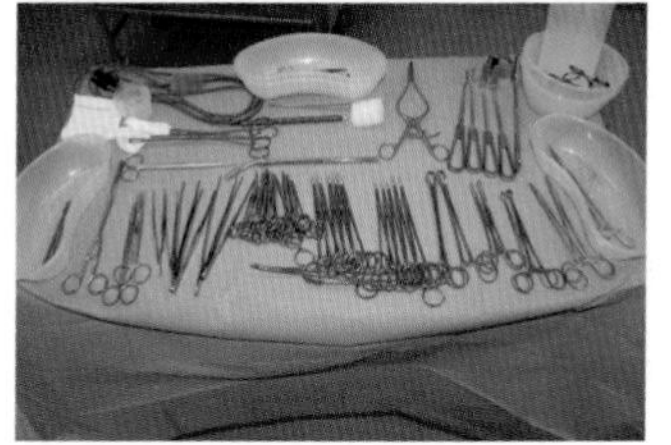

Figure 1.1 A minor basic general set.

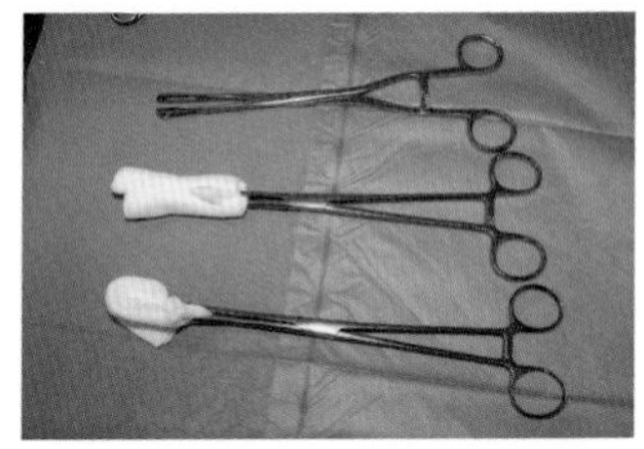

Figure 1.2 Top to bottom: the 'nude' Rampley; swab-on-a-stick; swab mounted for prepping.

Commonly used general instruments

Rampley sponge holder

The **Rampley sponge holder** is frequently used to hold a swab, which can be used to prep the skin and then discarded. You can also wrap a swab around its jaws and use this to dissect or dab blood – the so called **'swab-on-a-stick'**. It's also useful in its own right to grasp hold of the gallbladder and pull it this way and that.

Forceps

Forceps vary first on whether they are **toothed** or **non-toothed**. Toothed forceps are good to grasp the skin edge when closing the subcuticular layer, but never use them in the abdomen where you risk making an enterotomy – non-toothed forceps are much safer for this. They also vary dependent on their length and robustness. The average toothed forceps common to many sets are **Gillies forceps** (although you can get non-toothed versions), whereas **McIndoe forceps** (sometimes called **DeBakey forceps**) are common non-toothed options. **Lanes forceps** can be toothed or non-toothed and are a little larger. More robust tips, for grabbing hold of firmer material such as tendons or cartilage, are **Ramsey forceps**.

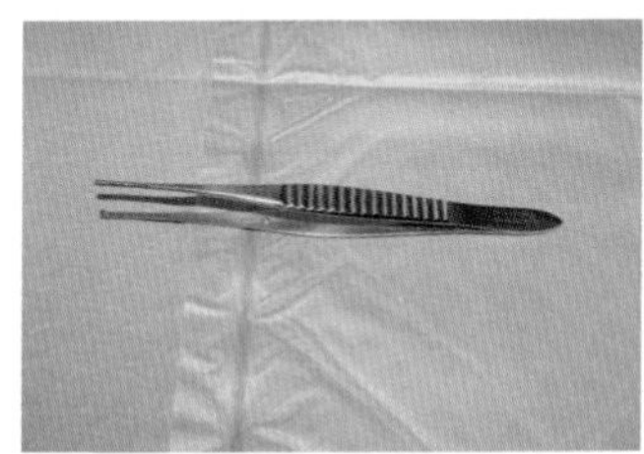

Figure 1.3 Gillies (toothed) forceps.

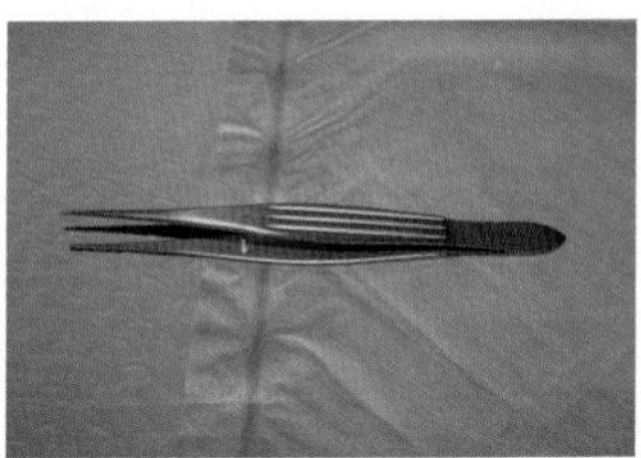

Figure 1.4 McIndoe (non-toothed) forceps.

Scissors

Scissors, broadly speaking, are divided into **dissecting scissors** (such as

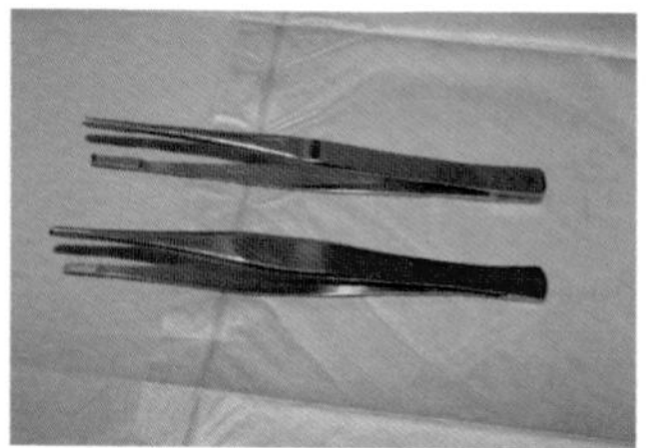

Figure 1.5 Lanes forceps.

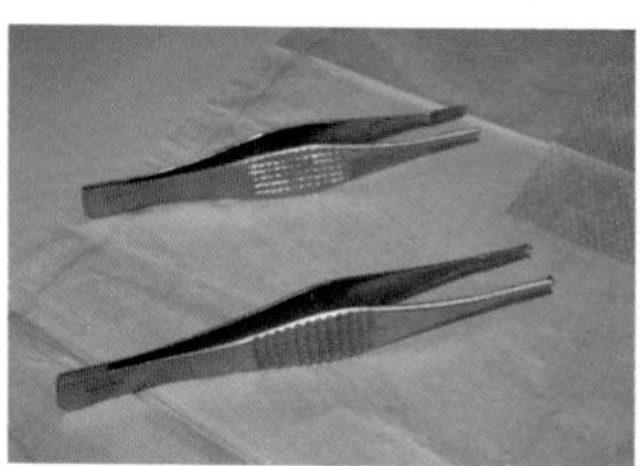

Figure 1.6 Ramsey forceps.

McIndoe scissors) and **stitch-cutting scissors** (such as **Mayo scissors**). You shouldn't use the former to cut stitches because it blunts the blades, and you shouldn't use the latter to dissect as they aren't delicate enough. Sometimes there is tough tissue to cut through, however, such as when opening the abdomen, and here using the Mayo scissors to chomp through the linea alba once the bowel is out of the way is the preferred method for some. They can also be used on tough scar tissue. Dissecting scissors are almost always curved, as this makes dissecting easier. Mayo scissors can be curved or straight.

Haemostatic clips

You'll need something to clamp off vessels, or bits of tissue in which you

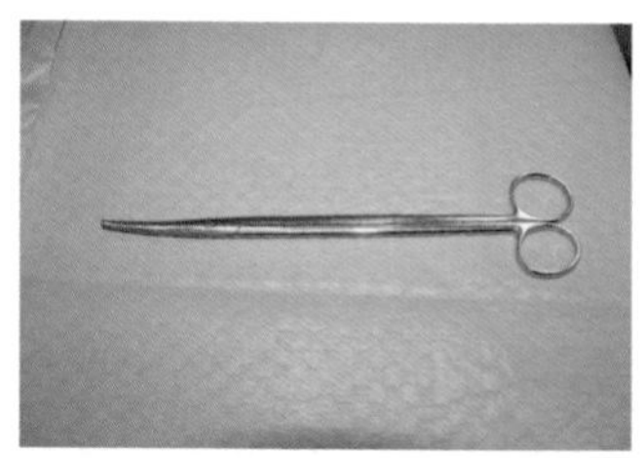

Figure 1.7 McIndoe dissecting scissors.

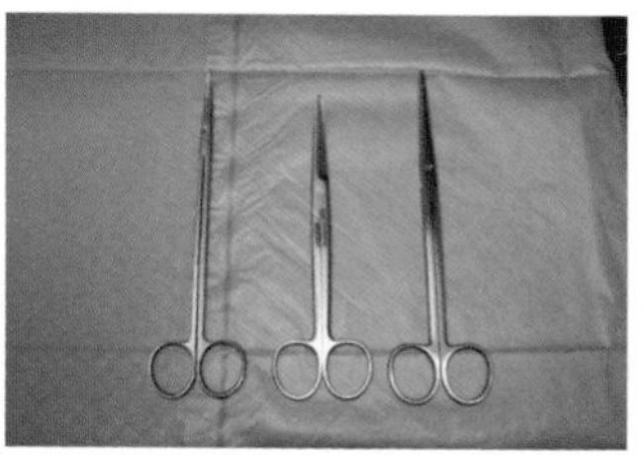

Figure 1.8 Left: McIndoe scissors; middle and right: different lengths of Mayo scissors

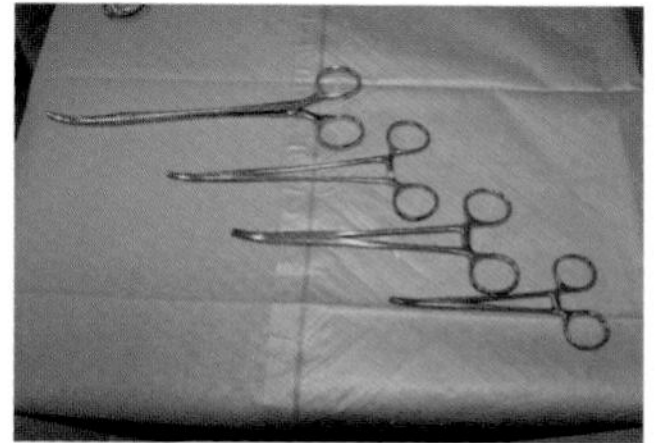

Figure 1.9 Top to bottom: Roberts, Spencer–Wells, Birkett and Dunhill artery forceps.

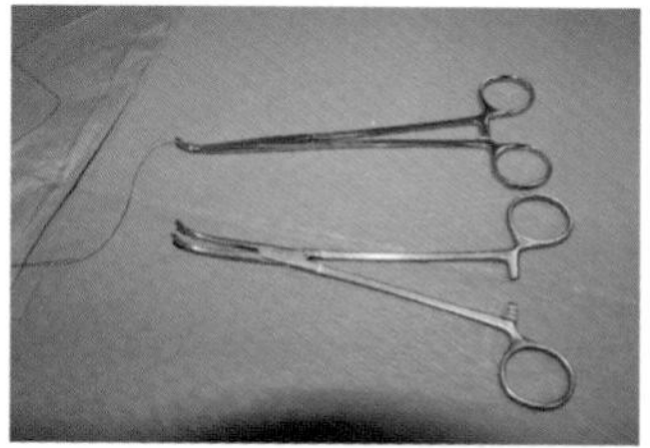

Figure 1.10 Lahey artery forceps.

think there is a vessel. You need a haemostatic clip, or clamp, more confusingly also generally called artery forceps. They range in size, can be straight or curved, and can be slender or thicker. **Mosquito** or **Dunhill artery forceps** are on the smaller side. **Spencer–Wells artery forceps** are average in length but quite slender, whereas **Birkett artery forceps** are fatter and more robust for grasping chunks of tissue. Going up in size are **Roberts artery forceps** and, even bigger for fat chunks of tissue deep in the abdomen for instance, **Moynihan artery forceps.**

Lahey artery forceps have a right-angle turn on their tips. This makes them very useful for dissecting around the back of vessels or ducts, and you can also mount a tie on them and pass it easily around an inaccessible vessel in order to ligate it.

Special tissue-holding forceps

There are three particularly special tissue-holding forceps (the names of which you'll be glad to know are usually quite consistent across the land and therefore worth memorising). **Babcock forceps** have atraumatic tips that are excellent for encircling the appendix or picking up bowel or other tissue. Atraumatic should really be in inverted commas – they **can** damage the serosal surface of the bowel, so when fishing around for the caecum in an appendicectomy you should still be careful. **Allis forceps** are perfect for picking up the subcuticular layer of skin to retract or lift it up, or to place on some tissue that you're resecting and want to draw up into the wound. Beware, however: these cannot be used on bowel – they will damage it. Then there are the **Lanes tissue-holding forceps** (not to be confused with Lane forceps). With very much traumatic tips, they will grasp anything firmly by biting into it, so these should only be used on structures such as the fascia of the abdominal wall – never inside the abdomen.

Needle holders

Needle holders, like everything else, vary depending in length and the robustness of the tip. Clearly a small needle requires a fine tip, a big needle requires a robust tip. A deep suture requires a long needle holder, a skin suture requires a shorter one. If the handles are golden,

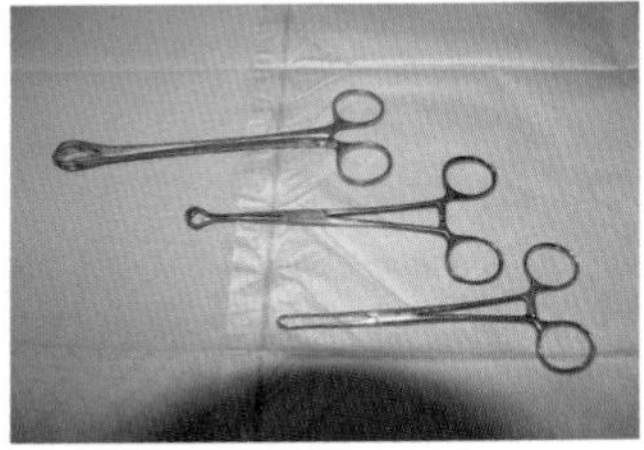

Figure 1.11 Top to bottom: Lanes tissue-holding forceps; Babcock forceps; Allis forceps.

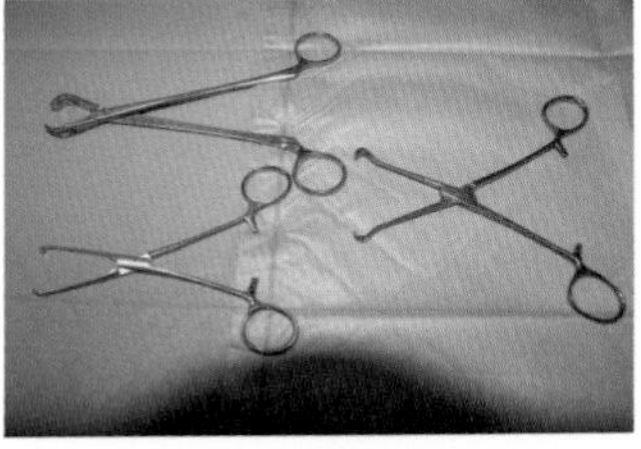

Figure 1.12 Top left: Lanes tissue-holding forceps; bottom left: Allis forceps; right: Babcock forceps.

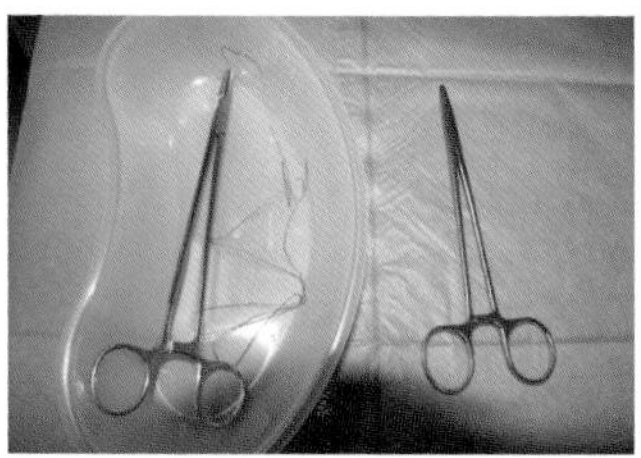

Figure 1.13 Needle holders.

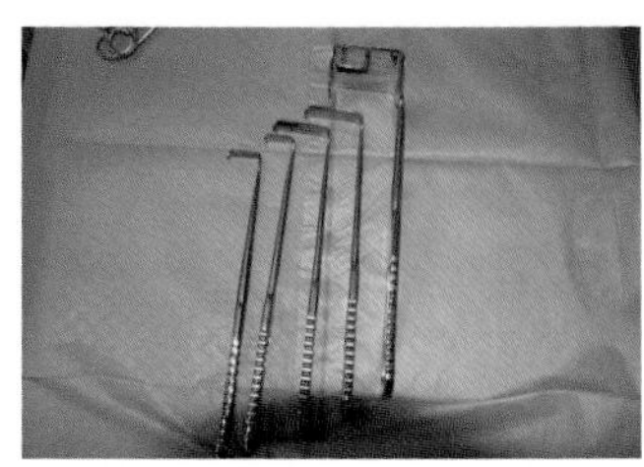

Figure 1.14 Increasing sizes of Langenbeck retractors from left to right, with a Morris retractor far right.

the tips are made from **tungsten carbide** – a very strong needle holder that won't slip.

Retractors

Retractors can be either of the kind that you pull on or the kind that holds itself apart, i.e. self-retaining. Probably the commonest example of the former is the **Langenbeck retractor** – excellent for retracting the edge of a wound – which come in a variety of sizes. An alternative is the **Czerny retractor**, which has two prongs to lift up the skin edge. To retract the abdominal wall you need something more robust like a **Morris retractor** or to retract deeper layers, a **Deaver retractor**.

Sometimes you only need to retract the skin edge, when creating a flap for instance in a mastectomy or thyroidectomy. An instrument with a single hook is a **Gillies skin hook**, and with two hooks a **McIndoe double-prong skin hook**.

The commonest and most 'middle-sized' **self-retaining retractor** is a **Travers retractor**. For a deeper wound, use a very similar instrument – the **Norfolk and Norwich retractor**. If you need a small version, for instance for a temporal artery biopsy, you can use a **West retractor**.

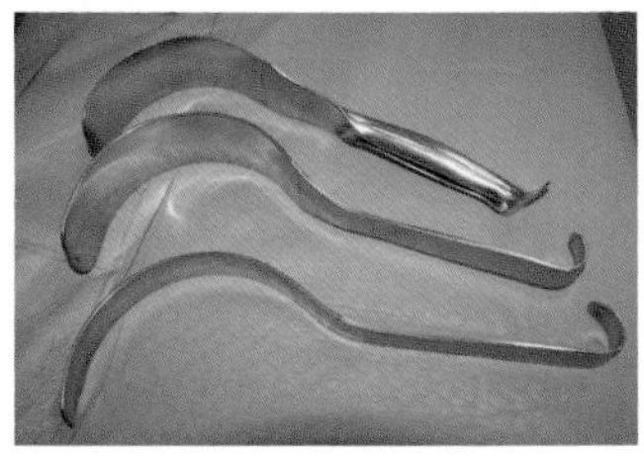

Figure 1.15 Varying shapes and sizes of Deaver retractor.

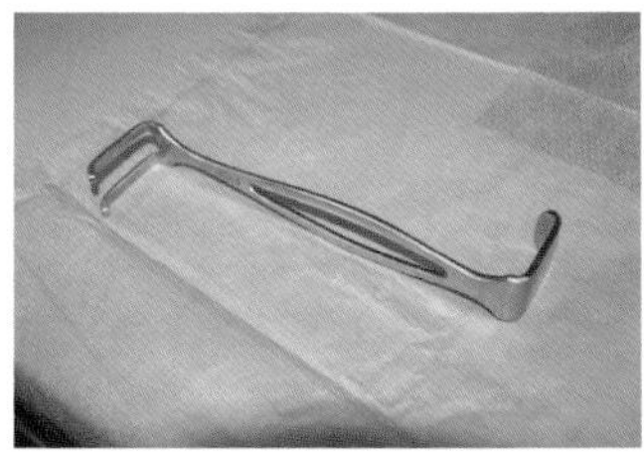

Figure 1.16 Czerny retractor.

Suckers

You're going to want to keep the operative site dry from all that blood you keep

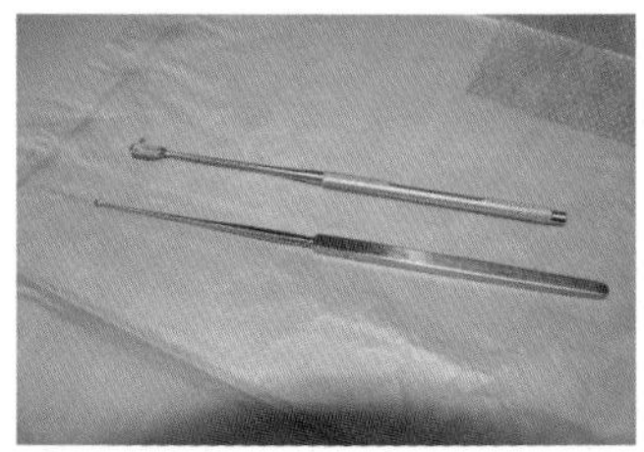

Figure 1.17 Top: McIndoe double-prong skin hook; bottom: Gillies skin hook.

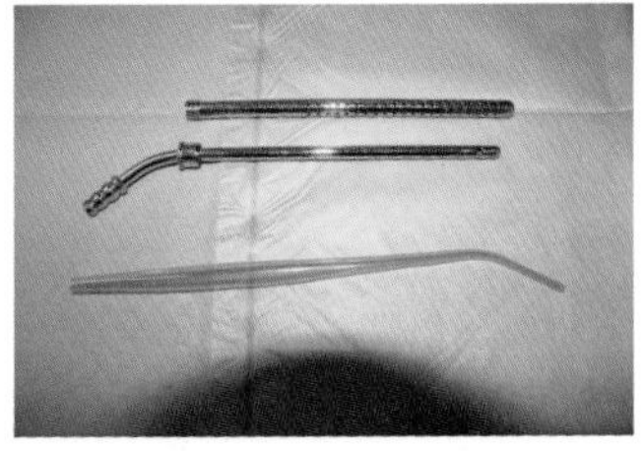

Figure 1.19 Top: Pooles sucker with guard; bottom: Yankauer sucker.

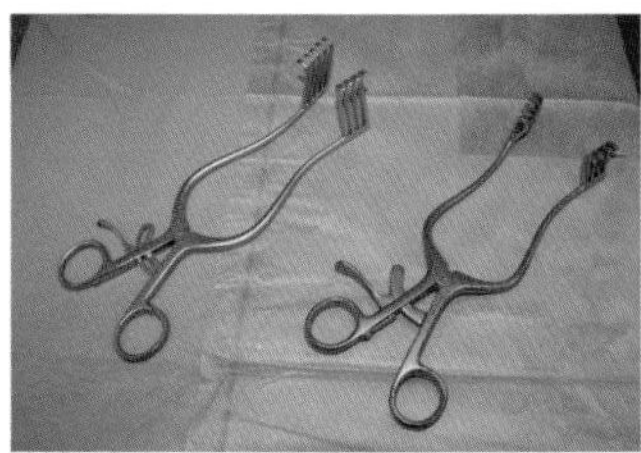

Figure 1.18 Left: Norfolk and Norwich retractor; right: Travers retractor.

spilling...A **Yankauer sucker** is a disposable plastic sucker that sucks from the tip and is thus useful when you want to suck in a particularly focal place. Often you may just want to suck more blindly in a pool of fluid, or if the tip keeps getting blocked with lumps of fat, in which case you can use a **Pooles sucker**, which has an inner piece and an outer guard that screws on to it. It sucks over a broad surface area. The inner piece on its own can be a useful instrument for doing blunt dissection.

Diathermy equipment

Sucking up the blood isn't going to stop it bleeding though, unfortunately; for that you may find the diathermy helpful. Diathermy comes in two broad kinds:

- **Monopolar** – the AC current passes from a diathermy machine through a lead to a diathermy instrument, usually forceps, a finger switch or point. It then passes through the tissue you want to coagulate or cut, through the patient's body, the earthing plate, a wire and back to the diathermy machine. Never use it on an extremity or the returning current to the earthing plate will concentrate at the narrowest point and heat up – a lot.
- **Bipolar** – the AC current passes between two metal components of the instrument, for example the tips of some forceps or the blades of scissors. It passes from one tip, through the tissue to be cut or coagulated and back up to the machine through the other tip (thus also having the advantage of going nowhere near the patient's pacemaker).

It is strongly recommended that you always ensure that the smoke produced from burning flesh, also known as the diathermy plume, is extracted by an evacuation device, because of the potentially oncogenic contents.

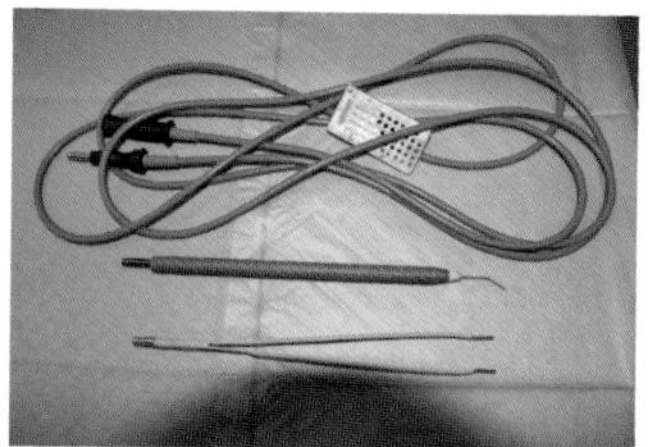

Figure 1.20 Top: diathermy lead; middle: diathermy point; bottom: diathermy forceps.

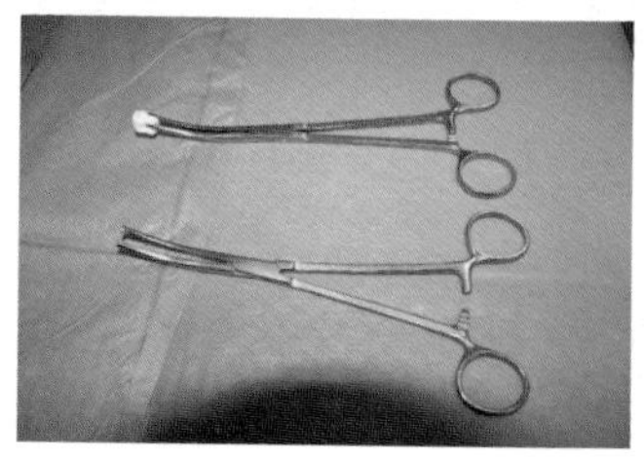

Figure 1.22 Kocher forceps with and without a pledget.

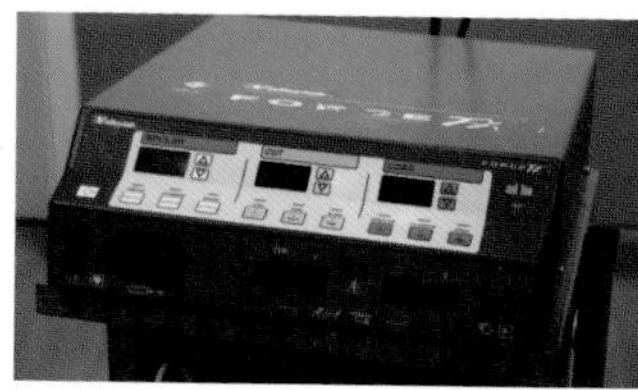

Figure 1.21 A diathermy machine.

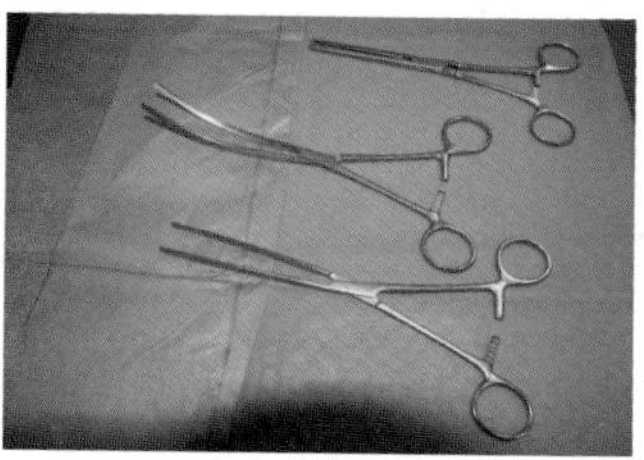

Figure 1.23 Top: crushing bowel clamp; middle and bottom: curved and straight non-crushing bowel clamps.

Miscellaneous general

Pledgets are small, almost pea-sized things, usually made of gauze, which can be grasped in the end of a **Kocher forceps** (one of the few useful roles for such forceps as they have an extremely traumatic bite to the tip). These can be very useful for fine blunt dissection, for instance when trying to define the structures in Calot's triangle or the axilla.

Bowel clamps can be **non-crushing** (**Doyen**) or **crushing** (**Stevens**), curved or straight. Never use crushing bowel clamps unless you're planning on removing whatever bit of bowel you're crushing, and sending it off to the lab.

Blades are mounted on **Bard–Parker handles**, or colloquially known as **BP handles**. They come in a variety of sizes.

The **Howarth elevator** and the **McDonald dissector** have a variety of uses. They can help in bluntly dissecting a plane, for instance during an endarterectomy, or lifting up the nasal mucosa.

The **Volkmann spoon** is a type of curette; they come in various sizes and can be used to scrape out the lining of an abscess cavity or sinus, for instance. Larger ones can be used to scrape out the femoral canal.

Orthopaedic

Bone spikes and **ring handled spikes** are useful to get control of fragments of bone when operating on a fracture site, for instance.

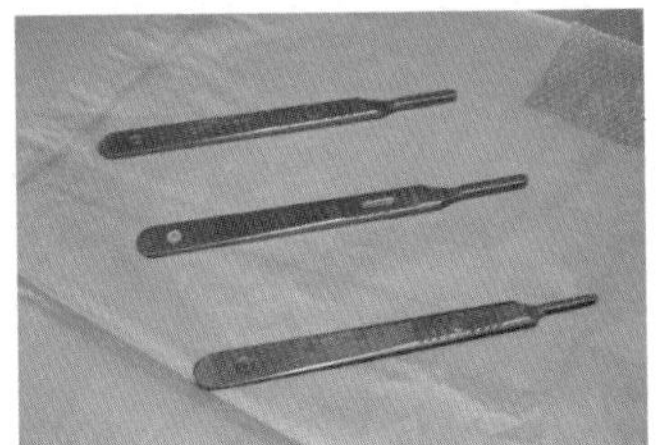

Figure 1.24 Bard Parker handles.

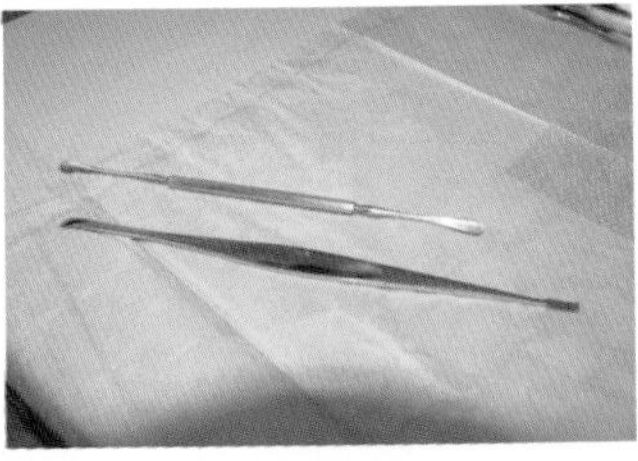

Figure 1.25 Top: Howarth elevator; bottom: McDonald dissector.

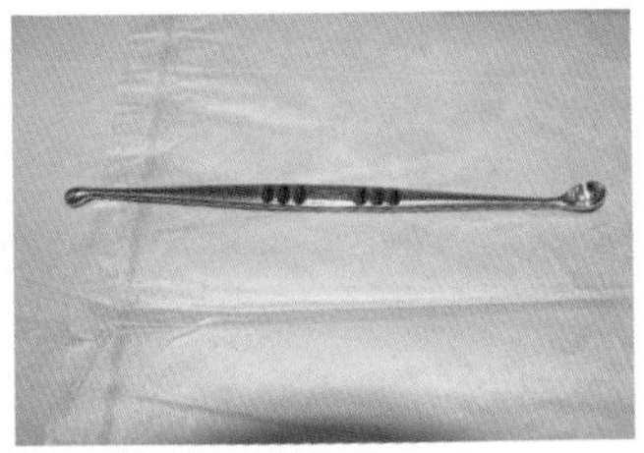

Figure 1.26 Volkmann spoon.

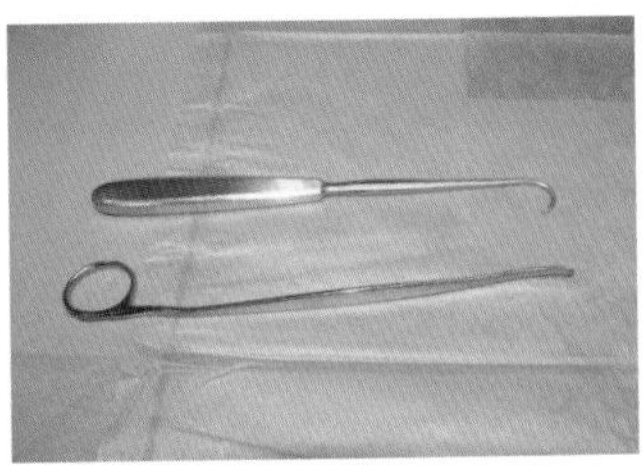

Figure 1.27 Top: bone spike; bottom: ring-handled spike.

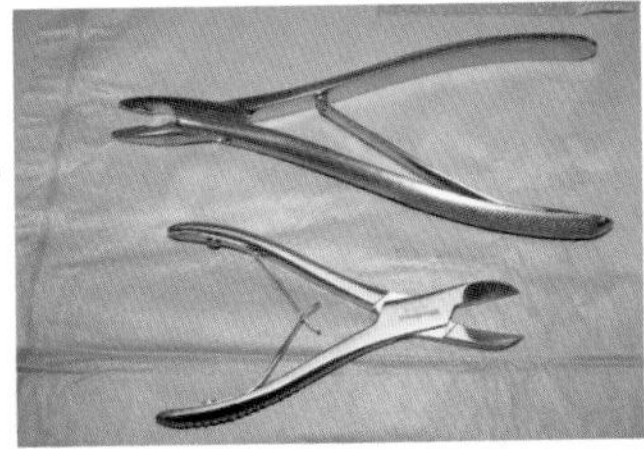

Figure 1.28 Top: Northfield bone nibbler; bottom: Bailey bone cutter.

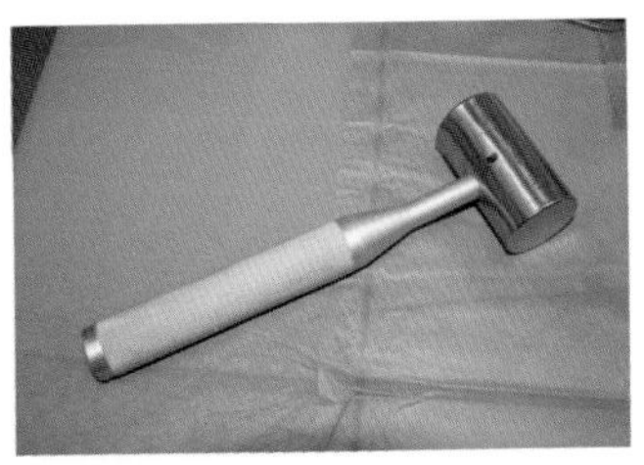

Figure 1.29 Orthopaedic mallet.

Northfield bone nibblers come in a variety of sizes and do the function you'd expect – nibble bits of bone – useful for anything from nibbling off osteophytes to removing residual bony spikes in a toe amputation. **Bailey bone cutters** are the bony version of scissors and also come in a variety of sizes.

An **orthopaedic mallet** can be used for chiseling, banging home prosthetic hips and generally making a lot of noise.

Remember, bone is covered in a layer of periosteum which you frequently need to peel off the bone cortex

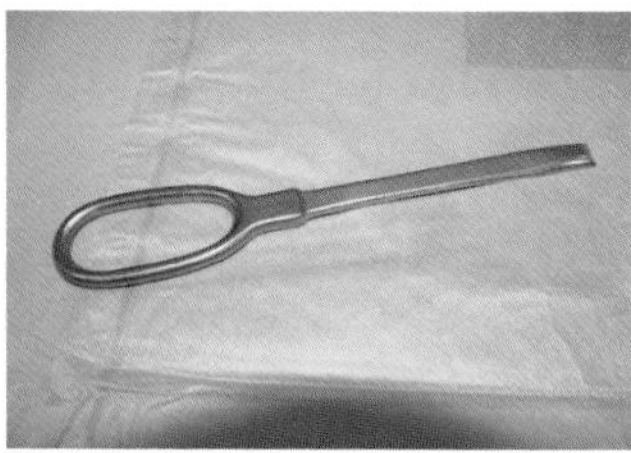

Figure 1.30 Bristow periosteal elevator.

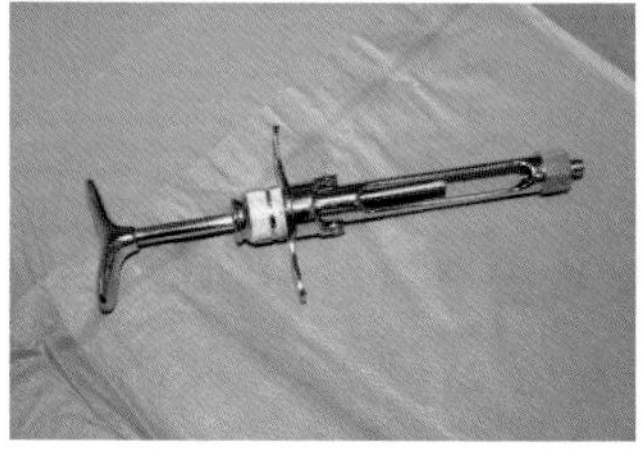

Figure 1.31 Dental syringe.

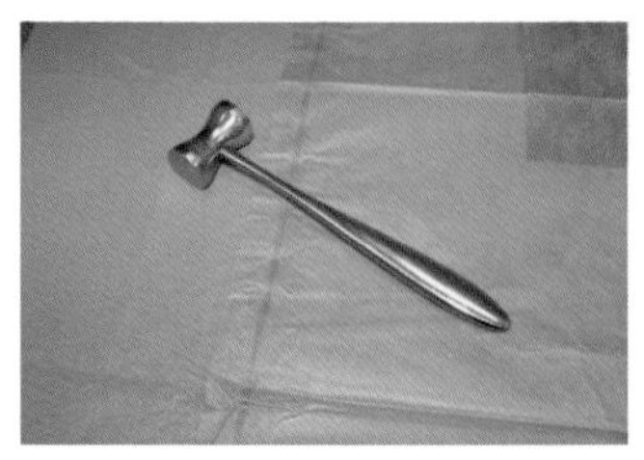

Figure 1.32 Toffee hammer.

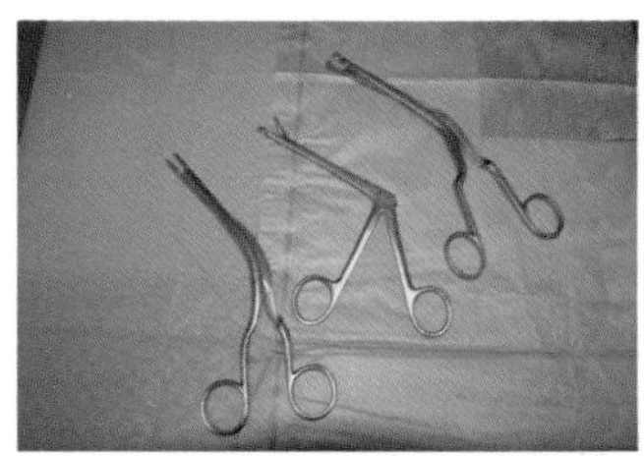

Figure 1.33 Left: nasal scissors; middle: Tilley Henkel forceps; right: nasal polyp forceps.

itself. The **Bristow periosteal elevator** will do this for you nicely.

ENT

The **dental syringe** has greater versatility than just invoking fear at a visit to the dentist. It stores a glass vial, the contents of which can be inserted into mucous membranes of the nose or mouth.

The **toffee hammer** is the much more genteel version of the orthopaedic mallet. It is light and easily handled, and can be used to chisel up the nasal carriage, for instance.

Tilley–Henkel forceps can be used to extract tissue deep within the nasal cavity and beyond. There are a variety of other **nasal polyp forceps** and **nasal scissors** to fit up the nose.

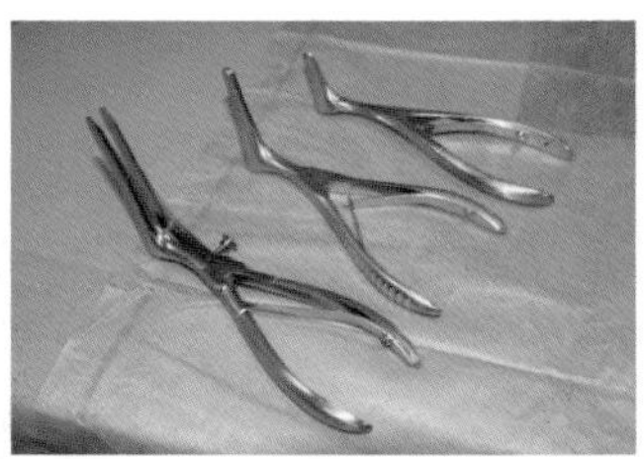

Figure 1.34 Killian nasal speculums.

Killian nasal speculums also come in a wide range of sizes and are obviously inserted into the nostril to gain access.

Sutures

Matt Stephenson and Cheryl Funnell

Introduction

There is a bewildering array of sutures, and because there are different manufacturers, there are different commonly used names for essentially the same sutures. In general, it is acceptable to use the trade name of a suture in exams, as long as you know what it is and why you'd use it. You're also more likely to get a blank look from your scrub person if you ask for Polyglactin 910 rather than Vicryl.

Two of the commoner suture manufacturers are **Ethicon** and **Covidien**. Your hospital may stock sutures from both suppliers, and there will therefore be a different trade name for each supplier for what is more or less the same suture, making it very frustrating to learn them all. We'll discuss the common attributes of sutures that you need to be aware of to help you choose which one to use, and then some examples of commonly used sutures.

If you really want to get into sutures though, there are many other characteristics to be aware of which aren't covered here, such as breaking strength (limit of tensile strength), capillarity (extent to which fluid is absorbed up its length), knot-pull tensile strength (tensile strength after knot tied), fluid absorption (amount of fluid absorbed after immersion), natural or synthetic, etc.

Absorbable versus non-absorbable

In a vascular anastomosis of Dacron graft to aorta, the join is never going to heal in the way a bowel anastomosis will.

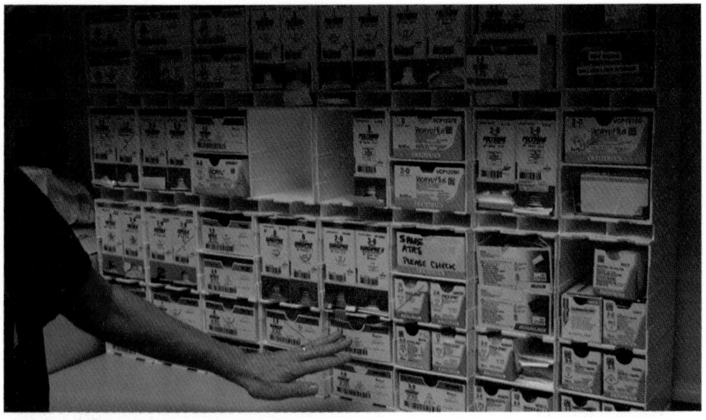

Figure 1.35 The average suture stack.

The suture must be as strong 20 years down the line as it is the day you put it in, so you need a **non-absorbable suture**. The same goes for hernia meshes. However, if what you're stitching together is eventually going to heal up, e.g. a bowel anastomosis, the linea alba, the fascia lata, etc., you can use an **absorbable suture**, so that there won't forever be a foreign body there to act as a nidus for infection, for instance. Some tissues take longer to heal, therefore you will want to use suture material that dissolves over a longer time period.

Monofilament vs braided (polyfilament)

Ideally all sutures would be **monofilament**, as there are fewer microscopic grooves and hiding places for organisms to fester and cause an infection. However, monofilament sutures have two significant disadvantages: first, they tend to have more **memory** (they keep recoiling to their awkward shape even if you stretch them out); and second, they are **less strong**.

Size (thickness)

Whoever came up with the sizing system for suture thickness should be ashamed of themself. It is of course a throwback to when sutures were much thicker. Originally they were numbered 1 to 6, 1 being the thinnest available, 6 the fattest. However, with great advances in suture manufacturing and materials technology, thinner sutures could be used instead with equivalent strength (and less foreign body). So they started numbering back to 0 and then 2-0, 3-0, 4-0, etc., down to 11-0, which is like trying to suture with a spider's web, and only used in ophthalmic surgery. In general, it's rare now to use a suture thicker than a 1.

Needle type

Some more mature theatre sisters will tell you how they used to have to thread the suture through a hole in the needle. Of course this has been superseded by sutures that are attached to the needle already (using a process called swaging). The former were necessarily more traumatic as there would be a tiny bulge at the site where the needle had been threaded. The latter are described as **atraumatic** needles. There is a variety of **shapes** of needle and they also vary in the **geometry** of the point. Shapes include straight, ¼ circle, ⅜ circle, ½ circle, ⅝ circle and J-shape, and they can be selected mainly based on the space you have available to put the stitch in. For instance, a J-shaped needle is ideal for getting down a deep dark laparoscopic porthole. Point geometry variations include the following.

- **Round body** – which smoothly tapers to the point; a commonly used standard needle. They make the smallest possible hole in the tissue, good for anastomoses but not really strong enough for tough skin.
- **Cutting** – triangular needle body with extra sharp cutting edge on the inside (i.e. on the side of the wound edge); for tougher tissues.

- **Reverse cutting** – again for tougher tissues but having the cutting edge on the outside, i.e. not the side of the wound edge, which means there's less likelihood of the needle cutting out through the tissue edge.
- **Tapercut** – a cutting needle body that also tapers to a diameter not exceeding that of the suture (ideally), thus attempting to combine the powers of both the round body and cutting needle,
- **Blunt** – no sharp point but can still be passed through some tissues, as in mass closure of the abdomen, with less risk of pranging bowel or your fingers.

Specific examples

The commonest absorbable sutures you are likely to come across in most surgical practice are **Vicryl** or **Polysorb** (roughly equivalent). They can be used for general ligating and transfixing of vessels or chunks of tissue, or closing layers of tissue in most cases. The average thickness is 2-0. So if in doubt in your exam, the answer is probably 2-0 Vicryl. For thicker leashes of tissue or bigger vessels, use a thicker thread such as 0 Vicryl. It's important to choose an appropriate thickness of thread for the tissue you're ligating. You wouldn't tie a boat to a dock with a fishing line, just as you wouldn't use a rope to go fishing. Vicryl and Polysorb can be used for closing skin too, although because skin heals quickly, many people prefer to use **Vicryl Rapide**, or **Monocryl** or **Caprosyn** (roughly equivalent), to minimise the time foreign material is in the wound. Also you wouldn't want to use Vicryl or Polysorb to close tissue that will take several weeks to heal – the linea alba after a laparotomy for instance. Here, **PDS** or **Maxon** (roughly equivalent) will do the job.

The main non-absorbable sutures in common use are **Prolene** or **Surgipro** (roughly equivalent), which are biologically inert and have good strength – use them for vascular anastomoses and hernia repairs. Again, 2-0 is the average for a hernia repair or a large vascular anastomosis such as the aorta to a graft, for instance; whereas 7-0 would be used for a radiocephalic fistula. **Nylon** sutures tend to be used mainly for interrupted sutures when closing skin, but are also useful for incisional or paraumbilical hernias where you want the tissue to be held together for as long as possible to give it time to heal. **Silk** sutures have disadvantages, mainly because they're braided and can cause a biological reaction in the tissue. They are generally reserved for stitching in the drain, marking a specimen or practising tying knots.

Theatre etiquette

Matt Stephenson and Ginny Bowbrick

Introduction

Theatre is a unique environment and one in which, as a surgeon, you will want to be most comfortable. Sometimes on entering a new theatre you find yourself entering a peculiar world filled with fragile egos, ambitious

Table 1.1 Commonly used sutures with some of their important characteristics

	Ethicon name	Covidien name	Half life and complete absorption	Mono or braided	Examples of use
Absorbable	*PDS* (polydioxanone)	*Maxon* (polytrimethylene carbonate)	T½: 21 A: 180	Mono	Mass closure
	Monocryl (poliglecaprone 25)	*Caprosyn* (polyglytone 6211)	T½: 5–7 A: 21	Mono	Subcuticular
	Vicryl (polyglactin 910)	*Polysorb* (lactomer copolymer)	T½: 14–21 A: 56–70	Braided	Very versatile, commonly used suture
	Vicryl Rapide (polyglactin 910)		T½: 5 A: 42	Braided	Subcuticular
Non-absorbable	*Prolene* (polypropylene)	*Surgipro* (polypropylene)	N/A	Mono	Vascular anastomoses, hernia repairs
	Ethilon (nylon)	*Monosof* (nylon)	N/A	Mono	Skin stitches
	Permahand silk (silk)	*Sofsilk* (silk)	N/A	Braided	Drain stitches

T½ = half life in days; A = complete absorption in days.

career climbers, clandestine political wrangling and complex power struggles. Patients also have operations there. For that reason, learning to grease your way through this often complicated domain is very important.

You might broadly divide the rules you should observe into **before**, **during** and **after** the operation. In general it is just common sense.

Before the operation

Few things are more like a red rag to a bull for a consultant than somebody turning up to his list without having done a bit of **groundwork beforehand**. Not going to **see the patient** before the operation, or at least having a good **read of the notes** and **review of the imaging** if applicable, is asking for trouble and you will have little or no chance of being allowed to operate on that particular patient. It is a good idea to bring up any relevant imaging such as computed tomography (CT) scans or arteriograms on the theatre computer and this can also turn into an impromptu teaching session with the boss while waiting for the patient to be anaesthetised. But it's not enough to know the patient; you need to have some idea of **what the operation is about**, too. Read about and watch the video the night before if you know what's on the next list. The sooner you show that you know and understand the operation, the sooner you'll be allowed to do it yourself.

It's a favourite pastime of all surgeons to conveniently forget that their **knowledge of anatomy** probably wasn't very good at your stage of training either, but still scoff and bemoan the demise in undergraduate anatomy education if you can't recall some obscure anatomical fact. In fairness, there is probably some truth in this – anatomy has taken a battering in many undergraduate courses. Make sure you've opened an anatomy textbook and/or atlas before the operation so that you can at least guess the answer to any questions fired at you.

If it's your first time in a particular theatre and you're not familiar with the theatre staff, **introduce yourself** before the list starts. With a theatre sister not known for her friendliness to new intruders, having a little one-to-one time in theatre will make it a lot more challenging for her to make your life more difficult. **Communication is key** to the successful running of a theatre list – if, for instance, you know of a change in circumstances that will affect the list, let the theatre staff know as soon as you can. **Respect the theatre staff** – they often have an extraordinary amount of knowledge and experience, which will help you out in times of trouble. If left to operate without the boss, an experienced scrub nurse may for instance suggest instruments that the boss uses at different steps of the operation, but if you have not made any effort to get to know them then they will not. Never underestimate the relationship between the long-standing theatre staff and your boss.

Dress appropriately. It's obvious what you should and shouldn't wear but it's surprising to see how many new students or trainees arrive in theatre with a big fringe hanging down from under their hat or bling jewellery dripping off their fingers. Some theatres have colour-coded hats such as green for students and blue for qualified staff, whether medical or nursing, so it pays to ask first if this applies in each hospital you work in. Don't wear your identification badge dangling somewhere near your genitals where people can only look at it by making themselves feel uncomfortable. If you need to speak to someone in theatre, it's always a good idea to get **changed into scrubs** and go inside, rather than trying to talk through a crack in the doorway. It's usually best to pass on a message via the scrub person who can then speak to the operating surgeon at an appropriate time. **Never ever** wear someone else's clogs or you may end up with an irate and barefoot consultant hunting you down from theatre to theatre.

When watching an operation, make a big show of taking great care of **preserving the sterile field**. Don't, for instance, walk between the scrub person's sterile trolley and the operating table, and avoid walking around the anaesthetic end of the table when scrubbed – remember all surgeons view anaesthetists as dirty.

You need to get the theatre staff on side. This is immeasurably important. **Make yourself useful** and show that you're happy to muck in with whatever needs to be done and that you have no airs and graces about doing so. If the phone is ringing in theatre answer it. If there's a dirty swab dropped on the floor pick it up. When the patient is transferred help. If there are no snacks or sugary treats in the preparation room buy some. Be ready to catheterise the male, or female, patients if required.

Leave your bleep wherever it's supposed to be left (often this is at the front desk of theatres) or, if you can, hand it to a colleague to cover. **Return the favour** for them another time. Don't screw your colleagues over. **Turn off your mobile phone**. Don't be shy about asking to scrub up. Obey the World Health Organization **(WHO) checklist** (see Patient safety section), or instigate it yourself.

During the operation

Get to know your consultant's **glove and gown size** and open theirs for them before the case, as well as your own. **Scrub thoroughly** in the usual way and always **scrub for slightly longer** than the next most senior person to you. Hold your hands together across your chest when walking from the sink towards the table, and maintain sterility at all times.

When assisting, look and **be attentive** but **don't grovel**. If and when it seems appropriate, try and **ask appropriate questions** but don't be too talkative, unless that's the way your boss is. Suggestions and discussion of technique and steps in the operation are welcome – criticisms or saying how much better your last boss did something are not. Don't yawn and don't gossip with the other staff. Try to **blend in** with whatever the mood and ethos of that theatre seems to be. **Make yourself as useful as possible** when assisting. Try to anticipate what the operating surgeon is about to do next, which often takes a lot of practice, as you may not yet know the next step, but if a knot's being tied for instance, you're likely to need to cut the suture soon, so have scissors ready.

But of course, you don't want to be assisting all your life. You want to **get your hands on the knife**. Your success in this depends on many things, not least the generosity, patience and self-confidence of your boss (perhaps the three most important characteristics to have in a trainer), and the relationship you develop with them. Make sure you **know the basics**: suture, tie knots, hold instruments, etc. The Basic Surgical Skills course helps with this. Many bosses will judge whether you can do the operation on whether you can assist well, so get the basics right. Borrow instruments from theatre to practise with in the coffee room and practise tying knots – there is many a surgical trainee's bag or theatre coffee room chair leg with Vicryl ties hanging from them used to practise knot tying until smoothly performed.

If you're not getting much operating time, **make it known** gently that you're very interested in getting your hands on such and such a case. Tell him or her you've assisted in x number of procedures before and demonstrate your knowledge of the steps, and hint at how hard you've been working on the wards. If this doesn't work, your options range from purposely finishing scrubbing before your boss and then standing on the operating side of the table, to snatching the knife out of his hand. The latter, in general, is not recommended. If all else fails talk to your surgical tutor about your predicament.

When the patient is **awake**, under local anaesthetic, the atmosphere in theatre is usually very different. Remember you are there purely for that patient. Their comfort should be the focus of everyone's attention. They should have someone available to talk to them (unless they are sedated) all the way through. Take great care to remember all the way through the operation that the patient is awake and refrain from discussing your plans for the weekend or a recent mess party. In some theatres, a large sign is placed in a highly visible place to remind everyone – it can be easily forgotten. Ask the patient if they would like to listen to music during the procedure and if so listen to what they would like, rather than your preference.

All consultants have their own way of doing things, such as a preferred skin suture, so if allowed to operate on one of their patients it is only polite to do what they prefer, otherwise you will find yourself no longer operating on their patients, and rest assured the theatre scrub nurse will tell them if you digress. If you also always do it your consultant's way while you're working for them, for example doing all the dissection with a knife or scissors rather than the diathermy pencil, it also allows you to build up a wider range of skills by the end of your training. Eventually, you'll be able to decide the way you prefer to do it.

After the operation

You haven't finished the operation until you have helped **transfer the patient back** on to the bed. **Clean up** any detritus on the floor or around the operating trolley – **make yourself useful**. Offer to make the boss a coffee or take the op notes through to recovery when written – an all-day list requires a lot of concentration and is tiring, so these things will help to enhance your relationship with your boss.

It is mandatory to **go and see your patient** afterwards and let them know how it went. Sometimes at the end of a late list that's very difficult to do, especially if it's anticipated they'll take a long time to wake up. Make sure that at least the nursing staff or on-call surgeon is well informed from your op note. Make the **op note as clear as possible** with your postoperative instructions (see How to write the operation note section). **Thank everyone** in theatre, especially if you've delayed the list because you were being trained. If you performed the operation, try to have a **debrief** with your trainer on what you did well and not so well, preferably in the format of a **procedure-based assessment (PBA).** Record the operation in your **logbook**.

Patient safety and the WHO surgical checklist

Matt Stephenson and Christopher M Butler

Introduction

A relatively new hot topic in surgery is **patient safety**. But what does that mean exactly? The true magnitude of adverse events for patients during their time in contact with healthcare services was underappreciated until the 1990s. Statistics such as '1 in 10 patients affected by an adverse event' during their inpatient stay raised a few eyebrows. In 2007 in England and Wales, a whopping 129,419 incidents relating to surgical specialties were reported to the **National Learning and Reporting Service** (a branch of the NPSA, see later) – including 271 deaths – and that's just the ones that were reported (bear in mind that reporting adverse events is now more than ever considered a crucial part of our duty as doctors). All sorts of factors impact on errors in patient care, from simple human errors to complex systemic failures. This is a growing discipline of healthcare science. But what is most relevant to our practice as surgeons now?

The **National Patient Safety Agency** (**NPSA**) is charged with the responsibility for patient safety within the NHS and a check of their website (www.npsa.nhs.uk) will reveal a wide variety of guidelines for aspects of surgical and anaesthetic care, from alerts about the use of throat packs to avoiding wrong side surgery for burr holes. Make yourself aware of these guidelines and advice – they're there for a reason. Serious problems have happened in the past, which have resulted in harm to patients. There's only one thing better than learning from your own mistakes, and that's learning from someone else's.

What's the worst thing that could happen to you in your career? Your patient's anastomosis breaks down? You get a complaint from a patient because they had to wait too long for their hip replacement? Your young RTA victim didn't survive their serious injuries despite your heroic efforts? How about taking out the **wrong kidney**? Or getting your **patients mixed up** and stripping someone's long saphenous vein when you were supposed to be fixing their hernia? Or performing major elective vascular surgery and realising too late that there's **no blood available** and they exsanguinate? In the first three, within reason there's probably nothing else you could have done. The latter examples are catastrophic, avoidable and violate the first rule of the Hippocratic Oath: **First, do no harm**.

The patient safety checklist

In June 2008, the **World Health Organization** launched a global initiative (as by no means is this problem peculiar to the UK) called **'Safe Surgery Saves Lives'**. At the core of this, is a **simple checklist**. The idea behind it is to partially ritualise the process of perioperative care to make certain that in every single case, the most significant errors are avoided. Some of these errors have been termed **never events** – in other words, they should in no circumstances ever occur because they are avoidable and disastrous.

The checklist (see page 21) comprises **three stages: sign in, time out and sign out**. One member of the theatre staff – and it can be anyone, including you – must read each of these steps out aloud to the team. They may vary slightly from hospital to hospital, but this is the blueprint.

Sign in

Before the patient is even induced, the first part of the checklist must be completed. **First**, has the patient **confirmed his or her identity** and **procedure**, and have they **signed the consent form**? This is probably the most crucial step of all and it's generally taken for granted by us as surgeons that the right patient will turn up on the operating table. But without this step, you are essentially entrusting your GMC registration to the quality of your hospital porters. **Second, is the site or side marked**? In **every** case, if the operation is planned on one side of the body, they **must** be marked preoperatively, with the patient awake and witnessing where you're marking them so they can correct you if you're wrong. It doesn't matter if it's the only foot that's gangrenous or the only groin with a massive lump poking out (which may reduce on lying down and muscle relaxation). **Third, is the anaesthesia machine and medication check complete**? Yes, well, presumably that would be important, but one doesn't want to trifle too much with what the anaesthetists do. **Fourth**, does the patient have a **known allergy**? The importance of this speaks for itself. Put away your betadine if it turns out they're allergic to iodine. **Fifth**, is there likely to be a **difficult airway or aspiration risk**? Should you have put a nasogastric tube into your bowel-obstructed patient before induction? **Sixth**, is the risk of **blood loss** likely to be **greater than 500 ml** (or in a **child 7 ml/kg**)? In which case make sure blood resources are available to you if necessary.

Time out

The patient is now asleep and on the table. The theatre team reassembles and **introduces themselves by name and role**. Obviously this is particularly important if you're new to the theatre, but even in theatres with consistent staff and a consultant who's been there for 30 years, think about how often there's an agency nurse or a new medical student. One infamous case of a 'wrong side' nephrectomy occurred despite the medical student noticing they were about to operate on the wrong side and flagging it up – she was ignored. The concept of **flattened hierarchy** is that no longer should anyone feel they're not important enough to raise a concern. The HCA should be able to tell the consultant she's noticed the patient has a pacemaker and that therefore monopolar diathermy is contraindicated, for instance. By getting everyone's names and roles clear at the start, **communication** between the team can then flow much better.

You must then check again – what is the **patient's name**, what **procedure** are you planning, on **which side**, and what **position** do you want the patient in? It may sound far-fetched, but cases have occurred when the patient who came into the anaesthetic room is not the one who comes on to the operating table. Imagine you are on call and this is the emergency list. Your patient was in the anaesthetic room and you were called off to A&E for an emergency. You return to theatre half an hour later to drain said patient's abscess, only in the time you were gone an urgent testicular torsion took precedence over your patient who's been returned to the ward. It has happened! Don't rely on everyone else to prevent your mistakes.

As doctors we don't tend to like protocols, but in some cases they can truly get you out of some very unpleasant situations. Put up with the fact that perhaps 99% of the time there are no hidden surprises in order to safeguard that one patient, and you, from those odd freakish out-of-nowhere events that will have life-changing consequences not only for your patient, but for you, too.

Next, you want to warn the team about any **critical events you anticipate**. This could range from needing a rigid sigmoidoscope to assess the rectal mucosa when draining a perianal abscess, to a crucial piece of equipment you might need should something go wrong. There is then the rather unfortunately phrased: 'Are there any **critical or unexpected steps** you want the team to know about?' It doesn't mean 'do you expect there to be any unexpected steps', which would indeed make no sense, it means are there any steps that you know might happen but the team weren't expecting (however, this question invariably invokes incomprehension and derision from theatre staff every single time it's mentioned)? How much **blood loss** are you anticipating? Of course it may be difficult to say, but you're best placed to make an educated guess. There are also some questions for the anaesthetist regarding their concerns and their American Association of Anesthesiologists (ASA) grade etc., and also for the scrub person.

If you haven't heard of the **surgical site infection bundle**, here it is. It comprises four aspects of care that have an evidence base to reduce the risk of surgical site infection. Quite why it's called a bundle is anybody's guess.

1 Has **hair removal** been performed adequately? Ideally it should be avoided altogether, but where necessary it should be done with clippers, not a razor, with minimal disruption of the skin and as close to the time of surgery as possible.

2 If **antibiotics** are indicated (always for instance when bowel may be opened, including **always** before an appendicectomy) have they been given within 60 minutes prior to the operation?

3 Has the patient's **blood glucose** been adequately normalised?

4 Has the patient's **temperature** been adequately normalised?

The morbidity from **venous thromboembolism** is very significant to us all in our surgical practice. All patients must be **assessed** for their need for low molecular weight heparin and intraoperative pneumatic calf compression or at least thromboembolic deterrent stockings (TEDS). Finally, are the relevant **images** up on the computer screen or X-ray box? If you need to see a mammogram to help guide you in your wide local excision, you don't want an added 10 minutes of anaesthetic time while someone runs around the ward trying to find it.

Sign out

Once the procedure has been completed there is a third and final step to the process. The **name of the procedure** needs to be clearly stated (it often seems strange, when you've been slaving away at a laparotomy for the past two hours, how no one else in the theatre actually knows quite what you've been doing – least of all the anaesthetist). This enables safe handover to the recovery staff and recording of the procedure in the log. The scrub person **must confirm that the final count of swabs, needles and instruments is correct** (by the way, when they tell you this don't just ignore it, thank them, it's also for your benefit – who do you think will be in court if a swab is left in the abdomen?). The **specimens** must be appropriately **labelled** and any **faulty equipment reported** and acted on. Finally, are there any **concerns for recovery** or the ward for the ongoing management of this patient? Do they, for instance, have palpable pulses at the end of the operation and would you want to know if they vanish?

Summary

The WHO surgical safety checklist is not a tick box exercise. OK, so it is in fact exactly a tick box exercise, but for it to have value, it must be much more than that. It is not simply the observance of these steps in order to get through them quickly to satisfy sister; much more important is the **spirit** in which the checklist is handled. It is there for **your benefit** as much as anyone else's. It is there to prevent a once-in-a-career event that could ruin your patient's life, and yours. It's there to help mitigate against our natural **human tendency to err**, even if we're so superhuman

WHO Surgical Safety Checklist
(adapted for England and Wales)

NHS
National Patient Safety Agency
National Reporting and Learning Service

SIGN IN (To be read out loud)

Before induction of anaesthesia

Has the patient confirmed his/her identity, site, procedure and consent?
☐ Yes

Is the surgical site marked?
☐ Yes/not applicable

Is the anaesthesia machine and medication check complete?
☐ Yes

Does the patient have a:
Known allergy?
☐ No
☐ Yes
Difficult airway/aspiration risk?
☐ No
☐ Yes, and equipment/assistance available
Risk of >500ml blood loss (7ml/kg in children)?
☐ No
☐ Yes, and adequate IV access/fluids planned

PATIENT DETAILS

Last name:
First name:
Date of birth:
NHS Number:*
Procedure:

TIME OUT (To be read out loud)

Before start of surgical intervention
for example, skin incision

Have all team members introduced themselves by name and role?
☐ Yes

Surgeon, Anaesthetist and Registered Practitioner verbally confirm:
☐ What is the patient's name?
☐ What procedure, site and position are planned?

Anticipated critical events
Surgeon:
☐ How much blood loss is anticipated?
☐ Are there any specific equipment requirements or special investigations?
☐ Are there any critical or unexpected steps you want the team to know about?
Anaesthetist:
☐ Are there any patient specific concerns?
☐ What is the patient's ASA grade?
☐ What monitoring equipment and other specific levels of support are required, for example blood?
Nurse/ODP:
☐ Has the sterility of the instrumentation been confirmed (including indicator results)?
☐ Are there any equipment issues or concerns?

Has the surgical site infection (SSI) bundle been undertaken?
☐ Yes/not applicable
- Antibiotic prophylaxis within the last 60 minutes
- Patient warming
- Hair removal
- Glycaemic control

Has VTE prophylaxis been undertaken?
☐ Yes/not applicable

Is essential imaging displayed?
☐ Yes/not applicable

SIGN OUT (To be read out loud)

Before any member of the team leaves the operating room

Registered Practitioner verbally confirms with the team:
☐ Has the name of the procedure been recorded?
☐ Has it been confirmed that instruments, swabs and sharps counts are complete (or not applicable)?
☐ Have the specimens been labelled (including patient name)?
☐ Have any equipment problems been identified that need to be addressed?

Surgeon, Anaesthetist and Registered Practitioner:
☐ What are the key concerns for recovery and management of this patient?

This checklist contains the core content for England and Wales

www.npsa.nhs.uk/nrls

THIS CHECKLIST IS NOT INTENDED TO BE COMPREHENSIVE. ADDITIONS AND MODIFICATIONS TO FIT LOCAL PRACTICE ARE ENCOURAGED.

Figure 1.36 WHO surgical safety checklist. This checklist is not intended to be comprehensive; additions and modifications to fit local practice are encouraged.

we only err once every few decades. What's more, there is an evidence base to it. Despite all of that, you will find that surgeons' opinions about its usefulness are split, in common with pretty much anything else 'new' that's ever been introduced to an established system, be it Ignez Semmelweiss's attempts to introduce hand washing in the 1840s or laparoscopic surgery in the 1970s. Get used to it, embrace it, it's here to stay.

How to write the operation note

Matt Stephenson and Petra Marsh

Writing the operation note is one of those things no one ever shows you how to do. In truth it's not difficult and you basically just write down what you did. But there are a few simple things to remember to include and a commonly used standard format adopted by many surgeons for most operations.

You want your operation note to be **easily found** in the notes, to **accurately answer** any questions a nurse or doctor might have when looking after your patient on their first postoperative night and to contain **all the useful information** that might be sought 10 years down the line. The more experienced you become and the more hospitals you travel around, and then back to years later, the more you come across your own operative record written years back – you can then judge your own work retrospectively.

It's obvious of course, but begin by putting the **patient details** at the top of the page – **name**, **hospital number** and **date of birth** as a minimum. Put the **date** in the left margin and the **time** of the operation – not so essential for elective cases but for emergency ones it's more important. Some people like to write the **start time** (knife to skin) and the **end time** (closed up) with an arrow between the two; it's often helpful to know how long the operation took.

So, on to the operation note itself. What **colour** do you write it in? Well you will doubtless have heard innumerable times that you mustn't write in the notes in **red ink**. This dates back to **pre-ancient times** when photocopiers struggled to copy red ink, in the event that your notes might be requested by the coroner or similar. Well if you can find a photocopier these days that can't photocopy red ink, hats off to you. The idea of using red ink is that when you're in a hurry leafing through vast volumes of notes, 95% of which are taken up by **completely superfluous paperwork**, you can more rapidly identify the important operation note. However if your trust condemns such practice, obviously one must submit and write it in black.

In some hospitals it's normal practice to **type** all operative notes. This is particularly helpful if your handwriting isn't up to scratch. The only caveat to this is make sure it is typed straight away, not dictated on to tape to be typed the next day. If your patient has a problem in the middle of the night and the team looking after them doesn't have the op note to find out what went on in theatre, you'll be in big trouble.

At the top of the page write:

OPERATION NOTE (if it's not preprinted)

And below this, the name of operation for instance:

RIGHT INGUINAL HERNIA REPAIR

Then put:

Surgeon: YOUR NAME
Assistant: SOMEONE ELSE'S NAME

Then the form of **anaesthesia** used, **who** did it, if any **antibiotics** were given and what **venous thromboembolism prophylaxis** measures were taken. For some situations it's also worth writing down the patient's ASA.

GA + ILIOINGUINAL NERVE BLOCK: DR GAS

You should then say whether this was an **elective** case or an **emergency** case done on the CEPOD list. Sometimes it's obvious, but occasionally it's not and that can be useful in the future and also helps the clinical coders (the people that break down all hospital episodes into codes, and codes mean prizes, for the hospital at least). In some hospitals you even have to look up the code yourself.

Do you know why the emergency list is called a **CEPOD** list by the way? In the olden days emergencies would go to theatre as and when, tacked on to the end of elective lists (as they still are sometimes) or carry through into the middle of the night. In 1982 there was a study – **Confidential Enquiry into Peri Operative Deaths** – looking at outcomes from surgery and anaesthesia dependent on various factors, including when it was performed. One of the outcomes was that it was best not to do non-life- or limb-threatening surgery in the middle of the night, and recommendations were made to create dedicated theatre space during the day to accommodate emergencies. This enquiry was the precursor to the formation of the National Confidential Enquiry into Patient Outcome and Death (NCEPOD), which has looked into many other clinical governance issues. We digress. So simply state:

EMERGENCY (CEPOD list)

Then write the **indication** for the surgery, although this isn't always necessary as it's often self-evident why you're doing the operation, but you might do a Hartmann's procedure for instance either because of bowel obstruction or perforation.

INDICATION: INCARCERATED INGUINAL HERNIA

So now to the nitty gritty of it. For most operations you can follow the same formula: **incision**, **findings**, **procedure**, **closure**, usually abbreviated to I, F, P and C. Generally move to lower case unless your handwriting is a real problem.

I: Right groin crease

Then tell them the punchline straight away, **what did you find**? After going through the skin, everybody gets to the hernia in roughly the same way, so you don't have to repeat every obvious step about going through fat, fascia, etc. **Diagrams** can be really useful; they don't have to be complex, but when trying to explain what vessel you anastomosed on to what, for instance, or what the configuration of the fracture and your plates and screws were, a picture tells a thousand words.

F: *Incarcerated indirect inguinal hernia*
Sac containing viable omentum, no bowel
No direct hernia

So **what did you do** about it?

P: *Sac dissected and opened*
Cord structures identified and preserved
Sac contents inspected and returned to abdomen
Sac transfixed and divided
Polypropylene mesh shaped and sutured in place
Haemostasis

Include any biopsies or microbiology samples taken. And then how did you **close the wound** and did you put in any more local anaesthetic?

C: *External oblique – Vicryl 2-1 continuous*
Fat/superficial fascia – Vicryl 2-0 interrupted
Skin – subcuticular continuous monocryl 3-0
Opsite dressing to skin

Finally, what are your **postoperative instructions**. It's really important to be as clear on this as possible. If you don't know when the drain should come out or when the patient should start mobilising on their fixed fracture, how will anyone else? Were there pulses in the affected limb at the end of the operation? Can they eat and drink?

Post op: *Can eat and drink when desires*
Routine ward observations
Aim for home tomorrow after review

Make sure that the **drug chart** has everything necessary prescribed – do they need antibiotic cover, for how many days and what is the indication? Do they need low molecular weight heparin deep vein thrombosis (DVT) prophylaxis? What analgesia is prescribed? If the patient is a day case it's usually best to write the **discharge letter** along with any medication to take out (TTOs) at the same time as the op note just to save time.

Of course not all operations conform to this system and you can adapt it as much as you see fit, as long as it's still clear. Just make sure you've included all the important things. It's a general rule of thumb when writing any notes that you write as much detail as you would want to have at your disposal in the unfortunate scenario of having to explain something to the coroner. So, for instance, if you changed the pre-arranged plan midway through an operation because of unforeseen circumstances and called your boss to discuss it, say so. If you carefully checked there was no bleeding at the end of the operation put it in.

Your operation is not over of course until you've helped **transfer** the patient back on to their bed. Then write the note. It's usually best, especially if it's been a long case, to leave the theatre for a few moments and **sit down** quietly in the coffee room to write all this out. Perching the notes on the edge of the catheter trolley while the anaesthetist's shouting at the patient to wake up and the floor's being mopped around you is not conducive to good note writing. Make sure that the op note is **filed in the right place** in the notes, not just tucked in the front to get lost, and then take the notes round to recovery.

South Forest NHS Trust
South River Hospital

Patient Name	Tom Thumb
Hosp No.	100546783
Date of birth	12/03/1985

Date	21/11/2010	Surgeon	T Best
Elective/emergency	emergency	Assistant	F Tryer
Consultant	Mr N Bottom	Anaesthetist	A Gassman
		Type of anaesthetic	GA

VTE prophylaxis	LMW heparin 20/11/10	WHO Safe surgery checklist	✓
	20.00	Position	supine
	TEDS	Start	14.00
Antibiotic prophylaxis	amoxicillin	Finish	14.35
	gentamicin		

Indication for surgery	pain & tenderness Mc Burney's point
Operation	Open appendicectomy
Operative Diagnosis	acute appendicitis
Operative Codes	E2341

Incision	Lanz, muscle-splitting
Findings	acutely inflamed appendix, no free peritoneal fluid or pus No fluid in pelvis
Procedure	Mesoappendix divided between clamps, ligated using 2/0 absorbable ties Appendix base crushed & clamp applied distally. 0 absorbable tie to base. Appendix excised leaving short stump and sent for histology
Closure	peritoneum closed under direct vision 2/0 absorbable continuous suture Then layered closure: TA & IO closed with loose apposition suture EO continuous closure 2/0 absorbable suture

Local anaesthetic	20ml 0.5% bupivacaine block to wound
Drains	none
Samples	appendix specimen to histopathology

Postoperative Instructions

Routine postoperative observations
Start eating and drinking as tolerated
2 more doses of antibiotics
LMW heparin and TEDS as prescribed

Figure 1.37 Example of an operation note. Source: WHO

Introduction to operative sections

To be a successful surgeon you need the eye of a hawk, the heart of a lion and the hands of a lady
Sir Lancelot Spratt, Doctor in the House (1954)

It isn't really the purpose of this book to show you how to operate. No book can show you briefly how to do many different operations, you need a minimum level of detail to be able to really get it. So instead we've focused on just three common operations that you're very likely to encounter, but in all the detail you'll ever need. You'll need a different product for more on operative technique – go to Wiley.com and search for *How to Operate*, which shows you just that including DVDs with videos of the operations.

Appendicectomy

Matt Stephenson and George HC Evans

Introduction

Older surgeons often like to wax lyrical about how they were sent off to do an appendicectomy on their first day of being a houseman without any supervision or prior training. They apparently did about 1,400 appendicectomies in their first year and by the end of two months they could finish one in five minutes and still have time to have a drag on their pipe, check the cricket score and arrange a date with the scrub nurse. Either rose tinted be their spectacles or they really were a breed apart back then. It's true to say that an appendicectomy can be very straightforward, but if you believe they're all like that, you probably haven't done enough or you're just using a giant wound every time.

Procedure

With the patient **supine** and under **general anaesthetic**, shave and prep the whole of the abdomen but **drape** just the right lower quadrant. Identify **McBurney's point**, which is two-thirds of the way from the **umbilicus** to the **anterior superior iliac spine** (**ASIS**). A **gridiron** incision is an incision centred on this point but running perpendicular to this line – this is rarely needed and is mainly of historical interest, back in the days when cosmesis was lower on the surgeon's agenda. Instead perform a **Lanz** incision, which is centred on the same point but in the line of the skin creases, so essentially horizontal. A **modified Lanz** is another option, which is the same incision, just slightly lower, for the cosmetic benefit.

Cut through **skin**, **superficial fascia** comprising the fatty-laden **Camper's fascia** and then the more clearly seen thin whitish layer of **Scarpa's fascia**. Then through **true fat** and look out for the fibres of the **external oblique**, which are coursing inferomedially. Here, insert a self-retaining retractor – such as a **Traver's**

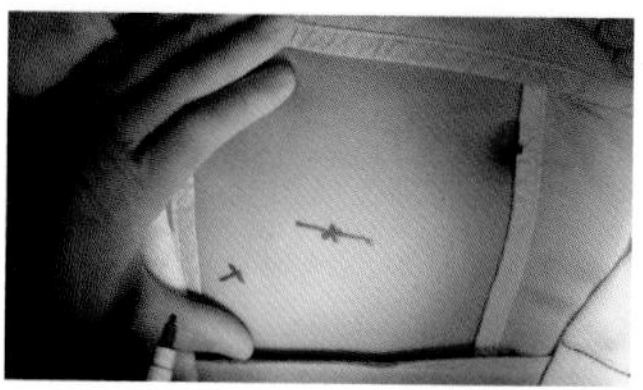

Figure 1.38 The landmarks of the ASIS and the umbilicus allow you to identify McBurney's point.

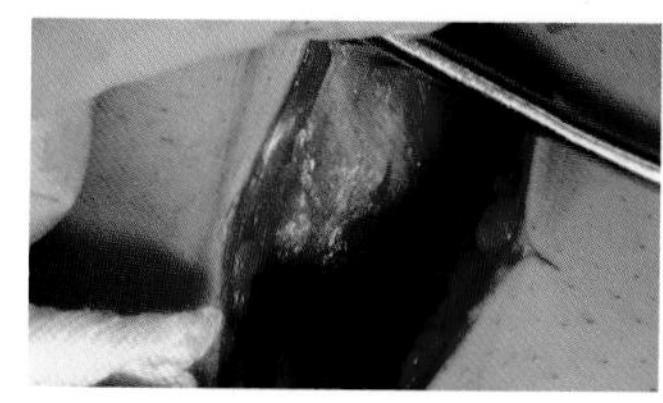

Figure 1.39 External oblique aponeurosis is exposed in the base of the wound.

retractor. Get **haemostasis** as you go with the diathermy.

Make a **small stab incision** in the external oblique and slide your dissecting scissors beneath that layer in both directions creating a space. Then cut the aponeurosis of external oblique with the scissors in both directions in the line of its fibres and insert your retractor into this space.

Next you have to open the **internal oblique** layer – there's a very thin layer of connective tissue around this which is usually easier to just incise, but then you need to split this muscle – here it runs perpendicular to the external oblique. You can open up a space initially with a clip but then it's easiest to use Langenbeck retractors. So this is a **muscle-splitting** technique. The same needs to be done for the next layer, the **transversus abdominus**, which runs transversely. If the patient is obese there's often a layer of fat in between each of these layers.

After you've opened the transversus abdominus you'll come to the **peritoneum** itself, which may be covered by an **extraperitoneal fat** layer. Here you can see the peritoneum as a whitish, often described as glistening, membrane. Put **two clips** on it and **feel** between finger and thumb to check you haven't caught any bowel. Then **snip** the peritoneum with your scissors and allow air to enter the peritoneal cavity – the bowel will then fall away to safety. Note any free fluid, and if there is any, take a **microbiology swab**; also note any free air, which you will see as a

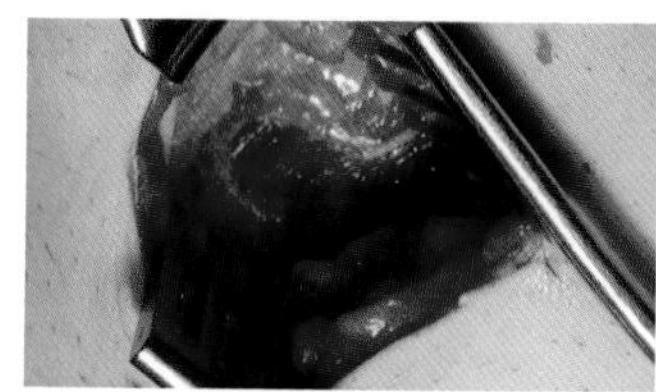

Figure 1.40 The next layer is the internal oblique with its fibres running at 90 degrees to external oblique.

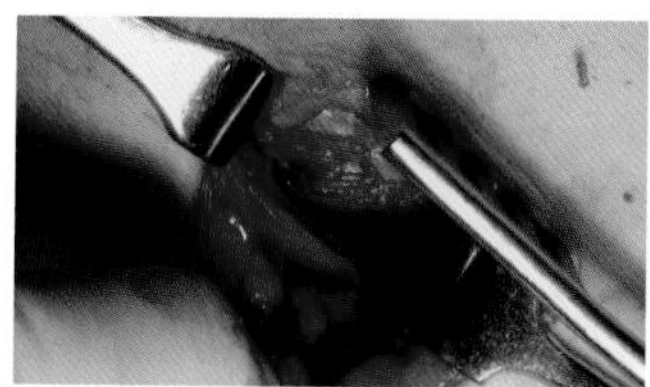

Figure 1.41 Here in the next layer the fibres are running transversely.

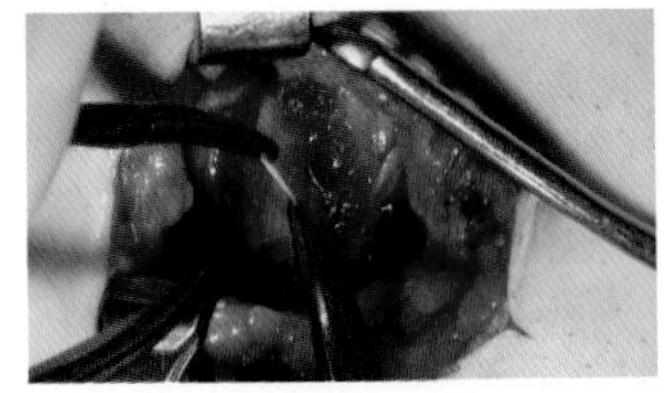

Figure 1.42 The shiny white peritoneum has been picked up in clips.

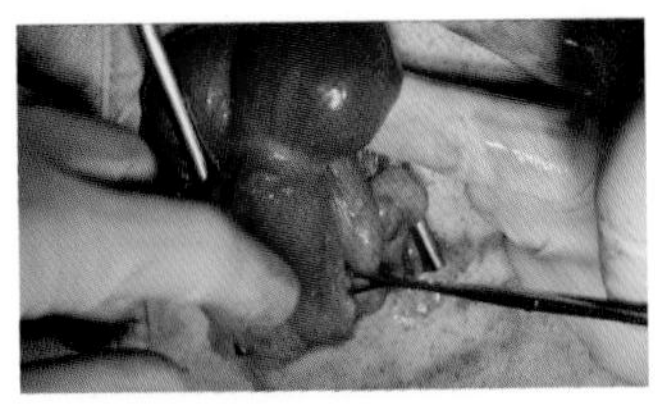

Figure 1.43 The caecum has been delivered and the appendix is becoming visible – Babcock forceps are now encircling it.

bubble under the peritoneum. Now **enlarge the hole** in the peritoneum with the scissors and then stretch it with your fingers.

So now we have to find the appendix, which is sometimes easier said than done. First of all, remove your retractor and clips as these just get in the way and put your finger into the peritoneal cavity. **Feel for the appendix** – a tubular structure, maybe there's a mass due to an inflamed appendix and adherent omentum. But the likelihood is you won't feel anything useful at all, at least until you're a bit more experienced at it.

You now need to deliver the appendix into the wound. **Non-traumatic forceps** such as **Dennis-Brown forceps** are very useful for this – some prefer using their fingers or **Babcock forceps**. Try to look for the caecum and deliver that out. When reaching in and delivering blindly, which to a certain extent you sometimes have to do, what you will deliver will be one of three things and none of them is the appendix: **omentum**, **small bowel** or **caecum**. It's the caecum you want. If you keep getting omentum or small bowel push it medially out of the way with a swab on

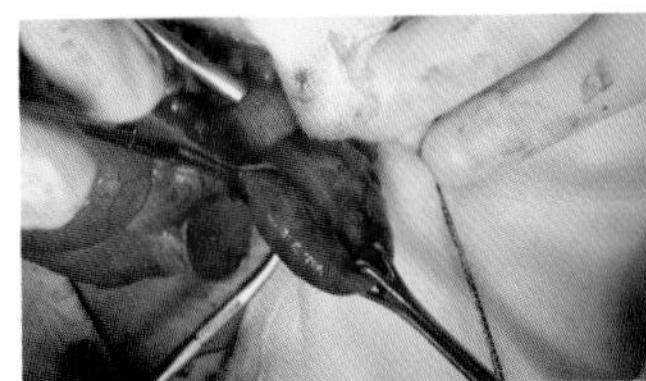

Figure 1.44 The inflamed appendix is controlled with two Babcock forceps to display the mesoappendix.

a stick. If you're really struggling with small bowel it sometimes helps to ask the anaesthetist to tilt the table to the left so gravity helps tilt the small bowel away. You will recognise the colon by its pale pink colour and presence of those longitudinal **taenia coli**. Once you've got it, trace the taenia coli inferiorly – they converge on the appendix. **Deliver** it into the wound using **Babcock forceps** around the proximal appendix, and another around the distal appendix to secure it.

First you need to **ligate and divide the mesoappendix**. Do this by clipping, cutting and tying, with absorbable ties like 2-0 Vicryl. Now crush the appendix base gently with a clip and then immediately replace the clip just distally

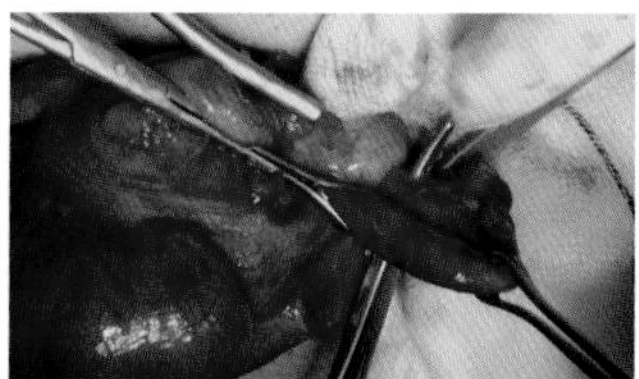

Figure 1.45 The mesoappendix is divided by creating a window with clips and then ties.

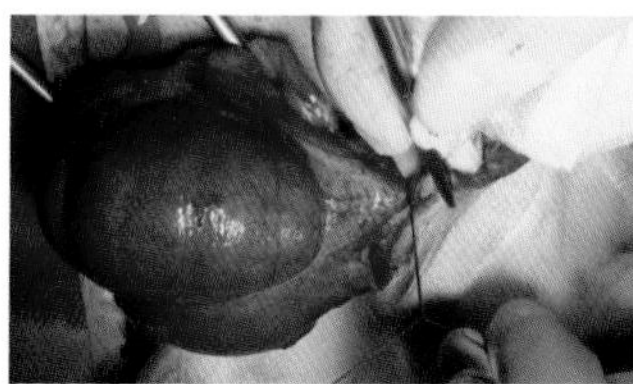

Figure 1.46 With the mesoappendix completely divided the appendix has been clipped and the base is tied and will then be divided.

to this. **Transfix or tie** the base of the appendix and cut the appendix off flush with the clip, leaving a short stump of appendix. Some people bury the stump with a purse string suture. Others diathermy the mucosa on the appendix stump. Others do neither of these and leave it as is. There is no strong evidence for any particular choice.

If the appendix was normal, **examine the rest** of the ascending colon, the distal small bowel for a Meckel's diverticulum, the reproductive organs in the woman and anything else you can reach through your small incision. If the appendix was really inflamed with contamination in the abdominal cavity, **wash** the peritoneal cavity out with normal saline. **Close the wound in layers** with absorbable sutures. You may find it helpful to close the peritoneal layer just because it keeps the bowel from interfering with the rest of the closure, but it's not imperative. Close the transversus and internal oblique together with a couple of interrupted stitches just to show them the way and then the external oblique with another continuous stitch. If you have any thread left you may try to close the fat and fascia layer altogether, but this isn't essential. If the appendix was normal or only mildly inflamed, close the skin with an absorbable **subcuticular continuous** suture. If it was gangrenous and there was lots of free pus, use **skin staples**, the rationale being that it's easier to remove one or two staples in the event of a wound infection than it is to open a wound that's been closed subcuticularly. Some do not agree and will always close using subcuticular stitches. Consider giving some **local anaesthetic** depending on whether the anaesthetist's already given a block. Apply a dry dressing like Mepore or Opsite.

Notes

So what do you do if you can't bring out the appendix just like that? Welcome to the club. Well first of all, the appendix may be **stuck** to some omentum and you will need to feel with your fingers to free it up, particularly if it's a pelvic appendix stuck, say, to the pelvic side wall. You need a little experience to know how much force you can use when blindly trying to free up adhesions, but most adhesions will come away with fairly gentle probing fingers, making it much easier to try again and deliver the appendix.

You'll regret thinking appendicectomies are easy when faced with a 35 stone patient with a high retrocaecal appendix. First, the obese patient will obviously mean that before you've even got to the external oblique, you're already looking down a very deep hole. Try using a **Norfolk and Norwich** self-retainer – like the Travers but with deeper scope. Second, always warn patients about this beforehand – you'll almost certainly need a longer incision. Third, there will probably be additional layers of fat in between all the muscle layers and in the preperitoneal space, just anticipate this and make your way through it. Fourth, even if the caecum and appendix are nicely mobile and easy to deliver out of the wound, in an obese patient that still only means at the bottom of a deep dark hole. You need **good retraction** from your assistant and a **generous-sized hole**.

More problematic is the **retrocaecal appendix.** In your exam you will probably get away with saying **'mobilise the caecum'**, which means dividing the peritoneum holding down the caecum. You'll need a bigger hole for that, so extend the wound. Alternatively, if you can get the base of the appendix but the tip seems to be vanishing off into the distance and you can't deliver it, consider starting by amputating it at the base before you divide the mesoappendix. You can then divide the mesoappendix in a retrograde direction. This can make the appendix much easier to deliver. Bear in mind, however, that the appendix or even just the tip of the appendix can be very friable – you need to take care not to leave chunks of it behind.

Even more problematic is the **sub-hepatic appendix**. In other words, you've hunted everywhere for it and eventually find that it's coursing up behind the ascending colon and its tip is nestled somewhere in the region of the hepatic flexure. Bummer. Again, there are no two ways about it – you need excellent assistance and a generous-sized wound. Many people advocate extending the wound laterally by curving the incision superiorly, creating what looks like a **hockey stick**, or even turning it into something heading towards being a **Rutherford-Morrison** incision, which is a continuation of the lateral end of the wound obliquely up towards the loin. You obviously can't keep to the gentler muscle separation technique you usually use for an appendicectomy – you'll need to just cut through the muscles en masse. With the right exposure, the rest of the operation becomes much easier whatever the position of the appendix.

Remember, if you're struggling, the likeliest problem is that you have inadequate access – make the hole bigger – much better a safe operation at the cost of a larger scar. In fact, if you call your boss, the first thing he'll do is extend the wound – you can always do the operation if the hole is big enough. **Remember, big mistakes through small holes**.

Summary

- The patient is **supine** under general anaesthetic **(GA)** with the abdomen **shaved** and **prepped** and the right lower quadrant **draped**

- Make a **Lanz** incision over McBurney's point
- **Cut** through **skin**, **superficial fascia**, **fat** and identify **external oblique**
- Incise **external oblique** and open with scissors
- Insert a **self-retaining retractor**
- Open **internal oblique** and **transversus abdominus** by a **muscle-splitting** technique
- Put clips on the **peritoneum** and **open** this with scissors
- Take a **swab** for M, C and S if there's pus
- **Examine** with a **finger**
- Try to **deliver the appendix** into the wound
- Once identified, use **two Babcock's forceps** to hold on to the appendix
- **Ligate** and **divide** the **mesoappendix**
- **Transfix** or **tie the stump** and amputate the appendix and send to histology
- **Examine** the small bowel, caecum, pelvic viscera and anything else you can lay your fingers on
- Consider a **washout**
- **Close in layers** with absorbable suture
- **Close the skin** either with **subcuticular** absorbable suture or **skin clips** if heavily infected
- Consider **local anaesthetic** infiltration
- **Remember, if you're struggling, you probably need a bigger wound**

Inguinal hernia repair

Matt Stephenson and Stephen Whitehead

Introduction

Inguinal hernia repairs are easy aren't they? Ermm…no, not really. Or at least not to begin with. The learning curve for an inguinal hernia is actually quite steep, probably because they can look so different every time you open the inguinal canal – it can be very frustrating. We've all been there. It never looks as clear as it does in the textbooks or atlases, it's almost as if the people who wrote those books had never seen one in real life. Like the appendicectomy, the inguinal hernia repair can be difficult for the beginner, yet these two operations are still left to the most junior surgeons, often without supervision.

Nevertheless, take heart that everyone struggles to begin with and that once you've seen and done a few it will become second nature. Here we describe the Lichtenstein mesh repair – the most commonly used technique in the UK.

Procedure

With the patient **supine** and under **general** or **local** anaesthesia, **shave**,

prep and **drape** the groin. Note the **bony landmarks** of the **anterior superior iliac spine (ASIS)** and the **pubic tubercle**. The **inguinal ligament** runs between these two. Your incision therefore needs to be a finger breadth or two **above and parallel** to the medial half to two-thirds of this.

Incise through **skin**, **Camper's fascia** and **Scarpa's fascia** (which is white and membranous) then through **fat**. It's likely you'll encounter a **chunky vein** running vertically in your wound – ligate and divide it if it's substantial enough, otherwise use diathermy. Keep incising down to **external oblique** maintaining **haemostasis** as you go. If the abdominal wall is quite thick, inserting a **Travers retractor** at this stage can be quite helpful.

You'll recognise the **aponeurosis** of external oblique by the fibrous strands running parallel to your wound. Once you've reached it, you need to decide the level at which you're going to open it. **Trace the fibres** down towards the pubic tubercle and look for where they **decussate**. That's what the **external ring** is, a triangular gap where the upper fibres plunge inferiorly to the lateral tip of the pubic tubercle and the lower fibres criss-cross over and leap over to attach more medially. You can actually see this decussation and it marks the apex of the external ring where the hernia may be popping out.

So make a **stab incision** in the line of the fibres at the level of the apex of the external ring. Take a small **clip** and clasp the upper leaf and the same with the lower leaf. Using closed dissecting scissors bluntly, **create a plane** below the external oblique in the line of the canal, thus separating off the cord or the **ilioinguinal nerve** which may be sticking to it just below the surface. **Score** with the scissors inferomedially down to the external ring and the same superolaterally. With upward traction on the external oblique clips gently **dissect** beneath external oblique, superiorly and then inferiorly, thus **creating a plane** beneath it. Insert the Travers retractors into this plane. **Congratulations**, you have now opened the inguinal canal. But I'm sorry you haven't fixed the patient yet, now comes the hard part. You look into the canal and unless you're very lucky, you'll just see a big, bulging, muscley, fatty, tissuey lump. What you're

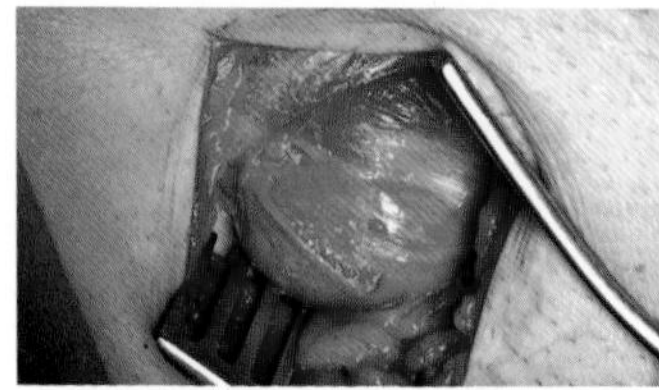

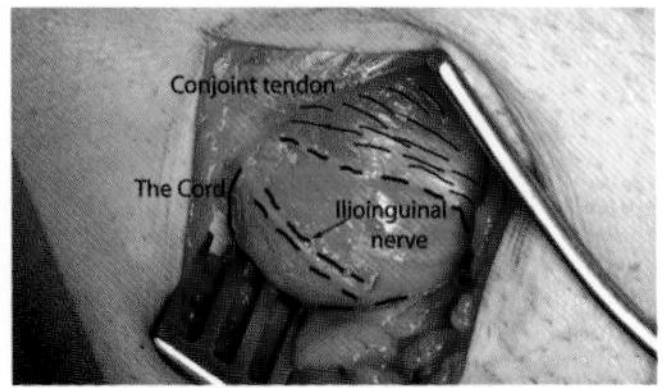

Figure 1.47 The bulging cord is shown outlined. Note the ilioinguinal nerve running over the front of it and the lower fibres of transversus abdominus which at their most inferior part form the conjoint tendon along with the internal oblique.

looking at is two things: the **cord** and the **sac** and they may be intimately entwined.

The first thing to do is separate the **cord (+/– sac)** from the **pubic tubercle**. Begin by **gently snipping** with the tips of your scissors any loose connective tissue that you can obviously see tethering the cord (+/– sac) down to the posterior wall of the inguinal canal. Next you need to **hook** the cord (+/– sac – that's getting boring, assume we mean potentially both for now) up **with your finger**. Insert your index finger into the inguinal canal with fingernail lying against the inside of the inguinal ligament and fingertip pointing to the pubic tubercle. Push your finger under the cord keeping your fingernail apposed to the pubic bone (there should be almost nothing between your fingernail and the bone; all the vessels, etc., arching over the tubercle are staying with the cord – you don't want to leave them behind). Hook up the cord with your finger and **gently probe** with the fingertip until you **see it emerge** on the medial side of the cord. There is a knack to it and it comes with practice. It helps if you keep the axis of your finger horizontal, i.e. in line with the superior edge of the pubic bone, rather than pointing it upwards, as you may just be pushing straight into a direct hernia.

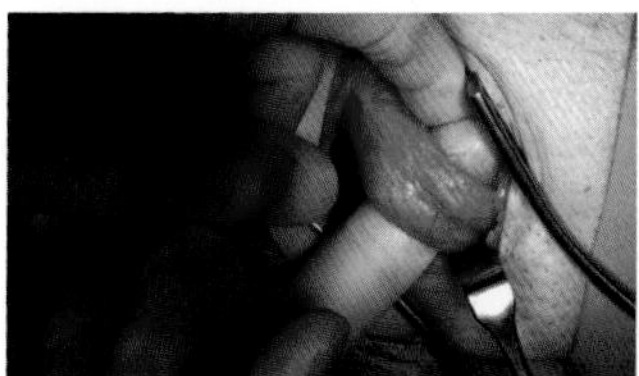

Figure 1.48 The cord has been hooked up by the index finger.

Once the cord is suspended over your hooked finger you need to work out **what's cord and what's sac**. First, is it an **indirect hernia** or a **direct hernia**? In an indirect hernia, the **whole cord is bulky** but it has a **relatively narrow base** (well, the same width as the rest of the cord) emerging from the deep ring and you can easily peel it off the posterior wall, which isn't bulging out. In a direct hernia, however, you will either feel a **thin cord** and behind it the **posterior wall is bulging out**, or more likely, the whole cord seems to be coming from a **very wide base** stretching out over the whole of the back wall. This is because the sac emerging from the posterior wall has **fused** with the cord structures running past it. If this is the case, hook the cord inferoanteriorly and you'll see the posterior wall tethered up to the back of it. **Dissect** the connecting strands with scissors all the way back to the deep ring and the direct hernia bulge will fall back into its rightful place on the posterior wall and the cord will thin out. You may of course find **both**.

So, for the indirect hernia the first part of this game is to find the **white edge** of the peritoneal sac. Everyone has their own favourite method of doing this. Here we show dissecting scissors gently peeling off the outer layers of the cord, all those cremasteric fibres, by firmly stroking the closed tips in the direction of the cord. Some people like to pinch the cord between finger and swab to firmly wipe off the outer layers and systematically go from one edge transversely across to the other, thinning out the cord as they go. However you do it, you're looking for a white edge somewhere within the cord.

Once you see it, **get a clip** on it, get two if you can. Lift them up and gently **dissect all the adjacent tissue away** from the white edge, keeping close to the white edge, until the white edge gets bigger and bigger and more and more separate from the rest of the cord. If you're not sure where it's going, for example if you think it's going all the way down into the scrotum, you can **open it** and put your **finger inside**. Get the whole sac dissected out down to the level of the deep ring.

Twist the sac several times thus pushing any contents back into the abdomen and **transfix it** at the base with an absorbable suture such as 2-0 Vicryl. **Cut the stalk** of the sac first, not the stitch, that way you can check it's not bleeding before it dives back into the abdomen. If the deep ring has been widened by this intruder a **simple stitch** or two, **medially** and/or **laterally**, to the ring will help.

Now what if you find a direct hernia? This is much easier, you could just go straight to the mesh step but it's usually easier to push the hernia back in with your finger, thus invaginating it, and then **plicate the posterior wall**. This stitch doesn't have much strength but it does make it easier to get the mesh down flat on the posterior wall. **Poke the hernia** back in with your index finger, this creates a **little ridge** of tissue (made of a bit of transversus abdominus and transversalis fascia) just above and below the tip of your finger in the medial part of the posterior wall – take a bite of the

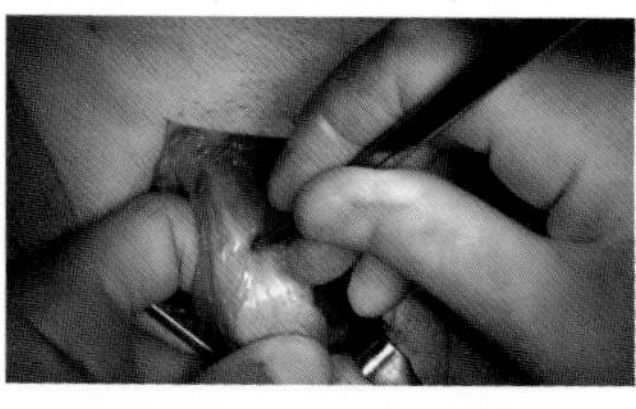

Figure 1.49 Dissection of the sac with the tips of the dissecting scissors.

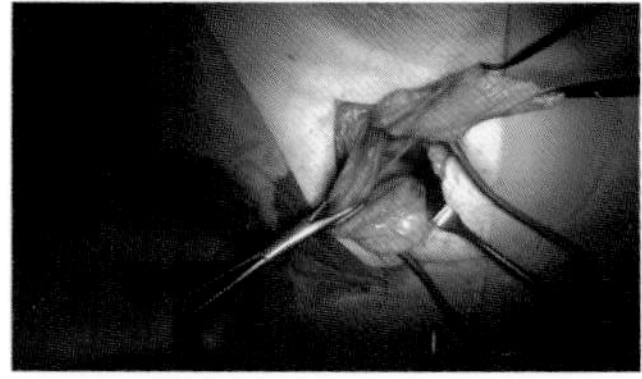

Figure 1.51 The sac has been dissected from the cord and is being retracted superiorly with clips while a Lane retractor is retracting the cord inferiorly. A Langenbeck retractor exposes the posterior wall.

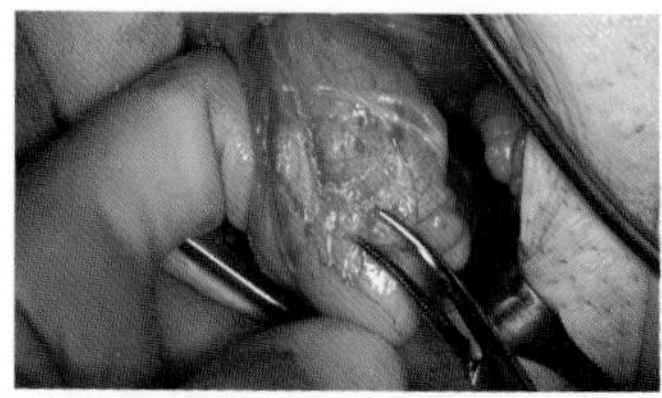

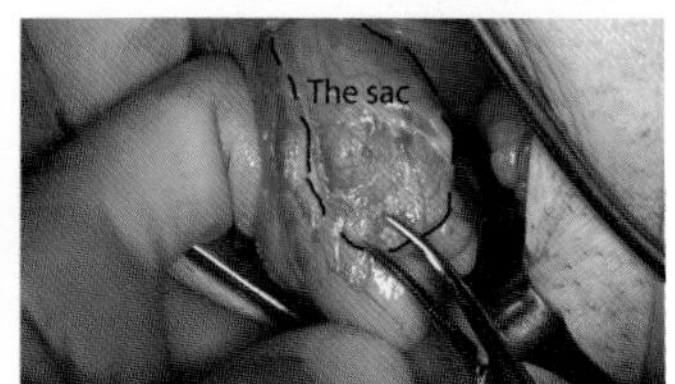

Figure 1.50 Identification of the sac.

bottom ridge and then the top ridge and tie a knot (obviously taking care not to include your finger in the stitch). Keep stitching bottom ridge to top ridge until the hernia is essentially **inverted** and the back wall looks flat. Don't be overly ambitious with those stitches, trying for example to stitch strong muscle all the way down to inguinal ligament – this is unnecessary and just creates tension, which is not what you want for wounds to heal. Also don't place the stitches too deep, don't forget that the **inferior epigastric vessels** aren't far behind.

Now for the **mesh**. **Shape** it roughly before inserting it. The corner that will lie over the pubic tubercle can be rounded off. **Create a slit** so that you can wrap it round the cord – and at the apex of the slit create a **V shape** so that the cord can fit through.

Stitch or **staple** the rounded corner to the tissue lying just over the **pubic tubercle**. It's very important that the mesh **overlaps the pubic tubercle** and, superiorly, extends well beyond it, ideally to the **midline** – this is where the hernia will recur if you don't. Hold the lower part of the mesh down so its lower edge is right over the inside of the **inguinal ligament**. Run a **continuous non-absorbable suture such as 2-0 Prolene**, suturing the two together, alternatively use staples. When you get to the deep ring, suture or staple the upper leaf to the lower leaf just lateral to the deep ring thus recreating a new deep ring. Stitch the upper leaf down to the inguinal ligament. Not much else needs to be done laterally. Medially you need to stitch the edge of the mesh down to the posterior wall, or staple it. **Stretch the mesh out** over the posterior wall so that it **isn't heaped up** or **too tight** and continue the suture or staples around the medial edge onto the superior edge. Take care to **avoid including a nerve** in your suture or staple.

If you've got this far and it's your first hernia, very well done to you. Now **close** up. Reapply **clips** to the upper and lower edges of external oblique and run a **continuous absorbable suture such as 2-0 Vicryl** from lateral to medial or medial to lateral, thus reconstructing the **external ring**. The **fascia** and **fat** can be closed with **continuous absorbable** suture and the **skin** with an **absorbable subcuticular suture**.

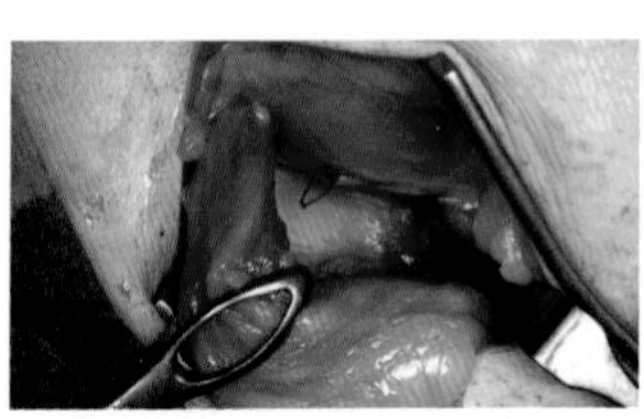

Figure 1.52 Gentle anteroinferior traction on the cord reveals the posterior wall – here it has been plicated.

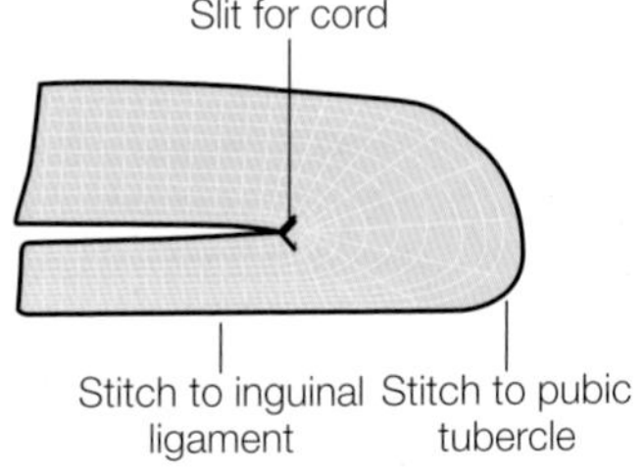

Figure 1.53 The shape to cut the mesh into for a right-sided inguinal hernia. On the left, obviously it's the mirror image.

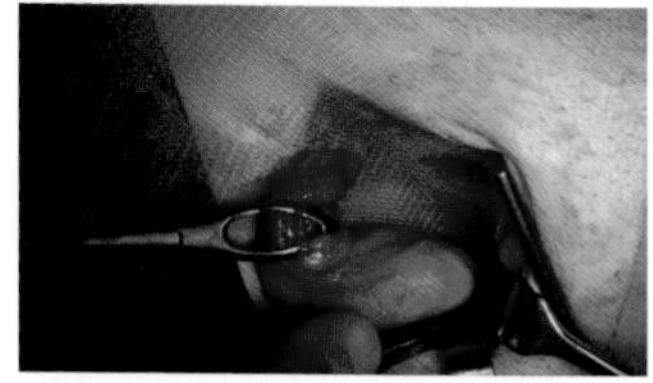

Figure 1.54 The mesh has been inserted with the upper and lower leaves wrapping around the base of the cord – the deep ring.

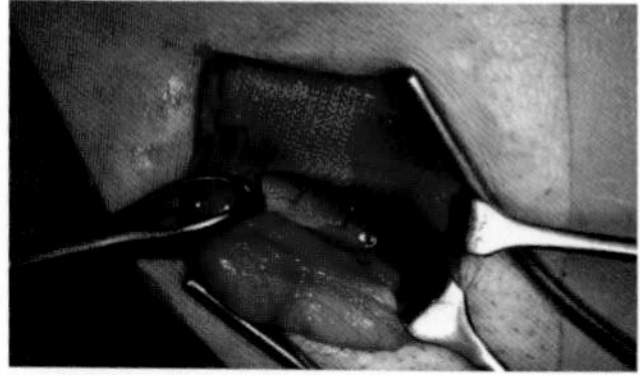

Figure 1.55 Completed mesh – note the inferior row of staples has been inserted onto the inside of the inguinal ligament.

Notes

In **women**, inguinal hernia repairs are considerably easier. They have only rudimentary structures, principally the round ligament, passing through their inguinal canal, and this can be simply **ligated and divided**. The hernia can then be invaginated back into the abdominal cavity and the posterior wall plicated as for a direct inguinal hernia. You can then apply a piece of mesh without the usual slit to accommodate the cord, directly on to the posterior wall and stitch or staple it in.

In **inguinoscrotal** hernias, the sac passes right through the canal into the scrotum, where it's usually firmly adherent. **Don't try and dissect** the sac out of the scrotum – this will just result in lots of bleeding and is unnecessary. Instead, dissect out the sac in the usual way from the cord and **transect it**, leaving the distal part in the scrotum undissected, and **leave it open**. Any fluid that builds up in the residual sac will drain out of the hole, so don't close it or you're effectively giving the patient a hydrocoele. Deal with the proximal side in the same way as you would for any indirect hernia.

Summary

- The patient is **supine** and under **general** or **local anaesthetic**
- The right groin is **shaved**, **prepped** and **draped**
- **Incise skin** above the medial half of the inguinal ligament
- Incise down to **external oblique**
- **Open** external oblique at the level of the external ring
- **Create a plane** beneath external oblique
- **Separate cord** +/– sac from the **pubic tubercle**
- Separate **cord from sac**
- **Transfix** and **amputate** indirect sacs
- **Plicate posterior wall** if bulging
- **Shape** and **insert** a mesh securing it, most importantly, medially
- **Close** the external oblique
- **Close** fascia then skin

Dynamic hip screw

Matt Stephenson and Lisa Leonard

Introduction

So when should you perform a **dynamic hip screw (DHS)** and when should you perform a **hemiarthroplasty** for a **fractured neck of femur**? The choice depends on whether or not the fracture is likely to compromise the blood supply to the femoral head, resulting in **avascular necrosis**. Remember that the **blood supply** to the femoral head comes from three principal sources:

1 through the **foveolar artery** in the ligamentum teres (not usually affected by a hip fracture and doesn't supply much blood anyway so clinically irrelevant, except in children)

2 the **nutrient artery** of the shaft

3 the **retinacular vessels** that run within the hip joint capsule, these are the most important ones.

Femoral neck fractures can be broadly divided into **intracapsular** and **extracapsular**. Remember that the capsule inserts **low down** on the femoral neck, perhaps lower than you might think.

Intracapsular fractures are then classified by the **Garden classification** into the following four stages.

Stage 1: A valgus impacted fracture, and undisplaced.

Stage 2: Complete fracture of the neck but undisplaced.

Stage 3: Complete fracture and partially displaced, because the femoral head is still hinged on to

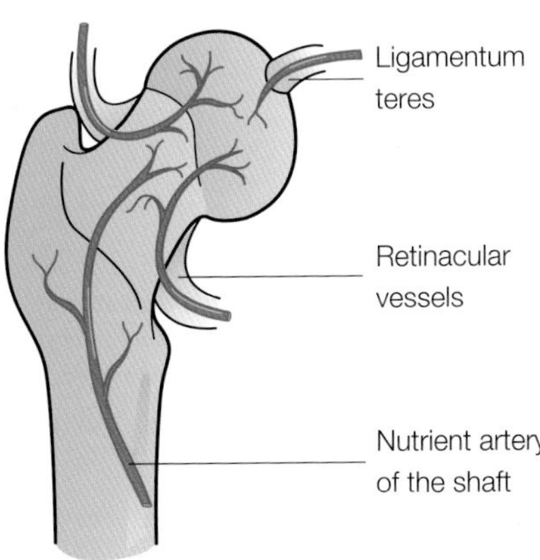

Figure 1.56 The blood supply of the femoral head.

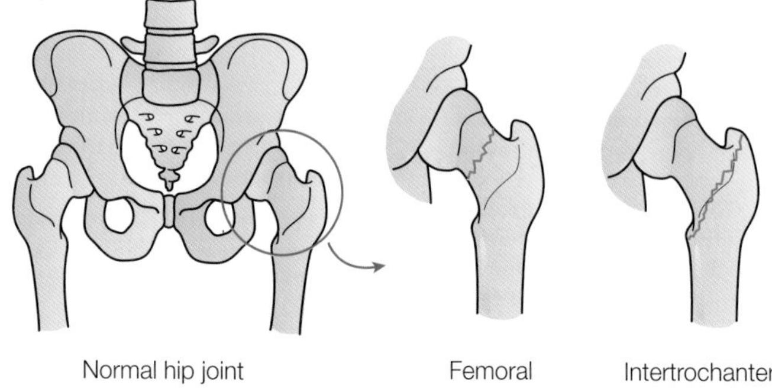

Figure 1.57 Types of hip fracture – extracapsular and intracapsular

the shaft to some extent, and the bony trabeculae of the femoral head no longer line up with those of the adjacent acetabulum.

Stage 4: Complete fracture and completely displaced, now the head is free to rotate back to the anatomical position in the acetabulum and the trabeculae lines now line up again.

In **Garden 1 and 2**, the femoral head should still be perfused by a combination principally of the retinacular vessels and to a lesser extent the nutrient artery. Therefore all that is required is to fix the fracture site to give it time to heal – a **dynamic hip screw** is indicated. If the head is displaced, however, i.e. **Garden 3 and 4**, then the nutrient artery will certainly have been torn, as almost certainly will the retinacular vessels because the capsule will also have been torn. The femoral head, even if you fix it in place, will die. Replacement of the femoral head is indicated – a **hemiarthroplasty**. You can use the mnemonic: **one, two: screw; three, four: Austin-Moore**. This is a slight oversimplification (see the Notes section).

In **extracapsular fractures**, the retinacular vessels will still be intact and all that is required is fixation of the fracture, hence a **dynamic hip screw** is needed in these patients.

Procedure

The patient is under either **general** or **spinal anaesthetic** and **supine** on an **orthopaedic traction table**. The **feet** are **secured in stirrups** allowing the legs to be manipulated into various positions. There are numerous joints and adaptable components on this equipment, making it very versatile. The first thing to do in a displaced fracture is to **reduce the fracture**, obviously

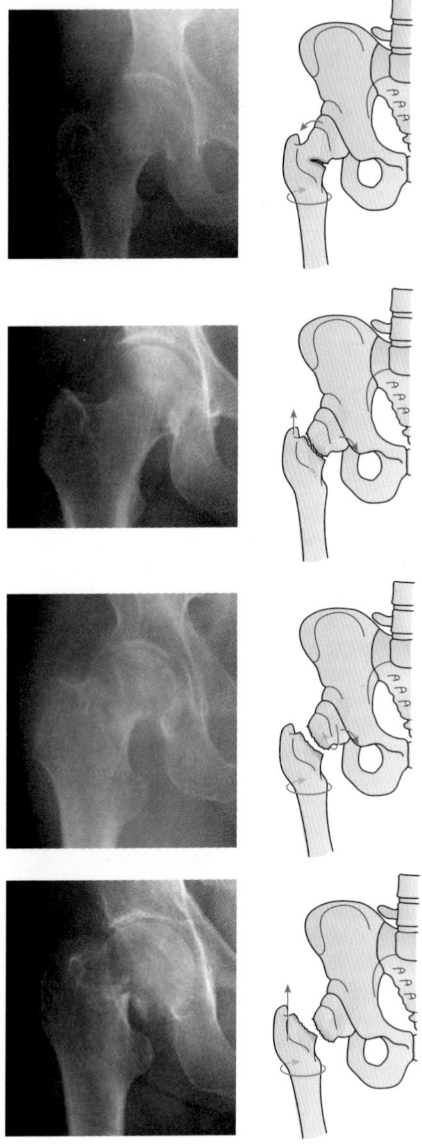

Figure 1.58 The Garden classification of intracapsular fractures.

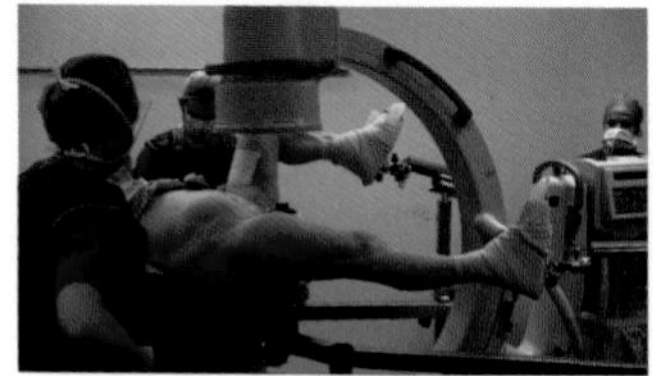

Figure 1.59 The patient is on an orthopaedic traction table with the affected leg on traction, abduction and internally rotated. The unaffected leg is abducted allowing the II to easily view the hip. Note the traction groin post between the patient's legs; this allows traction to be applied to the leg without the patient falling off the table – take care of the genitals though.

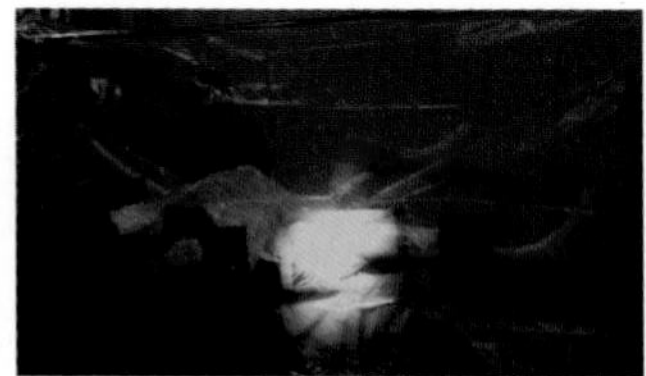

Figure 1.60 The operative site is draped with a large sterile drape attached to drip stands and an overhead bar.

you don't want to fix it into an abnormal position. To do this, put **traction** on the affected leg and apply **internal rotation** to it so that the patella is facing the ceiling.

Clearly you're going to need to have X-ray vision to see whether you've returned it to a satisfactory position. And that's what the **image intensifier** (affectionately known as the **II**) is there for. It is shaped like a large C, emitting X-rays from one end with an X-ray detector on the other end. By abducting the unaffected leg widely, you can get the II into position to view the fracture site in both **anteroposterior** (AP) and **lateral** views. Make sure that there's nothing obstructing the movement of the II so that it can be easily changed to the AP or lateral positions during the course of the operation. Of course, if the fracture is undisplaced, you can fix it where it is without any manipulation.

Once you're happy with the position **prep** the whole of the thigh and surrounding areas and apply a **drape** to the upper lateral thigh. This drape is pretty huge with a sticky bit for the operative site, and peripherally to this is a large transparent plastic sheet that can be fixed to some drip stands and an intervening horizontal bar or similar equipment to give a very large sterile wall from floor to above standing height. It also has a collecting pouch beneath the operative field that will help to collect any blood dripping out of the wound and stop it getting to the floor.

So now make the **skin incision**, this should be about 15 cm long, commencing just behind the palpable **greater trochanter and** continuing **longitudinally** down the thigh over the lateral femur (often easily palpable in thin old ladies). Cut straight down through **subcutaneous fat**, maintaining haemostasis as you go. The first obvious layer you see will be the **fascia lata** – a white fascial layer. Incise straight through this. Inserting a **self-retaining retractor** such as a Travers or in a deeper wound, a Norfolk and Norwich retractor (or even two), will help exposure.

The next layer is the **vastus lateralis**. This can be retracted anteriorly and approached from behind, but this can result in a lot of bleeding because of an abundance of perforating vessels posteriorly, so simply **split it** in line with its fibres. First **cut the fascial envelope** of the muscle with a knife and then **bluntly dissect** your way through the muscle. Replace the self-retaining retractor within the muscle and you will find yourself down on to the **periosteum**-covered **lateral femur**. There will be strands of muscle attached to the surface too, so **strip** all these off with a periosteal elevator, including the periosteum, to give a broad surface of upper lateral femur to later place the plate of the DHS device on to.

Apply an **angle guide** to the lateral femur and feel the anterior and posterior edges to make sure you're in the middle. Insert the guide pin through the appropriate hole, which will give you a 135 degree angle into the femoral neck, matching that on your plate. Once your guide and pin are laid against the bone take an X-ray to check the position.

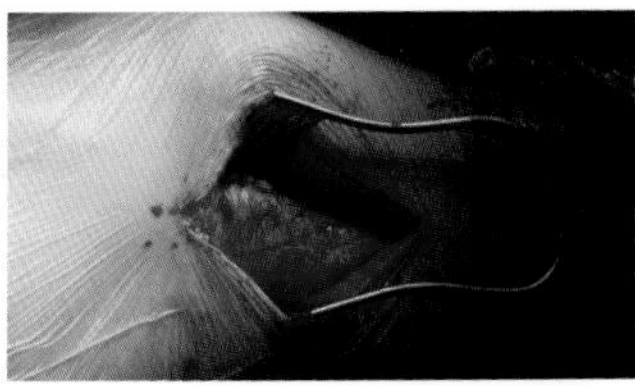

Figure 1.61 Fascial covering of vastus lateralis is exposed

Drill the guide pin into the femur a few centimetres, keeping the angle guide firmly pressed against the femoral shaft and directing it just very slightly anteriorly, as the head is usually slightly anteverted on the shaft (you can see this on the lateral film). **Take another X-ray** in the AP position and check that it's advancing in the right direction. If it is, keep drilling it into the femur with regular X-rays to check its position. You're aiming for dead centre within the femoral head. If it's going in the wrong direction, reposition the angle guide, checking that it's flat against the femoral shaft. Once you've gone some way in towards the femoral neck, **reposition the II** to check the **lateral view**. Sometimes you think you're doing a great job and the angle looks great in the AP view, and then you change to the lateral and realise you've gone out the back of the hip altogether. So the guide pin must be going directly up the axis of the femoral neck in both views. If not, correct it early by withdrawing,

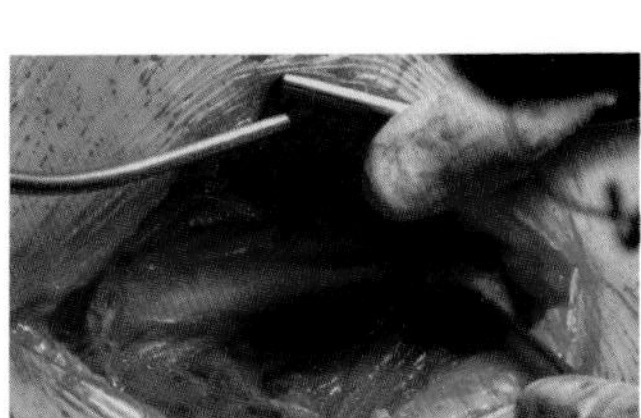

Figure 1.62 A periosteal elevator has scraped off the muscle to expose the lateral surface of femur.

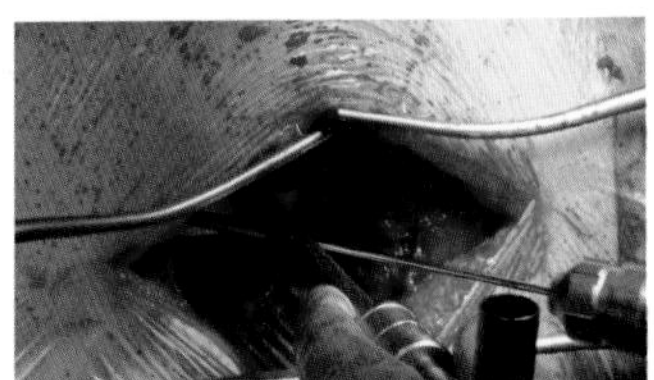

Figure 1.63 Angle guide is placed over the lateral surface of the femur. The guide pin is seen passing obliquely on to the femoral surface.

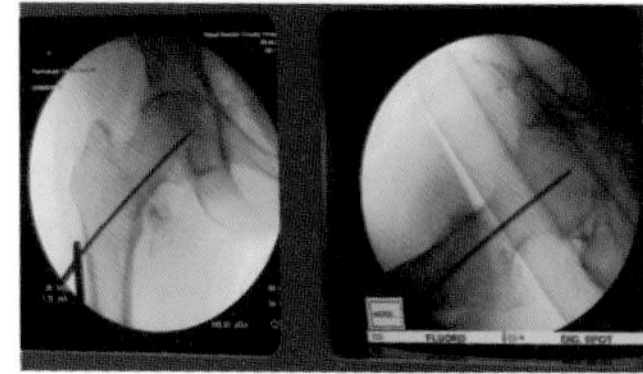

Figure 1.64 On the left, the AP view is seen, and on the right, the lateral view, with the guide pin in an acceptable position.

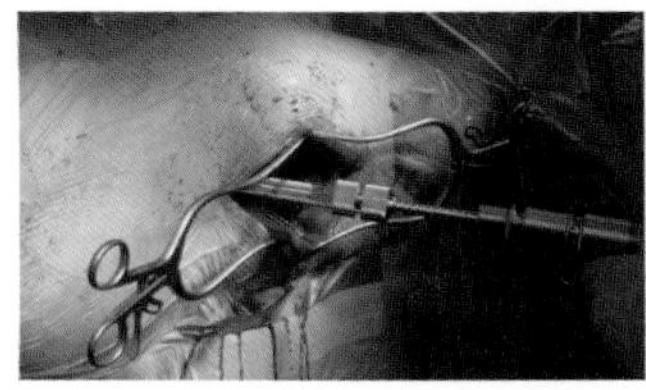

Figure 1.66 The reamer is threaded over the primary guide pin.

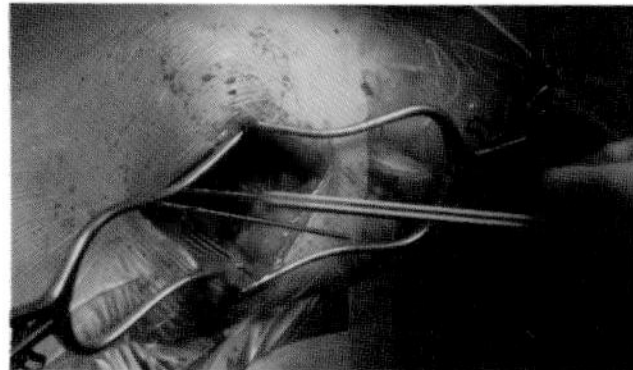

Figure 1.65 You can see two guide pins here, the second is to stop the femoral head from spinning when the screw is screwed in. The measuring device is being fed over the primary guide pin.

repositioning and re-drilling. Get the tip of the guide pin up to the **subchondral surface** of the femoral head. The crucial distance to estimate is the 'tip-apex' distance. This is the distance from the pin to the centre of the femoral head surface. Add this measurement from both the AP and lateral views and the total should come to less than 25 mm. This reduces the chance of the screw cutting out.

Once you're happy with the position in both views you may wish to insert an anti-rotation guide pin. The purpose of this is to prevent the femoral head from spinning around when you come to the next step: reaming. **Remove the angle guide**.

Once you've got a guide pin in the right position, you need to **measure the length** of screw you need. Slide a **measuring device** over the exposed guide pin down to where it vanishes inside the femur. This is specially calibrated to give the length of screw needed, determining how much guide pin is inside by subtracting how much is left outside. Ask for the screw at this stage at the same length as your measurement, but ask for the reamer to be set at 5–10 mm less than the measurement. Check the reamer length you are given and feed it over the guide pin and **ream out** the space for the screw to go in, checking on the II that the pin hasn't been pushed in through the acetabulum.

Now **insert the screw** into the reamed out space and **screw it in firmly** so that the screw engages deep within the femoral head. Once it's in position, the handle of the screwing device should be **parallel** with the axis of the femur. This is important because the end of the screw is shaped to engage with the plate in this orientation, thus preventing rotation of the femoral head once the plate is in place.

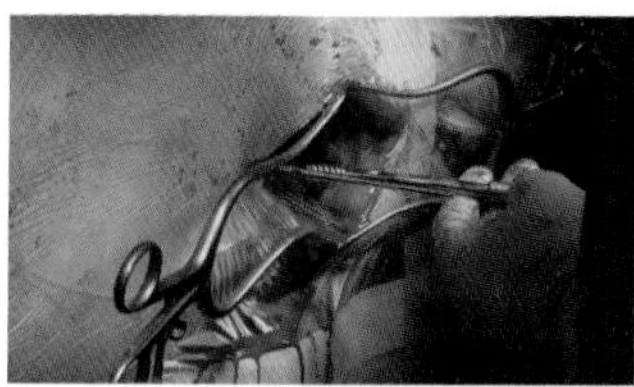

Figure 1.67 The dynamic hip screw is threaded over the guide pin and screwed into place.

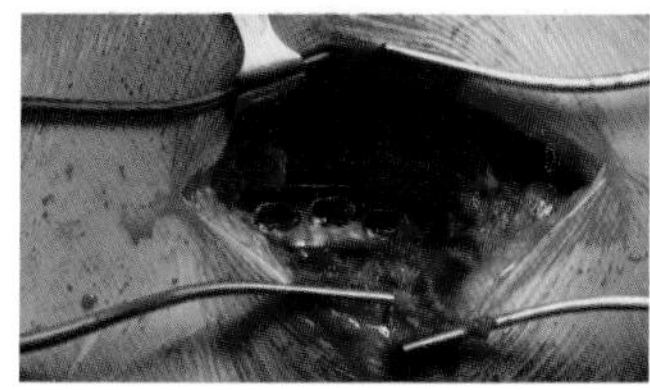

Figure 1.69 The plate lying against the femur – the holes are about to accommodate screws.

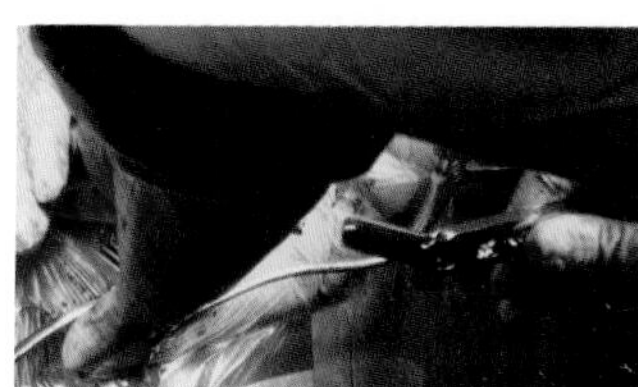

Figure 1.68 The barrel of the plate is about to be threaded over the screw.

Confirm the position throughout with the II.

Next, **slide the barrel** of the **plate** down over the distal end of the screw and lay it down along the long axis of the femur. Make sure there are no strands of muscle interposed between it and the femur. Because of the shape of the screw, the plate will fit on to it and not be able to rotate; however, the screw will be able to **slide in and out** of the buttress plate, hence the term dynamic, and this allows the fracture site to **collapse**, **compress** together and **unite**. Using an orthopaedic **mallet,** hammer the buttress plate firmly into position.

There are several holes along the plate to accommodate the screws. Check that the most distal screw hole lines up with the femur. The first thing to do is **drill a hole** all the way through the femur through the proximal plate hole. You'll feel the resistance in drilling while going through the **lateral cortex** and then a give as it passes through this because the drill passes easily through the soft **medullary canal**. There will then be another wall of resistance as it engages the **medial cortex**. Drill through this and there will be another give of overcoming resistance as you pass through the other side of the femur – obviously stop as soon as you feel this. Remove the drill and insert a **depth gauge**. This consists of a long central pin with a hooked end that you pass straight through your drill hole out the other side of the femur and then pull back allowing the hook to get caught on the outer surface of the medial cortex. There is then an outer component that slides down over the central pin to abut the surface of the buttress plate, allowing you to measure the depth the pin has gone in and thus the length of screw required.

Repeat this for all the screw holes and **screw** the appropriately sized screws into position. **Check the final position** of the dynamic hip screw, buttress plate and femoral screws with the II.

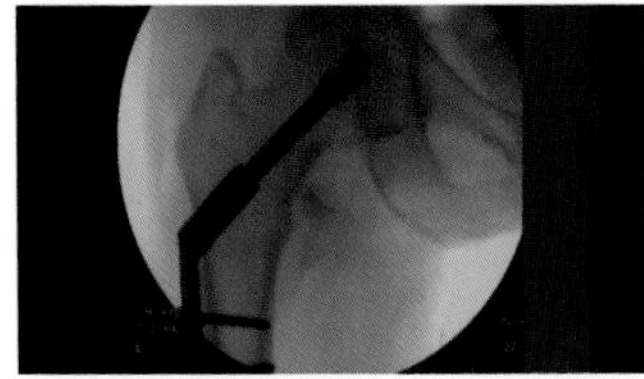

Figure 1.70 Final position of dynamic hip screw. A further image should be taken inferiorly to check the position of the other screws.

Irrigate the wound with normal saline to remove any fragments of bone that can act as a nidus for infection, and check for **haemostasis**. **Close the fascial envelope** of the vastus lateralis and then the **fascia lata** with absorbable sutures. Closing the fat layer is optional, but then **close the skin** with a subcuticular absorbable continuous suture.

Notes

In young and fit patients (for example under 40) with a displaced subcapital fracture you want to try to retain the femoral head if at all possible as an emergency, accepting the higher risk of avascular necrosis, with cannulated screws or a short dynamic hip screw with an anti-rotation screw. In a slightly older age group, but still fit, a total hip replacement might be a better option as these give better long-term functional results. Uncemented hemiarthroplasties are now usually reserved for medically unfit poorly mobile patients. Cemented hemiarthroplasty or bipolar prostheses are other options.

Summary

- The patient is under **GA** or **spinal, supine** on an **orthopaedic traction table**
- **Reduce the fracture** and abduct the unaffected leg
- **Position the II** and **confirm reduced position** in AP and lateral views
- Make **skin incision**
- **Incise** through **fat**, **fascia lata** and **vastus lateralis**
- **Scrape muscle** and **periosteum** off femur
- **Drill guide pin** using **angle guide**
- **Confirm position** with II in both dimensions
- Consider **inserting second pin** if risk of femoral head rotation
- **Measure size** of screw
- **Ream** appropriate size space for screw
- **Screw in dynamic hip screw**
- **Confirm position** with II
- Insert **buttress plate**
- **Drill holes** in femoral shaft and **measure depth**
- **Screw** in appropriately sized screws
- **Check position**
- **Irrigate** and **close in layers**

Reference

Stephenson M (2011) *How to Operate*. Oxford: John Wiley & Sons, Ltd.

Chapter 2
WARDS

Matt Stephenson

Surgical ward rounds, 45
Handover, 50
Drains and tubes, 53
Wounds and ulcers, 56
Managing complications, 60
Sick patients, 66
End of life care, 69
References, 70

The art of medicine consists in amusing the patient while nature cures the disease
Voltaire (1694–1778)

Surgical ward rounds

It's a universally accepted fact that **medics are lazier than surgeons** – this explains why they wake up so late and start their day at 9am, whereas surgeons begin at 8am or earlier. And because of our early, efficient starts we finish our ward rounds in a fraction of the time it takes the medics, who will occupy their whole day with a ward round. In fact many surgeons will cite the fact that surgical ward rounds don't last all day as the reason they went into surgery (although don't use this reason in any interviews).

However, **never underestimate the importance and value of the ward round**. Every day should begin and end with a ward round. And end? Yes, a lot can happen during the course of the day and a snapshot once every 24 hours is not enough in acute surgical patients – the patient list needs to at least be run through on paper with all members of the team at the end of the working day, even if not physically going back to the bedside.

The days of Sir Lancelot Spratt-style ward rounds are, alas, over (if you haven't seen the film *Doctor in the House* you should). **White coats** it seems, for now at least, are out. **Jackets** are left at the door. **Sleeves must be rolled up** above the elbow and cuff links dispensed with. **Ties** must also be consigned to the bin, or at least tucked in. In other words, turn up as if you've just walked in off the street and the powers that be are happy. In truth, patients want to see a doctor

The Hands-on Guide to Surgical Training, First Edition. Matthew Stephenson.

with an open collar no more than they want to see one with an open fly, but that's the way it is at the moment.

You will have already been on some terrible ward rounds at one time or another, when the ward round leader either spends so long **meandering inefficiently** around that you want to gouge your own eyes out, or worse, a **rushed sprint** such that significant problems are missed. How can you best **participate** in a ward round? As you begin to take on the mantle of **ward round leader**, and realise perhaps it's not quite as easy as you'd thought, how can you get the balance right?

Ward round participator

Ward rounds, whether there are two doctors or 15 doctors, are a **team effort**. Everyone involved needs to know what their role is. When it comes to ward rounds, too many cooks can definitely spoil the broth, with no one realising it's their responsibility to be doing something.

For **every patient** in **every ward round**, aside from the dialogue with the patient, the following 10 tasks must be fulfilled.

1 **Draw the curtains** around the bed.

2 Succinctly **summarise** the patient's condition and recent progress, for the benefit of the whole team.

3 Check the **notes** for any entries overnight.

4 Check the **observations chart**.

5 Check the **drug chart**.

6 Check for any **other relevant charts**, e.g. stool chart, blood sugars, etc.

7 Check the **recent blood results**.

8 **Write the outcome** of the round in the notes.

9 **Write down any jobs** generated from the round.

10 **Communicate with the nurse** looking after the patient.

All 10 of these must happen for **every** patient on **every** morning ward round.

At the start of the ward round, if you have been allocated to a specific role – stick to it. If you haven't – don't wait to be asked to do one of the above tasks. Standing by the bedside doing nothing, i.e. not checking a chart or writing in the notes, can make you feel like a lemon, and you're contributing nothing to the round. If there are only two of you, split up the tasks as appropriate. Other tasks that may be required depending on the case include the following.

1 **Peeling off dressings** – always be ready with gloves and some scissors, especially on vascular rounds.

2 Checking **peripheral pulses** with the Doppler probe.

3 Log into PACS (picture archiving and communications system) and **check any recent imaging**.

4 Write **discharge letters**.

5 Write out **request forms** for investigations.

Always carry a **stethoscope** with you, especially if you're a more junior member of the team – the registrar is less likely to have one. All good surgical trainees carry a **permanent marker pen** with them at all times to mark the side of surgery for any preoperative patient. Have to hand **consent forms** and **continuation sheets** for the notes.

Ward round leader

This isn't the **ward round navigator** who decides which patient the round is moving to next, this is the central decision maker and is usually the most senior member of the team, either the consultant or registrar. However, if you have the opportunity to take on this role at FY1 level, this is a valuable experience, even if your decisions are censored/modified somewhat by a senior member of the team. Certainly in FY2 and beyond there will be times it's just you and the FY1 +/– student.

You now must become a **manager of people**. The first key thing is to make sure someone, usually the FY1, knows where they're going – the ward round navigator – i.e. where all the patients are and what order you're seeing them in. This should be pre-planned to optimise efficiency and for this, in general, you need a printed patient list. Always start with patients you've been warned are sick, anticipate might be sick or have had recent major surgery.

Often it's helpful if you have plenty of people to **send someone in advance** to the next ward/bed to get the notes ready there. You should **allocate every member** of the team with a **clear responsibility** at the beginning, i.e. if you have enough people, one person always picks up the drug chart, one person always check the obs chart, etc.

Try to **encourage the most junior staff** to get involved as much as possible – presenting the patient's condition and progress is a particularly useful learning experience for medical students, for instance. Try as much as possible not to have to shoot off to theatre or clinic and to allow some time for **teaching**, even if it's just the smallest of points.

The very first thing on arriving at the patient's bedside is to **greet the patient** and organise for the **curtains to be drawn** around the bed to give the patient some privacy. Imagine how you'd feel if you were the patient and a team of doctors arrive and whisper to each other with the odd glance over to you, before finally acknowledging you. This is a bad practice to get into but is frequently seen. Even if you've never met the patient before, greet them and **introduce yourself** before explaining you're about to hear their story from a colleague. It's almost always best to hear the history **in front of the patient**, as they'll often be able to correct inaccurate points. Obviously sometimes this is inappropriate due to the sensitivity of some problems. **Listen carefully** to the history while observing the patient from the bedside and concentrate on trying to put the whole story together in your head. You must learn to enter an almost hypnotic state where nothing else should enter your mind, especially for those first few moments where often the most crucial hidden points may lurk. **The patient has 100% of your attention** and they should feel that.

Having listened without interruption, proceed with any **clarifying questions** and **examine** the patient as appropriate to the case. Ask for the most recent **physiological observations** from the nursing chart, and from any **other charts**, such as blood sugar monitoring. Have any comments been written in the **notes** over the course of the night? **Scrutinise the drug chart**.

If the patient develops a deep vein thrombosis (DVT) and you missed the fact they weren't written up for, or receiving, their low molecular weight heparin, you are responsible. Are there any antibiotics that should be stopped? If this isn't done now, no one else will do it. Ask for the results of **recent blood tests**. Make sure the **nurse** looking after the patient has voiced any concerns.

While all of this information is being directed to you, it gives you time to cogitate on the problem and consider what to do next. With each patient you see, the surgeon in you is asking three specific questions.

- Does the patient need an operation?
- What operation do they need?
- When do they need it?

Of course in many cases the answer to these three questions is an obvious 'no', so you need to decide what else to do.

Sometimes this is easy. The patient had their laparoscopic cholecystectomy yesterday and they're feeling fine, looking fine with completely normal observations, their bags are packed and they're ready for discharge. But let's be clear, **sometimes you haven't got a clue** what to do next. The patient, the other doctors and the nurses are looking at you patiently waiting. Your 24-year-old female patient came in two days ago with mild right iliac fossa pain and normal tests but it's not quite settling. Do you take her for a laparoscopy? Do you wait a little longer? Do you phone a friend? Perhaps there isn't a right answer, but you must **maintain the trust of the patient** and your team. **Look decisive**, even if you're only being decisive about procrastinating. **Allow yourself time to think** about it, you don't have to make a final decision there and then. Ask a senior or colleague for their opinion and come back to it later.

Sometimes we fool ourselves into thinking everything's OK when it isn't. Your patient is five days post right hemicolectomy and they don't look quite right with a fever of 38.0°C. It's probably just a bit of atelectasis isn't it? Or we'll dip the urine and review it tomorrow. It's all too easy to convince yourself that it's all OK because **you don't want there to be a problem**. Perhaps you did the right hemicolectomy yourself and if you ignore it for a while, the possibility of an anastomotic leak will disappear? Or perhaps you're not sure what to do to find out if they have had a leak or what to do about it if they have? Perhaps you don't have time for it? It's a natural human instinct to avoid problems. However, you must be aware of this, your own hidden agenda, and remember that on a ward round you're primarily **looking for things that have gone wrong** with a patient, not things that have gone right.

The principal way of knowing whether patients are well or ill on a ward round is: '**are they progressing appropriately for their stage?**' This comes with experience. For instance, you should expect a patient admitted with uncomplicated diverticulitis to be having less pain, less tenderness and fewer fevers within 48–72 hours of antibiotics. If not, why not? Are the antibiotics appropriate and is she receiving them? Was the diagnosis right? If so, is she developing a diverticular abscess? If a man is getting worsening abdominal pain over the first 48 hours post laparoscopic anterior resection, something is wrong. Was bowel injured during the procedure? Has there been a bleed? There is, of course, a range of rates of healing after surgery, or responses to treatment, but diversions from the usually trajectory should make you worry.

Everyone assesses the patient in their own way and it's sometimes helpful to have a system to follow, especially when you don't know where to start and especially for very complex patients who have been in for ages, or those in ITU who seem to be attached to dozens of tubes. SOAP is one such method.

- S = Subjective – how does the patient feel?
- O = Objective – what do the observations and examination findings show?
- A = Assessment – what's your summary of the situation?
- P = Plan.

However, this doesn't help you much with the detail of what you're actually supposed to be looking for, so an alternative is needed. One such method is to start from basics and assess each system in turn in order not to miss anything, although they won't necessarily all be relevant in all cases. It's particularly helpful if you've really no idea where to start.

Respiratory – What is their respiratory rate and saturations? Do you need to listen to their chest? Do they need a chest X-ray or arterial blood gas assessment? Atelectasis, pneumonia and pulmonary emboli can all occur in surgical patients and their early recognition is crucial.

Cardiovascular – What is the pulse and blood pressure? It's not sufficient to say that the 'obs are stable' when reading them out. If the blood pressure is consistently 60/30 it's stable, but not normal.

Neurological – Are you having a normal conversation or are they drowsy? How much morphine have you been giving them? Would it be worth knowing their CO_2?

Gastrointestinal – Are they eating and drinking, and if not why not? Is it that they don't have their dentures or they've been nil by mouth for the past 10 days getting no nutrition? Should you be thinking about organising some TPN (total parenteral nutrition)? Has your post-dynamic hip screw patient had their bowels open lately? Could they do with some laxatives?

Metabolic – Loosely fit the temperature in here – are they pyrexial? Hypothermic? Are you worrying about sepsis? How are their BMs in the diabetic? How are the electrolytes (including magnesium)?

Renal/Urological – What is the renal function? What is the urine output? What is the fluid balance? Do they still need their urinary catheter?

Musculoskeletal/Soft tissue – Where appropriate, is the patient getting as much opportunity as possible to mobilise? Have they developed any pressure sores?

Operative site – Does the wound look healthy (don't remove the dressing in the early days though unless really necessary, this just risks introducing infection)?

Drains and tubes – Do they still need their intravenous (IV) cannula? Could their chest drain come out?

Psychological – Don't underestimate how far honest words of comfort and reassurance, especially from a doctor, can go. Be aware of the psychological trauma of illness, not just the physical that you can cut out.

It's always recommended where possible to regularly remind your team of the prospect of a cup of tea as the light at the end of a long ward round.

Drug charts

Drug charts must be reviewed on every morning ward round, even if you looked at them the day before – you don't know if someone overnight has changed something. Specifically check the following.

1 **DVT prophylaxis** – Usually a minimum of TEDS (thromboembolic deterrent stockings) and low molecular weight heparin, e.g dalteparin 5000 units, enoxaparin 20 mg, tinzaparin 3500 units. TEDS are contraindicated in peripheral vascular disease.

2 **Antibiotics** – Which antibiotics? Are they appropriate? Is the indication written in the drug chart (increasingly checked in hospital audits with antibiotic rationing)? Should they be stopped? Remember that you aren't a GP. You don't see your patient and prescribe a seven-day course of antibiotics because you may not get to see that patient again for another seven days. You have the advantage of seeing the patient daily and can review the appropriateness of them daily. There's nothing magic about seven or 10 days.

3 **Regular medications** – Were any medications missed or inaccurately dosed on admission?

4 **Fluids** – If nil by mouth or requiring additional IV fluids, make sure they're written up for the next 24 hours unless further assessment will be needed later in the day. This should not be left to the on-call evening/night team.

5 **Anticoagulants** – If the patient is preoperative, should they have stopped their warfarin? Should they be restarting it?

6 **Analgesia** – Surgical conditions, and the recovery from surgery is often painful. Do they have appropriate regular and as required analgesia written up?

Paper rounds

It's essential to do a bedside ward round each morning, but at the end of the day, and sometimes even at the middle of the day if there's a lot going on, it's often sufficient to run through the patients on paper with all the members of the team present. If the plan from the morning ward round was written on the patient list, you can use it to check the jobs have been done, check any bloods or X-rays done during the day. It also highlights whether any patients need to be reviewed again at the bedside at the end of the day and whether anyone should be handed over to the on-call team.

Handover

There was a time when junior surgeons were on call continuously for their

Patient lists

Patient lists should always be updated regularly so if for whatever reason you failed to make it to work one day, the list would give an accurate summary of your current patients. It should include all basic details, such as name, date of birth and hospital number, and a summary of the diagnosis and any surgery or other interventions, with the date performed. All recent blood and imaging results should be included and what the plan for the patient is.

The most important thing however about patient lists is that you should never underestimate the importance of keeping them confidential. Just imagine the disaster that would ensue if all of that information fell into the wrong hands. It's happened before and health professionals have faced serious consequences. Never leave the hospital with them – drop them in the confidential waste bin before you go home. If you have a collection of them at the bottom of your bag, take them to work tomorrow and dispose of them . . .

patients for days on end (in fact in many countries that remains the case). There was no need to hand anything over to anyone else about your patients – you were 'it'. The downside to the more modern development of giving doctors a life of their own has been this loss of continuity, for doctors and patients. In general surgery in particular, this has resulted in widespread, often unpopular, shift work.

To mitigate against the effects of changing from one shift to the next, a meticulous handover from the outgoing team to the incoming team is absolutely crucial. It is the most critical point in a patient's care where the new team may miss important details about a particular case, or worse, a sick patient may not be handed over at all.

If you are a patient admitted at 3pm on Friday with ongoing problems, you will potentially be handed over up to seven times over the weekend: 5pm Friday (if there is a separate evening on-call team), 8pm Friday, 8am Saturday, 8pm Saturday, 8am Sunday, 8pm Sunday, 8am Monday. Only by excellent handover can the Chinese whispers effect be controlled.

Handovers can take a number of forms, and their format will vary as appropriate to the situation, but can be divided largely into whether they are for new admissions (take handovers) or already admitted inpatients (non-take handovers).

Take handovers

Night handover – the outgoing on-call day team hands over to the night team all of the acute admissions and any patients of concern on the wards.
Morning handover – the night team hands over to the admitting team/s (which may be multiple, for instance if you have been on call for general, urology and vascular, you may have to hand over to three different teams) all the new admissions and any problems on the wards.

These handovers occur outside '9-to-5 hours', where there is only a skeleton of the usual hospital staff, all the diabetic specialist nurses, managers and dermatologists are safely tucked up in bed drinking their Horlicks. Why did you choose surgery again?

There are some key overarching principles to remember for safe handover:

- it should consist of a structured team discussion
- it should be led by an appropriate, usually most senior, member of the outgoing team
- all members of the team should be able to voice concerns
- all members of the team should be present if not deep in someone's abdomen
- it should be at a fixed time in a fixed convenient place conducive to confidential conversation
- it should be bleep free (yeah, right)
- it should be during working, i.e. paid, time.

If you are leading the handover, how can you make handover structured? The following is an example of a system to use. By keeping to this general order for all handovers, nothing should be missed. Points 2 to 9 specifically should be not only in verbal form but written/printed too.

1 Make sure everyone in the incoming and outgoing teams **knows who's who** and which consultant/s is/are on call.

2 Discuss any **patients who are currently very sick** and may require a lot of input, possibly immediately, both new admissions and current inpatients.

3 Discuss all the **patients who have been admitted** during the take.

4 Discuss all the patients who have been seen on the take but **have been discharged** if it's possible that they may re-attend.

5 Discuss all the **patients who are to be seen** or who are expected but have not yet arrived in the hospital.

6 Discuss all the **patients who have been operated on** as emergencies that day and are therefore in the early postoperative period.

7 Discuss all the **patients who are due for emergency theatre** on that shift.

8 Discuss any **non-acute admissions that require review** or to be made aware of.

9 Any **other specific jobs** outstanding or **pending investigations**.

10 Encourage any other members of staff to raise any concerns, i.e. **any other business**.

How much information should be included about each of the cases? The Royal College of Surgeons issued guidance in 2007 on the minimum information to include:

- patient name and age
- date of admission
- location (ward and bed)
- responsible consultant surgeon
- current diagnosis
- results of significant or pending investigations.

And to also include where relevant:

- the patient's condition
- urgency and frequency of review required

- management plan including what to do if a particular foreseeable event occurs
- resuscitation plan
- consultant surgeon contact details and availability
- operational issues (e.g. how many ITU beds are available)
- outstanding tasks.

Non-take handovers

Weekend handover – the regular team hands over the care of their patients to the weekend on-call team, flagging up any patients of particular concern.
Holiday handover – you pass the baton to a colleague while you're sunning yourself in Spain.
Job handover – when changing from one job to another you hand your inpatients over to your successor.
Postoperative handover – usually expressed in the form of a detailed operative note for the recovery and ward staff.

Clearly it's not usually possible to hand over verbally an entire surgical department's current inpatients to the weekend team – no one could possibly remember everything about 100 patients they've never seen. So handover of patients on the weekend needs to be more selective. All the patient lists for the different teams must be accurately updated on Friday to include all the relevant information that the weekend team may find helpful. These then become the handover sheets for those patients. If patients have been in for 6 months, you must include a summary somewhere on the sheet of their progress. Put yourself in the shoes of the person who has to quickly put all the facts together in the event of an emergency over the weekend.

Drains and tubes

Surgical patients frequently have tubes sticking into them or drains coming out of them, placed perioperatively, for monitoring or as adjunctive or definitive treatment (often radiologically). They can be a source of some confusion for doctors and nurses alike, and the main question you'll be asked is 'when can it come out'? This confusion is usually because no one quite knows what this mysterious tube coming out of the belly, or wherever, is doing. So the first thing to do is check the notes and ask the following questions.

1 **Where is the tip of the drain lying?** This can be very different from where it's coming out. Is it in the left paracolic gutter, the pleural cavity or a superficial wound space?

2 **Why was it placed?** Was it placed prophylactically in case of early haemorrhage or to drain an abscess cavity?

3 **When was it placed and how long did the person placing it want it to be in?** Check the record of its insertion, often for instance there will be an instruction saying remove when output < 30 ml/h, for example.

4 What is it draining? If a drain in the pelvis placed intraoperatively to drain excess fluid following an anterior resection starts draining faeces, you have a problem.

The short answer about when can a drain come out, is 'when it's finished doing its job'. So as a general rule, if 24 hours have passed and a negligible amount has passed, it's usually OK to pull it out. However, give some thought to the chance it's blocked – does it need a quick flush with 10 ml of normal saline? Do you need to perform any imaging to check whatever it was draining has resolved, for instance repeat a computed tomography (CT) scan of the abdomen to check an abscess cavity has reduced in size? Perhaps it would be working better if you withdrew it a few centimetres.

Chest drains

Chest drains may be placed in surgical patients due to trauma causing a pneumothorax, haemothorax or haemopneumothorax. They are always placed prophylactically during thoracic surgery, such as in an oesophagectomy.

To assess chest drains: ask the patient to take a big breath in and then out – does the level of water suspended in the tube get sucked upwards on inspiration and fall down on expiration? If so, the tube is 'swinging', which means it is correctly placed in the pleural cavity and isn't blocked. If it isn't swinging, it's doing precious little and can probably come out. If bubbles are appearing in the water when the patient coughs, the tube is 'bubbling' – leave it in, it's still draining air. It's always best to repeat a chest X-ray before and after removing a chest drain.

Abdominal drains

T-tubes – these are placed (in the common hepatic or common bile duct) with one end of the horizontal limb of the T passing up towards the liver and the other end pointing down towards the ampulla. The vertical limb is much longer and passes out through a hole in the main bile duct, and out through the abdominal wall usually into the right flank. Bile can pass down from the liver through the horizontal limb of the T down the natural route to the ampulla, but if there is a blockage there, it can also drain out of the body through the vertical limb.

They are placed because there is a hole in the main bile duct. Why is there a hole in the main bile duct? It was either made by accident during a cholecystectomy for instance – oops. – or on purpose to get a choledochoscope into the ducts to explore them. So why not just stitch up the hole in the duct? Occasionally you can, but you don't want to risk narrowing the duct; late biliary strictures are a real problem. Also, if there may be a stone in the duct distally, the pressure of bile will blow the stitch. So instead you create a controlled fistula between the duct and the outside world. If you leave the T-tube in for a month, the body will have magically formed a track around it – you can pull it out and there will be a fistulous connection between skin and bile duct and no bile will leak into the peritoneal cavity. Provided there is no blockage to the bile duct distally, the fistulous track will close up in a matter of days. To confirm that there is no blockage, you can ask for a T-tube cholangiogram – an image taken after injection of contrast through the T-tube – prior to removal.

Abscess drains – remove when no longer draining pus and the patient's condition has improved. For very viscous pus, prescribe twice daily flushes with normal saline. If the patient is still spiking temperatures/tachycardic despite no pus draining, request imaging to confirm the abscess has resolved. If not, the drain may need to be resited or flushed more.

Post-laparotomy drains – often placed following a laparotomy where there has been contamination. Check the op note that it's not there for a particular purpose, for example it may be placed in the gall bladder bed after a difficult cholecystectomy where there has been injury to the common bile duct and a T-tube has been placed. In this setting, leaving it in a few days to make sure that there is no leak around the T-tube is sensible. Otherwise, these rather non-specific contentious drains can be removed if only draining small amounts of haemoserous fluid after about day two.

Pancreatic drains – for pseudocysts and post-necrosectomy. These get blocked frequently by large chunks of necrotic pancreas, are usually very large bore and often multiple. It's usually best to leave decisions about these up to the boss.

Wound drains

For tight compartments, e.g. the neck following a thyroidectomy. Usually placed prophylactically in case of early haemorrhage, because haemorrhage into such a space can be catastrophic due to airway compression. If drainage is minimal after 24 hours, it can come out.

For large compartments, e.g. mastectomy wounds or incisional hernia repairs. Usually placed because the large surface area of raw tissue forms lots of fluid and hence a seroma. Usually remove when drainage is <30 ml/day.

Enteric tubes and drains

Nasogastric (NG)

For drainage – usually wide bore. Placed in mechanical bowel obstruction, paralytic ileus and often in upper gastrointestinal (GI) surgery. After obstruction is relieved or paralytic ileus is resolving as evidenced by hunger, passage of flatus, restoration of bowel sounds and diminished nasogastric output, try spiggoting the tube (taking the bag away and sticking a plug on the end of the tube) rendering it functionless but easily restorable by reconnecting to the bag. If no nausea or vomiting after 24 hours you can take the tube out.

For feeding – when the patient can use their GI tract but can't eat. Higher rates of aspiration than with a nasojejunal feeding tube so aim to change to nasojejunal tube if longer term.

Nasojejunal

When the patient can use their GI tract but can't eat. It is best placed endoscopically.

Percutaneous endoscopic gastrostomy (PEG)

Placed for longer-term enteral feeding where the GI tract may be used.

Flatus tube

Placed in the sigmoid colon during rigid or flexible sigmoidoscopy for sigmoid volvulus or pseudo-obstruction. Gets blocked by faecal matter quickly. Once the abdomen is decompressed and the patient is passing good volumes of flatus and faeces it can come out.

Other

Epidurals

Highly variable and dependent on user preference how long these stay in, ranging from removal on the first post operative day to several days. When removing, ensure there is adequate alternative analgesia on the drug chart.

Intravenous

As a general rule, to reduce the risk of line sepsis, remove IV lines as soon as they are no longer needed. Do not leave IV cannulae in patients on the off chance they might need it again; remove it and put a new one in if necessary.

Central

Used for central venous pressure (CVP) monitoring intraoperatively. Aim to remove early postoperatively when the patient is stable.

Peripheral

Obey local protocols about how long these should stay in for, but aim to get them out early.

Urinary catheter

Usually placed for monitoring perioperatively. Remove as soon as the patient is stable enough for you to not need hourly urine outputs, and they are able to wee in a bedpan or bottle. Beware older men whose prostates you suspect are large, and make sure they don't go into retention. If they do, the catheter needs to go back in.

Wounds and ulcers

Assessing the state of surgical wounds is a staple part of ward work. Wounds may either be closed at the time of surgery or left open. Assessing the former is usually straightforward, the latter can require a little more thought. Similar principles apply as to when assessing other non-surgically created wounds such as ulcers.

- **Primary closure**: the skin edges have been closed in apposition.
- **Secondary closure**: the skin edges have been left apart, or have since fallen apart and the defect will close from the base upwards. This is usually done when there is sepsis within the compartment to be closed and obviously you don't want to close infection in.

Primary closure

The majority of surgical wounds are closed primarily. There are three common complications that can occur in the early postoperative period that you need to know how to manage and these are covered in the Managing complications section. In general, however, it's best to leave the dressings covering a wound for the first few postop days to reduce the risk of organisms entering the surgical site – so don't go looking for trouble if there's no suspicion of it.

Secondary closure

Distinguishing between a healthy, healing open wound and one that isn't healthy is a crucial skill you'll need, because at first they can all look like a dog's dinner. Similar principles apply as to when looking at leg ulcers and debridements to assess whether they appear to be healing.

1 **Presence of granulation tissue**. This combination of angiogenesis and fibroblasts provides the basis for wound healing when closing by secondary intention. Look for a reddy/pink shiny moist layer in the base of the wound. It's often covered by a thin layer of sloughy (usually white or yellow) material that looks like it would wash off.

2 **Absence of necrotic tissue**. Especially after a foot debridement, for instance where non-viable ischaemic tissue has been excised. Necrotic skin or necrotic tendons at the base of the wound will prevent healing and mandate a further debridement back to healthy tissue.

3 **Absence of pus** – thick yellow-green goo, so distinguish this from slough. If pressure at the edge of a wound results in pus pouring out, there is almost certainly deep sepsis and the wound must be explored to open it up, often requiring a return to theatre.

4 **Reduction in cavity size** over time.

5 **No undermining**. Inspect the wound to ensure the skin is not closing up too fast, leaving a cavity. If the skin closes over a cavity, the fluid produced by the healing surface of the cavity still needs somewhere to drain and this is likely to become a sinus.

6 **Absence of offensive smell**. Many organisms produce characteristic smells, as does necrosis. This may just be from colonisation rather than infection, but lower your threshold of suspicion that the wound is infected.

7 **Healthy skin edges**. Usually with a reddish hue, but a larger red area or stripes of red leading away from the wound raises the likelihood of spreading cellulitis or lymphangitis.

8 **In the case of foot ulcers**, adequate circulation to support healing. The patient must have their circulation assessed by clinical examination, ankle-brachial pressure indices (ABPIs) and where necessary further imaging and revascularisation.

Pressure sores

Be particularly mindful about pressure areas in your surgical patient. Bedsores are a very unpleasant consequence of inadequate attention to them, particularly in theatre if you don't take measures to protect prone areas. Make sure you know their classification so that you don't look foolish in front of the tissue viability nurse. Assess them in the same way as described for wounds and ulcers, and intervene where there is necrosis or infection.

Grade 1: Non-blanching erythema caused by damage to capillaries. Remember this can develop in just hours on a hard trolley in A&E in susceptible patients.

Grade 2: Partial-thickness skin loss.

Grade 3: Full-thickness skin loss but not extending to the underlying fascia.

Grade 4: Full-thickness skin loss with extensive underlying soft tissue destruction.

Dressings

The array of wound dressings coming to market over the past 30 years is baffling and their availability across hospitals is inconsistent. Local units usually prefer one dressing over another, often for entirely incomprehensible reasons. What's more, it's a developing industry, so products are often waxing and waning in popularity – there's no better example than the recent recovery in popularity of maggots ('larval therapy'), of course. So get used to what you have available to you, and understand the broad categories of types of dressing and where certain ones are most appropriate. Your local tissue viability nurse can be an invaluable source of help with difficult wounds. See if they'll give you a short tutorial on wound dressings.

In general, wound dressings are there to provide the right environment to promote healing, and it's usually best if this is a moist, but not wet, environment. This stimulates cell proliferation and encourages epithelial migration. Some dressings can also promote autolytic debridement. It should act as a barrier to the ingress of microorganisms but still allow exchange of oxygen and carbon dioxide. It should absorb the exudate and slough without soaking through the whole of the dressing ('strike through').

If you're struggling to get a wound to heal despite inspection of the wound revealing no local problems requiring debridement, ask yourself why it **DIDN'T HEAL** and treat appropriately.

D = Diabetes

I = infection

D = drugs (e.g. steroids)

N = nutritional deficiency

T = tissue necrosis

H = hypoxia (especially for leg ulcers – is there sufficient arterial and venous flow?)

E = excessive tension or other strain

A = another competing wound

L = low temperature (slower healing when less than core temperature)

The following table gives some of the characteristics and examples of some of the popular types of dressing in current use.

Negative pressure wound therapy

The other type of specialised dressing you'll probably come across a lot is the ubiquitously popular VAC (vacuum-assisted closure) dressing. This is essentially a foam dressing applied to a wound or cavity, covered in a transparent film with a hole in it. The hole in the film is then attached to a tube, which in turn is attached to a machine that applies a constant negative pressure through the tube to the wound. This has the purported benefits of removing excess wound fluid, protecting from infection and increasing local blood flow.

Larval therapy

This medieval treatment for necrotic wounds resurfaced in the 20th century, and it's not for the faint hearted. Disinfected maggots are placed either directly on to a necrotic wound with a special dressing to limit their movements or into a permeable pouch directly in contact with the wound, with a dressing

Table 2.1 Characteristics and examples of dressings in current use

Category	Notes	Uses	Examples
Alginate	Made of seaweed extract. High absorptive capacity. Need another covering layer usually	Where there is copious exudate, also desloughs	Kaltostat Sorbisan Algisite
Hydrofibre	Combines with wound exudate to create a gel. Aquacel-Ag is impregnated with silver, inferring antimicrobial properties	Where there is copious exudate	Aquacel Aquacel-Ag (silver)
Foam	Polyurethane foam	For granulating wounds with less exudate	Allevyn Lyofoam
Hydrocolloid	Microgranular suspension of natural or synthetic polymers, e.g. gelatin in an adhesive matrix	For dry wounds with minimal exudate. Avoid in anaerobic infections as it's occlusive	Granuflex
Hydrogel	Water-based or glycerin-based semipermeable hydrophilic polymers. They can regulate the level of hydration of a wound	Will moisten dry or sloughy wounds, aiding autolysis. Not for heavy exudate wounds	DuoDerm Aquasorb
Transparent films	Comfortable and simple but no absorptive capacity	Clean dry wounds	Opsite Tegaderm
Low-adherence dressings	Removed easily without damaging the skin. Dry dressings	Simple non-infected wounds	Mepore

placed over them. The maggots digest the necrotic tissue, getting very plump in the process. They can't escape from the pouch or dressings and they can't breed (they're too immature). The dressing must allow them to breath or they'll quickly suffocate, poor things.

Managing complications

Unfortunately, sometimes not everything goes well after an operation, not necessarily because of technical incompetence but often just bad luck. On a basic level, humans weren't designed/evolved to be operated on. Cutting out the right hemicolon or sticking a titanium rod down someone's fractured femoral shaft goes against the grain of nature. Surgery is a constant battle against the forces of nature. It's not surprising then that if you're operating on old, frail, co-morbid protoplasm, nature will sometimes conspire to dehisce your wound, block your graft or dislocate your prosthesis – however well you've sewn it together, anastomosed it or cemented it in.

It's important that patients and their loved ones understand this concept, too, and before they have their operation (see Appendix 2). Unfortunately, however, some complications are caused by surgeons: leaving a swab inside or operating on the wrong limb are quite another matter (see Chapter 1, Patient safety). But, in general, complications are usually quite excusable. Missing them, and managing them inappropriately, however, is not. Look for complications – anticipate the problems.

Managing complications can be extremely difficult and often requires very senior advice. What is important is recognising that something's not right, initiating appropriate, timely management and summoning senior help.

Problem-based approach

Hypoxia

Assess the ABCs first and give the patient high-flow oxygen to allow yourself time to think. Remind yourself of the patient's pre-admission co-morbidities – are they known to have chronic obstructive pulmonary disease (COPD) for instance? If so, treat for this. Examine the patient thoroughly and decide if they need arterial blood gas analysis and/or a chest X-ray.

The commonest cause of hypoxia in surgical patients is **atelectasis** – collapse of alveoli, usually at the bases of the lungs, due to inadequate amounts of deep breathing (due to a painful wound or excessive opiates for example), patient position (slouching in the bed) or diaphragmatic splinting from a distended abdomen. It may also occur due to plugs of mucus blocking the airways, especially when the patient hasn't been coughing stuff up due to pain. So, first, get the patient to take several deep breaths in and out and cough anything up that's rattling. Recheck the sats, this usually makes an immediately noticeable difference. If it does, prescribe some saline nebulisers to clear mucus plugs, give adequate analgesia and instruct the patient about deep breathing. Where possible, consider requesting chest physiotherapy.

Other common causes of postoperative hypoxia to consider include the following.

- **Pulmonary embolus** – tachycardia, tachypnoea and pleuritic pain in the context of risk factors for PE. IF there's a reasonably high suspicion of PE, it's usually best to start treatment dose low molecular weight heparin or unfractionated heparin, but in recently postoperative patients this can be a difficult decision as the risk needs to be balanced with surgical site bleeding. Organise an urgent computed tomography pulmonary angiogram (CTPA) to confirm or refute the diagnosis. Consider an inferior vena cava (IVC) filter in those with recurrent PEs despite adequate anticoagulation.

- **Lower respiratory tract infection** – hypoxia with evidence of sepsis and clinical or radiological signs in the chest. Consider whether this could be due to aspiration – if so, this affects the antibiotics prescribed and the preventative measures to take to reduce the risk of it happening again. Organise a chest X-ray, venous bloods, arterial blood gas analysis, antibiotics and consider chest physiotherapy.
- **Left ventricular failure** – treat usually with IV frusemide +/– a glyceryl trinitrate (GTN) infusion. Ensure you establish the cause, i.e. exclude an acute dysrhythmia, myocardial infarction or sepsis.
- **Pleural effusion**.
- **Adult respiratory distress syndrome**.
- Less commonly – **pneumothorax**.
- **Pre-existing lung pathology**, e.g. COPD, asthma, fibrosing alveolitis, bronchiectasis.

Pyrexia

The upper limit of normal for core temperature is 37.1°C, although the precise level considered to be a significant pyrexia is somewhat contentious. As a general rule, 37.5–38.0° is considered a low-grade pyrexia, while > 38.1° is a high-grade pyrexia.

Fever is a manifestation of cytokine release, and this occurs as a response to a number of stimuli. In the first 24–48 hours after surgery, fever is usually a normal systemic response simply to the trauma of surgery. At later stages, the timing of the pyrexia is sometimes a useful clue as to the potential cause, thus was christened the famous four Ws mnemonic.

Often the cause is obvious, but take a thorough, focused history anyway, and examine the patient carefully. When no

Table 2.2 The four Ws

Wind	Day 1–2	Respiratory causes such as pneumonia and PE (interestingly, atelectasis, which traditionally has been taught as a cause of pyrexia, is, in fact, not one)
Water	Day 3–5	Urinary tract infection, usually due to a catheter
Wound	Day 5–7	Surgical site infection, not just the wound – this could also be the anastomosis or other deep infection
Walking	Day 7–10	Deep vein thrombosis or PE

obvious cause is forthcoming, a septic screen should be performed. This should include venous bloods and blood cultures, a chest X-ray and mid-stream urine (MSU). In more occult cases, you should give the patient a top-to-toe examination, thinking outside the box. For example, does the patient need an echocardiogram to exclude infective endocarditis? Patients with long-term NG tubes in situ can develop associated sinusitis. Some medications can cause pyrexia.

Hypotension

A low blood pressure in a surgical patient makes you think the following.

1 Have they **bled postoperatively**? Is there frank surgical-site bleeding? If the surgery was deep in the abdomen this may not be immediately obvious. Keep this high in your list of things to rule out.

2 Are they **dehydrated**? Probably the commonest reason – assess the fluid intake and output over the **past** 24 hours.

3 Do they have an epidural in situ? This is a very common cause of hypotension, secondary to the vasodilatory effects of the epidural.

4 Are they **septic**? Especially relevant if there's an anastomosis that could have fallen apart, for instance.

5 Are they overloaded with **opiates**? How much morphine have they had? Look for other signs of opiate toxicity – bradypnoea, reduced consciousness, pin point pupils.

But remember the other less common but by no means less important causes.

1 **Cardiac** – the physiological demand of recovery from surgery can push an unhealthy ticker over the edge to coronary ischaemia.

2 A **massive pulmonary embolus** should be obvious by its respiratory effect also.

3 **Anaphylaxis** from any of the new drugs received perioperatively, especially antibiotics.

4 **Tension pneumothorax** – an unusual complication of being ventilated on a machine during an anaesthetic is a pneumothorax.

Tachycardia

Don't ignore an isolated tachycardia, especially if the patient is not progressing appropriately. Tachycardia in a surgical patient makes you think the following.

1 Have they bled?

2 Are they dehydrated?

3 Are they in pain?

4 Are they septic? Especially if they have developed fast atrial fibrillation.

5 Have they had a PE?

Complication-specific approach

Wound problems

Infection

Wounds heal by a process that includes inflammation, so the wound edges are usually slightly red, but if they are more than slightly red and especially if it is spreading away from the edge of the skin, it suggests infection. Also note increased wound pain, swelling, local heat, systemic pyrexia and pus leaking out. In the most mild form, cellulitis, it usually responds to antibiotics. Remember to treat the likely pathogen. Flucloxacillin and benzylpenicillin may be the antibiotics of choice for leg cellulitis, but if this is an appendicectomy wound, there will almost certainly be coliforms and anaerobes, so co-amoxiclav may be a better choice. However, if there's any suggestion of pus under the wound it must be opened up promptly. In addition, give antibiotics if the patient is immunocompromised (HIV+, diabetic, cancer, elderly, etc.) or if there is also significant cellulitis. If they are not immunocompromised and there is no cellulitis, opening up the wound is usually all that's needed, with no antibiotics.

Opening up a surgical wound

Take to the bedside:

- sterile pack
- sterile gloves
- skin prep
- two microbiology swabs
- normal saline
- 20 ml syringe
- clip/suture remover
- optional – wound packing material to keep wound open, such as Aquacel
- a new dressing with absorbent qualities such as a Surgipad taped on with Mefix.

Local anaesthetic won't help but giving the patient some oramorph 20 minutes before will.

Under aseptic conditions:

- set up your aseptic tray and don your gloves
- prep the skin over and around the wound
- remove as many staples/sutures as necessary over the most infected area to provide an adequate hole to drain
- use the first microbiology swab to bluntly separate the skin edges and probe into the cavity – dispose of it
- use the second microbiology swab to take a sample for microbiology (the first will have contaminated itself on the skin edges)
- irrigate the cavity with copious amounts of normal saline
- insert some porous packing material to prevent the skin edges from closing over too early and allow drainage
- apply new dressing
- give instructions to the nurses to repeat irrigation and repacking in 24 hours and continue until infection resolved.

Haematoma or bleeding

This presents as a swelling under the wound often with overlying bruising. It usually results from some bleeding in the superficial wound space and is usually self-limiting and will be reabsorbed. The exception is an expanding haematoma – one that is getting bigger in front of your eyes. This is ongoing bleeding and requires firm pressure and usually a return to theatre to find the bleeding point.

If the wound is simply bleeding, firm pressure for several minutes, reapplied if necessary, is usually sufficient. Otherwise, a stitch placed under local anaesthetic into the bleeding area may stop it if the bleeding is from the wound edge. As a last resort the patient may have to return to theatre. Check for coagulopathy.

Dehiscence

Superficial – the skin closure can come apart due to an inadequate closure technique or due to infection. In the former, this either needs reclosure in theatre if there's a gaping wound, or consider some stitches under local anaesthetic on the ward, or alternatively Steristrips or skin glue such as Dermabond. If due to infection, it is better it is left open to drain.

Deep – where a wound is over the abdominal cavity, there are two layers: superficial for skin (and sometimes one for fat) and deep for the linea alba. This deep layer can come apart either due to poor surgical technique or poor patient protoplasm (e.g. malignancy, on steroids, malnourished, etc). Classically, the early warning sign is that the wound starts to leak serous fluid around day seven. Eventually bowel starts poking out. This is a major complication with high mortality. If called to see a patient with eviscerated bowel on the ward, don't panic. Cover the bowel in a large swab soaked in normal saline, make them nil by mouth, resuscitate them with fluids (they will have lost fluid through the dehiscence) and get them into the next available slot in theatre to have the wound reclosed.

Haemorrhage

There are three types of haemorrhage to consider in the postoperative patient.

Primary haemorrhage – you cut into tissue and a vessel bleeds. This is stopped at the time of surgery – hopefully.

Reactionary haemorrhage – the operation is finished and the patient is in the recovery room or back in the ward. After waking from the anaesthetic, blood pressure rises or the patient moves or coughs, which can cause inadequately tied ligatures to come off vessels.

Secondary haemorrhage – bleeding occurring a week or so down the line due to infection eroding through vessels.

Where haemorrhage is superficial, pressure is the best remedy. When haemorrhage is from somewhere you can't physically put your finger on, you're in trouble unless you act quickly. The first key is recognising it; it may be subtle in the early stages, and, particularly in the young and fit, may suddenly with little warning result in decompensation.

- Note the physiological parameters in Table 2.3.
- Look for blood in drains if there are any.

Table 2.3 Classification of degrees of haemorrhage

Parameter	**Class**			
	I	**II**	**III**	**IV**
Blood loss (ml)	<750	750–1500	1500–2000	>2000
Blood loss (%)	<15	15–30	30–40	>40
Pulse rate (beats/min)	<100	>100	>120	>140
Blood pressure	Normal	Decreased	Decreased	Decreased
Respiratory rate (beats/min)	14–20	20–30	30–40	>35
Urine ouput (ml/h)	>30	20–30	5–15	Negligible
Central nervous system (CNS) symptoms	Normal	Anxious	Confused	Lethargic

- Examine the wound for swelling, or the abdomen for distension and tenderness.
- Examine the conjunctivae.

Get an urgent venous blood assessment for haemoglobin, clotting and cross match. Often the quickest way to estimate the haemoglobin is using venous blood in an arterial blood gas analyser, which will give an almost instant result. Institute treatment immediately, in the form of high-flow oxygen to maximally oxygenate the remaining haemoglobin, and ensure that there are two working IV cannulae and give IV fluids. Colloids such as gelofusin usually give a quicker, albeit short-lived, rise in blood pressure. If the patient has had a significant bleed postoperatively, which has resulted in cardiovascular decompensation, they need to be returned to theatre urgently to find the bleeding point and stop it. Occasionally, in less severe bleeds, where there is rapid improvement with basic measures, it may be suitable to watch and wait.

Anastomotic dehiscence

A leak of bowel content from a gut anastomosis is usually obvious, with abdominal pain, pyrexia and cardiovascular disturbance between five and nine days postoperatively. Any one individual symptom, such as an isolated pyrexia, however, around this time must make you concerned to exclude a leak. Do not ignore the patient who 'just isn't quite right' after a colonic resection and anastomosis.

Where a leak is clinically obvious, the patient needs resuscitation with oxygen, IV fluids, correction of electrolytes and antibiotics, and an urgent return to theatre for a re-look laparotomy or laparoscopy for wash out and exteriorisation of the two leaking ends, usually as a double-barrelled stoma.

When uncertain, gather more information in the form of inflammatory markers such as the white cell count and C-reactive protein (CRP) and come back and re-examine the patient after a short interval. A CT of the abdomen is a useful tool for picking up a dehiscence. But particularly if the operation has been done laparoscopically, a re-look just with the laparoscope minimises the trauma of a second operation.

Paralytic ileus

Any operation on the abdomen is likely to disturb the small bowel, which generally doesn't take kindly to such intrusion. The abdomen tends to distend with swallowed air, which isn't propelled through to the colon, and the patient feels bloated and nauseated. The bowels don't work and the bowel sounds are absent. In general, the only way to stop this is to allow nature to take its course. In major abdominal surgery, this stage can last up to 10 days. Ensure, however, that the electrolytes aren't abnormal and that you have excluded sepsis in the abdominal cavity as these will retard the restoration of normal bowel activity. The patient must be adequately hydrated (by monitoring urine output with a urinary catheter), and their gastric distension relieved with a nasogastric tube if nausea or hiccupping are a particular problem. Early mobilisation out of bed can also be helpful in restoring normal bowel activity.

Essentially, it is ileus that is responsible for the now somewhat old-fashioned tendency to put all patients nil by mouth for several days after abdominal surgery, not just concern that food will cause an anastomosis to leak. However, not every patient gets an ileus and early tentative reintroduction of oral diet is possible in most, meaning fewer patients starving unnecessarily for days after their surgery. In fact, the enhanced recovery programme after colorectal surgery has revolutionised this in many hospitals.

Sick patients

Being a surgeon is not just about cutting, it's about looking after all of our patients' medical needs, and unfortunately sometimes they can be very sick indeed. The Care of the Critically Ill Surgical Patient (CCrISP) course organised by the Royal College of Surgeons is an excellent programme to teach you an approach to dealing with such cases; it really is a must. This section can by no means replace that, but if you haven't yet done the course, or you did it a long time ago, it will give you a basic approach to managing an acutely unwell patient.

You are bleeped to the ward to see one of your patients who has 'gone off'. What are you going do? Broadly speaking you can divide it into the following.

1 Before you arrive at the patient's bedside.

2 What you do once you arrive and

3 What is your assessment of the situation and plan of action?

1 Before you arrive

■ Before hanging up. give the caller some basic instructions, such as put them on high-flow oxygen, arrange an electrocardiogram (ECG) or whatever seems appropriate (which means by the time you're there you should have some more results to look at).

- As you're walking down the corridor, plan in your head the first things you're going to do when you arrive.
- Does it sound like you'll need to call senior help immediately?

2 Once you arrive

- Attend to the ABCs (see below).
- Try to establish what system is failing – are they hypoxic, hypotensive, etc.
- Request further observations.

3 Assessment and plan

- How critical is this case and how quickly do I need to do something about it?
- What is the diagnosis, or at least a summary assessment of the problem?
- What help do I need?
- What definitive treatment does this patient need?

The crux of the issue begins with a fairly rapid process of information gathering, and then acting on that information, i.e. **assessment** and **management**, and these should be synchronous but progress in a logical order. There are

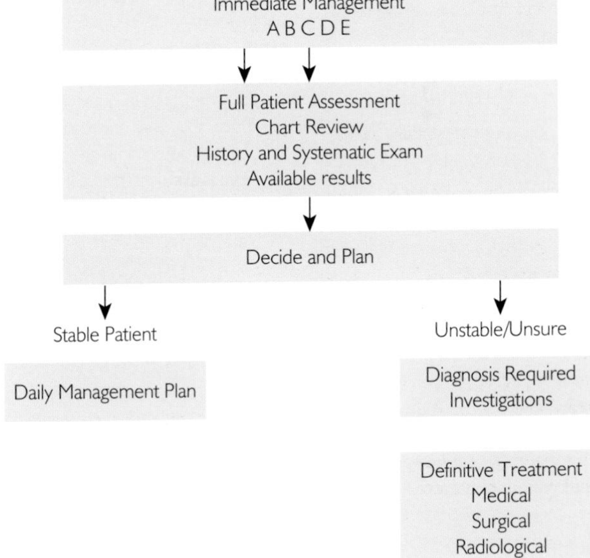

Figure 2.1 Algorithm for managing critically ill surgical patients used on the Care of the Critically Ill Surgical Patient Course.

strong similarities with the Advanced Trauma Life Support (ATLS) protocol. You do not, for instance, arrive, take a history and then examine the patient, neither do you find that the airway is compromised by your drowsy patient's tongue and move on to B without getting someone to do a jaw thrust.

A – Airway

- In the obtunded, will need airway support.
- Post-thyroidectomy stridor suggests postoperative bleed – remove the stitches immediately.

B – Breathing

- Assess the respiratory system in the usual way: repiratory rate, sats, cyanosis, auscultation, etc.
- Provide O_2, in the first instance 100% via a re-breather to all.
- Look for problems that require immediate treatment, such as a needle decompression for a tension pneumothorax.

C – Circulation

- Look for hypovolaemia.
- Don't miss a postoperative bleed, which may of course be concealed.
- If the patient is obviously bleeding and needs to go back to theatre, don't delay the inevitable just hoping they will get better with blood transfusions.

D – Disability

A = Alert,

V = Responds to verbal stimuli,

P = Responds to verbal stimuli

U = Unresponsive

E – Exposure

- A general inspection of the whole body is essential – have they developed widespread petechial haemorrhages – have they gone into DIC (disseminated intravascular coagulation)?
- Don't, however, allow them to become hypothermic – cover up again afterwards.

During all of this you need to institute basic care, including oxygen, IV access with fluids, draw blood, organise blood transfusions (if they've bled) and arrange basic investigations: a portable chest X-ray, arterial blood gases, ECGs, etc. If things seem to deteriorate at any stage, **start again** with the ABCDE assessment. If you haven't already called them, do you need HDU/ITU review?

Once this first run-through of the ABCDE has been completed, stand back and **reassess** – is the patient getting better? If not, start again at A. If so, you've got a bit of time to stand back and get the bigger picture. You now want to do a **full assessment** of the patient. This usually begins with the patient's **charts**, **notes** and **recent bloods**. Have there in fact been warning signs on the patient's chart all day, with a rising pulse and gradually declining urine output? Has their white cell count been rising over the past couple of days?

Get a detailed picture of the patient's recent history.

- What **operation** have they had?
- **When** was it? Read the operation note.

- What **co-morbidities** does the patient have?
- What **medications** are they on?

Go back to the patient and take a more detailed history from them. If at any time the patient starts to deteriorate, go back to ABCDE.

You may decide at the end of all this that you've established what was wrong with the patient – they were a little overloaded with fluid and their shortness of breath has abated, they're much more comfortable, you've adjusted their fluid regime – well done doctor, the patient is now **stable** and can be reviewed on the daily ward round as per usual. However, you may decide that despite your best efforts the diagnosis is not clear, or they're still **unstable**. It sounds like **further investigations** and **definitive treatment** is needed. This will involve more people than just you – phone a friend (senior/intensivist/radiologist).

End of life care

We must accept that not all cases will end with a living patient. Death is a natural process, and prolonging life can often be cruel and not in anyone's best interests. There are those lucid patients who choose not to accept life-saving treatment for a potentially surgically curable problem, preferring to die. In these circumstances, it is mandatory to accept their wishes without coercing them into operations that we feel would be best, and provide the best possible end of life care for them – regardless of the fact we don't operate on them.

There are other patients who don't have that capacity but it is obvious that their outlook is dismal and treatment options are fraught with likely pain and indignity. These patients need us, as doctors, to have the courage and wisdom to say when enough is enough and allow them a dignified death. Again, just because we don't operate on these patients doesn't mean they should be ignored and relegated to being just a row on a patient list hidden away in a side room. It is our duty as doctors to ensure we manage their symptoms, communicate with their relatives and comfort them as fellow humans.

DNAR orders

If you can picture a scenario in the middle of the night where one of your patients might unexpectedly find themselves in a peri-arrest situation, it is essential to make a decision during daylight hours about whether that patient should or shouldn't be for resuscitation in the event of a cardiopulmonary arrest. Few things are as vexing as a 3am cardiac arrest call to an 80-year-old patient you've never met, who from her clerking, probably has dementia, might have a history of severe cardiac disease and possibly also has breast cancer. If this patient does in fact have all three of these co-morbidities, it is unlikely that cardiopulmonary resuscitation (CPR) is in her best interests, and therefore a decision should be made by the team looking after her, not the on-call team. Ideally, and where appropriate, such decisions should be discussed with the patient and/or the family.

Liverpool Care Pathway

A big stride forward for palliative care in recent years has been the popularisation of the Liverpool Care Pathway (LCP). Its aim is to help identify patients who are in the terminal stages of life and optimise their treatment through a helpful system of protocols. It is often felt that hitherto, symptom relief was often patchy and substandard, with patients in their final days still receiving a bowl full of unnecessary medications and ungenerous pain relief, while offers of spiritual support were less than forthcoming. Learn about the LCP and what it can offer your patient. As the very accurate cliché goes: when it comes to death, you only have one chance of getting it right.

References

Anderson ID (Care of the Critically Ill Surgical Patient (2e). London: Hodder Arnold.

British Medical Association (2004) *Safe Handover: safe patients. Guidance on clinical handover for clinicians and managers*. London: British Medical Association.

Royal College of Surgeons (2007) *Safe Handover: guidance from the Working Time Directive working party*. London: The Royal College of Surgeons of England.

Chapter 3
CLINICS

Matt Stephenson

Seeing new patients, 71
Seeing follow-up patients, 72
Dictating the letter, 72
Keeping track of serious cases, 73
Specialty-specific investigations and procedures, 73

To study the phenomenon of disease without books is to sail an uncharted sea, while to study books without patients is not to go to sea at all.
Sir William Osler (Physician, 1849–1919)

At the earliest opportunity start going to surgical clinics to see patients for yourself. Don't wait to be invited. They are a hotbed of surgical pathology and offer an opportunity to see disease from its earliest stages to its resolution. They are helpful for seeing plenty of signs to prepare you for looking slick in exams and it's a chance to get some one-to-one teaching from the boss. So from foundation year 1 you should be going to surgical clinics.

Seeing patients in clinic requires new skills compared with A&E or the wards.

- **Time can be limited** to as little as 10 minutes per patient.
- A **definitive plan** must be reached for each patient (unlike in A&E where you're sometimes fire fighting just to get someone home safely).
- The patient and their relatives may have waited weeks or months to see you, **expectations may be far higher**.
- You have the full range of the hospital's **diagnostic tools** available to you.
- Your notes must be **more succinct but comprehensive**.
- You have to **dictate a letter** to the GP.

Seeing new patients

Begin, of course, by establishing the presenting complaint in the usual way, but then proceed to a mini-clerking – all new patients need this. It should be a focused history (mainly of relevant past medical and surgical history and risk factors, etc.)

The Hands-on Guide to Surgical Training, First Edition. Matthew Stephenson.

and clinical examination relevant to the problem you're dealing with. There are some specific investigations to consider and skills to learn for each specialty – see below (the common investigations common to so many pathologies such as computed tomography [CT] and ultrasound scans [USS] have not been included as you're likely to be familiar with those already).

Reach a differential diagnosis and formulate a plan. To begin with, most consultants will generally want to discuss all the patients you've seen. This will help you to become adept at succinctly summarising and determining how close your approach has been to your consultant's.

Seeing follow-up patients

This is usually quicker; the patient has already been 'clerked' into the clinic the first time and is now back either to receive the results of an investigation or to check on progress after a treatment has been commenced. Always make sure you've read the results of any investigations before seeing the patient. It doesn't look good to welcome the patient into the room with a big smile, only to then check the histology and realise you're supposed to be delivering some bad news.

Hospitals are under financial pressure not to follow up too many patients, they are, in fact, usually only paid to see them once. Any extra visits are a bonus; however, an extra visit is often clinically essential and this is the most important factor to consider. In many cases, you can write to the patient with the result of a normal investigation to save them the trouble of coming back.

Dictating the letter

In an effort to cut costs, many trusts have outsourced dictation to cheaper countries, so the audio files from your tape may be emailed to India and returned in an hour or so as document files. It's quite possible therefore that whoever transcribes your tape has never come within 4,000 miles of you, and it makes clarifying points very difficult, so be clear and spell out anything that may be equivocal.

Start each tape by saying:

- your name (spell it if you want it written accurately)
- your title
- your designation
- date of the clinic
- consultant in charge of the clinic

Before beginning the letter on each patient, state the patient's:

- full name
- date of birth
- hospital number

You'll develop your own style. Many people begin each letter with something like 'Dear Dr X, Thank you for referring Mrs Bloggs to the vascular clinic'. Then proceed with a summary of the presenting complaint, history of presenting complaint and so on. The letter then becomes an invaluable resource when reviewing notes later on, of the patient's succinct and relevant medical record. It is far better in fact than the 15 computer-generated pages of everything from years of repeat prescriptions to incomplete information about smoking history, that make up the GP records often sent with the GP referral letter.

Never ever be rude, even covertly, about either the referrer or the patient. Not only is it unprofessional, but the hospital receives its income from seeing referrals, and these days GPs often have the choice to send patients elsewhere. Also, the patient can request to see the letter at any time, and in some trusts it's normal practice for the patient to receive a copy of the letter, too. In fact, in some trusts you are expected to write the letter **to** the patient with a copy to the GP. Say at the end of the letter whether you want anyone else involved in the patient's care to be copied into the letter.

Keeping track of serious cases

You will see patients in whom you strongly suspect cancer – a palpable mucosal mass on digital rectal examination (DRE), an irregular hard lump in the breast or a highly suspicious mole. You request your urgent investigations and organise follow-up. The moment the patient walks out the door there is the risk that the forms you've written will get lost, the appointment sent to the patient doesn't arrive or some other cosmological event transpires to lose the patient to follow-up. This is a disaster and happens more often than you would think. You won't remember every patient like this you see and unlike ward patients, there isn't the constant reminder of facing them on the wards.

For this reason many clinics will have a special book in which you write all patients awaiting investigations in whom a cancer diagnosis is expected. Failing this, you must keep a record yourself, perhaps at the end of the inpatient list, to remind you to look out for the results for these patients.

Specialty-specific investigations and procedures

You'll be familiar already with common generic investigations such as X-ray, USS and CT, but here are a few specialty-specific investigations or procedures you may want to know about before starting an attachment in one of these subspecialties.

Colorectal

Investigations

Anorectal manometry – to assess functional disorders of the sphincter complex – useful in faecal incontinence and resistant constipation.

Flexible sigmoidoscopy – for bright red rectal bleeding and sometimes altered bowel habit, but only sees as far as the splenic flexure so will miss more proximal disease.

Colonoscopy – full endoluminal assessment of the colonic mucosa from anus to ileocaecal valve. Particularly for PR bleeding, altered bowel habit, iron deficiency anaemia and other colonic problems.

CT colonography – a CT giving dedicated, exceptionally clear views of the colorectal mucosa. Relatively less invasive than a colonoscopy, only requires a small insufflation catheter per anus. Radiation dose and inability to take biopsies of lesions seen is a disadvantage. Requires bowel prep.

MRI pelvis – magnetic resonance imaging for staging of rectal cancers and also for establishing the course of complex anal fistulae and sepsis.

EUA (examination under anaesthetic) – usually of the anorectum. A cross between an operation and an investigation. Useful when examination in clinic is too painful, for instance when trying to distinguish between a fissure and chronic perianal sepsis.

Procedures

Proctoscopy – examination of the anal canal using a proctoscope. Lay the patient in the left lateral position with knees tucked up to the chest, bottom at the edge of the bed and feet placed well away. Perform a DRE first; this helps to lubricate the canal. Attach the light source to the proctoscope and check it works. Insert the inner introducer into the proctoscope. Lubricate the proctoscope generously. Gently introduce, asking the patient to simultaneously take a deep breath. Once inside, remove introducer. At full depth you will be looking at the lower rectum, so slowly withdraw, pausing when necessary, and inspect the anal canal circumferentially.

Rigid sigmoidoscopy – position and DRE as for proctoscopy. Attach the light source and check it's working. Attach the bellows (a rubber balloon contraption that allows you to insufflate air). Insert the inner introducer to the sigmoidoscope and lubricate generously. Gently introduce while the patient takes a deep breath (mainly because it distracts the patient). Insert approximately 5–7 cm blindly, withdraw introducer and close the see-through lid of the sigmoidoscope so you can insufflate air without it escaping in the direction of your face. Inspect rectal mucosa and insufflate some air. Push sigmoidoscope under direct vision through the rectum; it's easier in some than others. If there are a lot of faeces present it can be very difficult or impossible. It's often possible to reach 20 cm.

Banding of piles – position and DRE as above. Perform proctoscopy to establish the diagnosis of first- or second-degree haemorrhoids. It won't help if third degree. Using the same proctoscope (or a specialised one with an angled tip if available) held in position with your non-dominant hand to reveal the base of a haemorrhoid (not the most protuberant bit), take the banding device in the other. The banding device is a suction tube, the tip of which, if held against the haemorrhoidal mucosa, will suck it into it. The tiny rubber band has been mounted around the tip of the suction tube, using your thumb you can press a switch, which pushes the band off the tip of the suction tube, and this will spring around the base of the tissue sucked into the tube. Repeat for all haemorrhoids. Make sure you are applying the bands above the dentate line. Warn the patient that while it's not painful, it can be uncomfortable for 24–48 hours as the haemorrhoid swells;

it also may not work, and it may bleed, especially around day 10.

Upper gastrointestinal tract

Investigations

Oesophagogastroduodenoscopy **(OGD)** – upper gastrointestinal endoscopy as far as the duodenum, particularly for upper gastrointestinal (GI) bleeding, iron deficiency anaemia, persistent dyspepsia in the over-45s and dysphagia. Can also take a duodenal biopsy for coeliac disease. Wide variety of therapeutic options.

Barium swallow – similar indications as OGD and now less commonly used, but may be performed as an adjunct.

Oesophageal manometry and pH testing – investigation of reflux.

Radionuclide study – where symptoms sound typical of gallstones but no gallstones are found, a hepatobiliary iminodiacetic acid (HIDA) scan may help by showing the gall bladder is non-functional – if so a cholecystectomy may, but is by no means guaranteed to, help.

Endoscopic retrograde cholangiopancreatography (ERCP) – for the treatment of stones in the main ducts or to place a stent for a biliary stricture. Also diagnostic in idiopathic pancreatitis or to take brushings for cytology in abnormally appearing ducts.

Procedure

Removal of T-tube – allow a month post insertion to allow fistula formation, cut any stitch and just pull it out. Consider taking a cholangiogram prior to removal if you want to confirm the absence of stones in the common bile duct.

General

Investigation

Herniography – when unsure of whether a patient has a hernia (usually only works well for groin hernias). In the radiology department the patient's peritoneal cavity is injected with a radioopaque solution which naturally moves down with gravity. The patient coughs while X-rays are taken. Watch to see if the contrast enters a hernia sac.

Procedures

Punch biopsy – for suspicious areas of skin such as on an ulcer edge where full excision will be an overkill for something that may not be malignant. Under aseptic conditions, inject lignocaine into the area. Take a biopsy punch. They come in various diameters, the average being 4 mm. It is simply a very sharp hollow tube, which, if pressed against the skin, with a little rotation will cut straight through it allowing a cylinder of skin into the biopsy tube. Withdraw once it's through skin, using a knife cut off any attachments. Remove cylinder of skin from the biopsy punch and put in a formalin pot and send to histology. The wound usually doesn't bleed much and pressure will stop it. Usually you can just close with a Steristrip.

Injection of ilioinguinal nerve – for chronic nerve pain post inguinal hernia repair. Only do this if there is a specific trigger point that you can press and reproduce the symptoms. It doesn't help just for general groin ache post hernia repair. Inject a mixture of lignocaine with hydrocortisone directly to the trigger point.

Vascular

Investigations

Arterial duplex – an excellent non-invasive radiation free assessment of the arterial system, looking for occlusions and stenoses, and also, by using velocity assessments, the haemodynamic effects of those blockages. Also for sizing aortic aneurysms.

Venous duplex – to look for sites of superficial to deep venous incompetence and the anatomy of the superficial venous system to help guide surgery for varicose veins. Also excludes deep venous occlusion or reflux, which is a contraindication to varicose vein surgery.

Computed tomography angiography (CTA)/magnetic resonance angiography (MRA)/digital subtraction angiography (DSA) – all used to assess the arterial system in high detail, usually used if duplex has found an occlusion/stenosis and you are considering intervention and need a detailed roadmap. The advantage of digital subtraction angiography is that you already have a catheter in the femoral artery so you can proceed to intervention at the same sitting if appropriate; the disadvantage is the risks of such an invasive procedure, which include embolisation to the foot, with a roughly 1% risk of limb loss.

Procedures

Ankle-brachial pressure index (ABPIs) – actually part of the examination. Inflate a manual sphygmomanometer around the upper arm while using a Doppler probe on the brachial artery. Inflate to above systolic pressure and document the pressure at which the signal reappears. Repeat around the ankle while listening to the dorsalis pedis (DP) and the posterior tibial (PT), and again note the systolic at which the signal reappears. Divide whichever pressure in the foot was higher by the brachial pressure, e.g. Rt brachial pressure = 140, Rt DP pressure = 50, Rt PT pressure = 70, Rt ABPI = 70/140 = 0.5.

Interpretation of Doppler signals – It's one thing to note that there is a Doppler signal in an artery, it's another to describe it. Normal arteries give a triphasic signal: three separate whooshes. This suggests an elastic artery with no occlusion. Biphasic signals may suggest some narrowing of the artery upstream but may be normal. Monophasic signals suggest significant upstream disease.

MRI thoracic outlet – to look for a cervical rib in thoracic outlet obstruction.

CT aortogram – once an USS has shown the aorta to be more than 5.5 cm, and surgery is countenanced, a CT aortogram allows accurate assessment of morphology to determine operability – as open surgery or endovascular repair.

Fistulogram – for renal dialysis arteriovenous fistulae to assess patency, aneurysms or strictures.

Breast

Investigations

Mammography – assessment of breast lumps, pain or discharge in women over 35.

USS – assessment of all breast lumps in all ages (women over 35 get both a mammogram and an USS).

MRI – occasionally used to assess complex breast problems.

Ductography – occasionally used to assess cause of nipple discharge.

Procedures

Fine needle aspiration (FNA) – to assess breast lumps, especially if your pathology service is driven mainly by cytologists and for same-day one-stop clinics. Under aseptic conditions without local anaesthetic, insert a butterfly needle attached to a 10 ml syringe into the lump. Pass the needle several times through the lump in different directions while pulling the plunger of the syringe – this will suck up tiny pieces of the tissue into the needle and first part of the tube. Remove the needle from the patient and spray the tiny pieces of tissue onto a microscope slide. Ensure they are accurately labelled and send to the cytologist for immediate reporting.

Core biopsy – under aseptic conditions, inject lignocaine into the skin overlying the lump. Make a tiny nick in the skin with a blade. Prime the core biopsy needle and introduce through the nick you've made into the lump and fire the trigger of the core biopsy needle. Withdraw and press on the breast with a swab to stop bleeding. Using a hypodermic needle remove the specimen from the core biopsy needle and drop into formalin. If it floats it may just be fat. Try to take a few more samples from different parts of the lump.

Punch biopsy – see General. Especially used when suspecting Paget's of the nipple.

Drainage of cysts – under aseptic conditions, without local anaesthetic, introduce a green needle attached to a 20 ml syringe into the cyst and drain to dryness. Send to histology if there is any suspicion of cancer. If no fluid comes out, treat as a solid lump and continue as for FNA or if highly likely to be a cyst, try using a white needle as the contents may be highly viscous.

Chapter 4 ON CALL

Matt Stephenson

Some practicalities, 78
Referrals, 79
Resuscitation essentials, 80
Trauma, 83
References, 88

Rule IV: There is no body cavity that cannot be reached with a #14 needle and a good strong arm.
Samuel Shem, *The House of God (1979)*

Some practicalities

Your on calls provide an irreplaceable opportunity to acquire the essential skills required of a surgeon. With your on call approaching, don't wish for a quiet day in the mess – you gain nothing but a risk of DVT. Hope for a busy day with lots of interesting pathology and hopefully lots of operating.

Many people find on calls extremely stressful, in fact everyone does at one time or another, and there are few things more stressful than feeling out of your depth. Always remember that you're not expected to have the answer to every problem you encounter. Consultants, as much as anyone else, can be foxed by a complex patient or struggle with a difficult appendix (although they'll never admit it). Try not to be too hard on yourself if at the beginning of your time in surgical training you seem to be floundering or often asking for help. The more you see and the more you do, the easier everything becomes.

As part of your surgical training, and also as part of service provision for the hospital, you will be required to participate in the on-call rota. Depending mainly on the size of the surgical department, the average general surgical on-call team is likely to consist of an FY1 doctor, an old-style senior house officer (SHO) grade (FY2-CT2), a registrar and a consultant. In the less busy specialties such as orthopaedics, urology and ENT, it's likely to be just an FY2-CT2, a registrar at home on the end of a phone and, of course, a consultant.

It's important to check at the start of any placement precisely what your role in the team will be, both during the day on-call shifts and the night on-call shifts.

The Hands-on Guide to Surgical Training, First Edition. Matthew Stephenson.

So at induction into the department, or at least before your first on call, ask the following questions.

- **Which specialties are you covering?** During the day you're probably covering only the specialty in which you normally work, but after 5pm do you cross-cover urology or orthopaedics for instance?
- **Are you principally responsible for ward patients, acute referrals or both?**
- **Who is your direct point of contact for senior advice?** Usually for an FY2-CT2 this would be the registrar, but in some units it goes straight to the consultant.
- **Who else do you have to help you?** Is there an FY1 on call with you? Are there night practitioners available to cannulate ward patients and deal with other ward problems?
- **Is there an on-call room?**
- **Where does handover take place?** Both in the morning and at night.
- **Where is the handover patient information kept?** This is sometimes on a dedicated computer in a specific office; at worst, it's kept on someone's USB stick.
- **Who admits minor head injuries when necessary?** It may be general surgery, orthopaedics or neurosurgery if you have it on site.
- **Where is your local referral centre for head injuries/burns/hand injuries/spinal injuries/vascular?** Depending on what you're covering and assuming you don't have them on site.
- **How do you book a patient for emergency theatre?**

Referrals

As much as it might angst and frustrate you, GPs are always right. In as much as the customer is always right at least. During your career you will receive some diabolical referrals and you will receive some spot-on referrals. Unfortunately, although it may seem like it, you usually can't tell which until you see the patient yourself.

That's the first reason you have to be nice to GPs when they call you up – as far-fetched or peculiar as their referral may sound, it just might be appropriate. The second reason is that the hospital receives its income from providing a service to primary care. The third, and most important, reason is you never know who that GP knows. They may very well be married to your boss.

So be nice to GPs and in general accept any referral they make. The only exception is if they're making a referral that should obviously go to a different specialty, for instance they're referring you a patient with knee pain and you're on for general surgery. In which case, politely ask them to speak to the orthopaedic team. However, it can be complicated when the presentation isn't a clear-cut referral to either team and the GP has already tried referring to the other team. For instance he's tried referring a 25-year-old woman with low abdominal pain to the gynae team but they refused and suggested you. This GP will have probably spent half an hour on the phone already trying to get through to switchboard, then the other registrar and now you. Just accept the patient. You can argue it out with the gynaecologists as to who will see the patient when you've finished speaking to the GP. Don't send the GP on a wild goose chase ringing all manner of people, because they may end up ringing your boss and you'll look like a prat.

Remember that A&E is under huge pressure to get their patients through the department. Remember that A&E doctors, especially in the middle of the night, might well be working outside their comfort zone with little support. Remember that these are your colleagues, and you're going to bump into them in the coffee room or the corridor or the department. As a consequence, don't submit to the patronising, obstructive manner some doctors have a tendency to take on in their role as the receiver of referrals. Listen carefully to the referral, ask questions and if obviously appropriate accept the patient. Don't be awkward. You don't necessarily need to wait for the LDH result in an acute pancreatitic or the abdominal X-ray in an acute abdomen, you're only delaying the inevitable – that you'll need to see the patient. But obviously if the result of an investigation could crucially affect whether you'll admit the patient under yourself, it's fair to request it before accepting. A negative HCG result in a young woman with abdominal pain, for example.

Resuscitation essentials

The first few minutes and hours of a sick patient's time in hospital is crucial. Ensuring adequate oxygenation, fluid resuscitation, blood transfusions, correction of electrolytes, judicious antibiotic use and pain relief is all you need to focus on primarily. Yet it is startling how often patients have been through the door for 6 hours and are still on their first bag of fluid and their pain is insufficiently controlled. Basic medicine comes before sophisticated diagnosis.

Fluids

Probably the thing done worst of all by admitting surgical teams is fluid resuscitation. Surgical patients almost invariably come into hospital dry. They've been vomiting, had diarrhoea, bled, sweated from fever, had third space losses from some intra-abdominal sepsis, not been drinking, or all of the above. What does the admitting doctor so often do? Make them nil by mouth and give them an 8-hour bag of fluid. That equates to 125 ml/h. The next time you wake up dying of a hangover, try going without water all day and then allow yourself to start drinking water again only in the evening, but only a thimble containing 125 ml every hour and see how you like it. While 125 ml/h is a reasonable maintenance speed of fluids for somebody who is already normovolaemic, these patients need fluid fast to correct their deficits. In the majority of patients, especially the young, it's reasonable to give 1 litre of crystalloid stat to almost everyone. One litre of fluid is like downing almost 2 pints of water, which is what you would want to do with your hangover (if only you could be sure you weren't going to bring it back up). Further litres of fluid can then be given based on how dry the patient looks, but they may need another litre stat, or over 2 hours and then another over 4 hours. This must be decided based on a clinical assessment of how dry they are and, where appropriate, after assessing the urine output following insertion of a urinary catheter.

Bleeding

Patients who have bled may of course also require a blood transfusion. If you are an FY1 who has just done a rotation on a care of the elderly ward you might be quite used to giving a dose of frusemide with your blood transfusions. Please, please, please, please, please do not give frusemide with blood transfusions for surgical patients. First, the idea of giving frusemide along with a blood transfusion is largely an old-fashioned idea from when whole blood was transfused rather than packed red cells. This was a far greater volume and osmotic load and pushed some elderly folk with dodgy tickers into heart failure. Packed red cells are a far smaller volume and have been used for years, but in medicine old habits die hard. Second, giving frusemide to an elderly patient who is having a blood transfusion because of a chronic anaemia when they are already normovolaemic or hypervolaemic, is a very different thing to giving it to an acutely hypovolaemic bleeding patient.

Also, remember that just because a patient's haemoglobin is normal doesn't mean they haven't necessarily had a major bleed. Haemoglobin is a concentration, g/dl, not an absolute volume. Once you've bled, fluid moves out of tissues into the circulating volume, diluting it but allowing maintenance of blood pressure to perfuse the brain. If, therefore, you check the haemoglobin too soon after a bleed, fluid won't have shifted yet to dilute the haemoglobin. If you can see that they've bled a lot, have a low threshold for transfusing despite a normal haemoglobin.

How quickly do you give blood to a patient who is bleeding? Because the maximum length of time over which you can transfuse blood before it spoils is 4 hours, that seems to be the magic number set in many doctors' heads for how long to run a transfusion over. Give it stat in the patient who has recently bled! It makes no sense to watch someone lose a proportion of their circulating volume but restore it only slowly. In the highly unlikely event that you push one of these patients into pulmonary oedema because of giving blood or crystalloids in this manner, remember that pulmonary oedema is far easier to treat than acute tubular necrosis or a PEA (pulseless electrical activity) arrest.

Electrolytes

Remember to check not only the urea and creatinine of your patient, but also their sodium, potassium and, where appropriate, magnesium. We aren't renal physicians who spend their day ensuring the sodium is between 139 and 141 mEq/l, but don't go giving litres of 5% dextrose to a patient with a sodium level of 120 mEq/l. While debate seems to rage endlessly about the best fluids for resuscitation, Hartmann's is probably the safest bet, especially when you don't know what the electrolytes are, because it is roughly physiological. However, don't give it if you know the patient is hyperkalaemic as it contains potassium. Try to correct the electrolytes, especially the potassium, early, particularly if the patient may need to go to theatre, because potassium abnormalities put the patient into significant anaesthetic risk.

Pain

Giving early adequate analgesia to patients in pain is good for everyone. The patient is happy, the relatives are reassured, the nurses are calmed, and you can make a proper assessment of the patient and are more likely to be able to discharge them. Many patients will imagine that they shouldn't take painkillers before coming to hospital so that you can examine them properly. Unfortunately, some frontline staff still have the notion that giving morphine will mask peritonism. It's much easier to assess a patient who isn't rolling around the bed in agony, and morphine doesn't mask peritonism. In general, pain that is made better by analgesia is reassuring. Do not follow the WHO analgesia ladder from the bottom upwards, start at the appropriate level. If the patient is in considerable pain give them morphine. Give pretty much everyone paracetamol (ideally in the intravenous form), but think twice in severe liver failure and alleged history of paracetamol allergy. In between paracetamol and morphine, trusts vary on the availability of weaker opioids such as codeine, dihydrocodeine and tramadol. Do not give non-steroidal anti-inflammatory drugs (NSAIDs) to octogenarians or older (there is a much higher risk of renal failure, peptic ulceration and a lower chance they'll work) or those with suspected peptic ulceration. They can work well in other painful conditions as an adjunct. Antispasmodics such as buscopan can work a treat for conditions where smooth muscle contraction is the cause of the pain, such as in ureteric colic or biliary colic.

Oxygen

For very non-specifically sick patients, the best starting point is to give 100% oxygen via a non-rebreather mask, particularly if they've lost blood, because it means the blood will be maximally oxygenated. There is the ubiquitous concern among medical students that if you give high-flow oxygen to a patient with chronic obstructive pulmonary disease (COPD), you will remove their hypoxic drive to breathe and make them stop breathing. While this is certainly the case in some patients, it is far rarer than the reach of this particular fact would suggest. Unfortunately, it can mean that patients who really need to be given high-flow oxygen don't receive it, just in case they might be a COPD CO_2 retainer. Always give high-flow oxygen in the early stages of resuscitation of a sick patient – you can always lower the oxygen delivered a few minutes later if you're concerned about it, or if you can see the patient obviously doesn't need such high inspired oxygen. CO_2 retainers aren't suddenly going to fall off their perch at the merest whiff of oxygen.

Antibiotics

Patients who arrive frankly septic should be given antibiotics as early as possible after the other basic resuscitation steps have been completed. Where the source is unknown, they should be broad spectrum and taken after cultures (blood, urine and anything else that looks culturable, such as sputum) are taken. Early antibiotics can make a difference to survival from sepsis. But antibiotics should not be used indiscriminately. Where there is doubt about the diagnosis and the patient is well, you don't need to jump in with a tonne of antimicrobials. For instance, if a man comes in with abdominal pain, a little tenderness, mildly raised inflammatory markers and a low grade fever, and you're not quite sure what's up, watching and waiting is often a perfectly reasonable thing to do, and withholding antibiotics can be part of the watching and waiting. If you suspect appendicitis, for example, but you're not sure and the patient is well enough and you plan to review him in the morning, you absolutely should not give antibiotics. If you give them he will probably get better, you'll be reassured when you see him in the morning and you'll let him go home. But his appendicitis will surface slowly but surely once the antibiotics stop and you will then have a delayed presentation of appendicitis often with an appendix mass that is more difficult to treat.

Alcoholics

If the patient's history or examination suggest a strong history of excessive boozing, the patient may be at high risk of developing delirium tremens, arrhythmias and Wernicke's encephalopathy, the former two particularly, as a result of withdrawal of alcohol. Many units have a standard protocol for these circumstances, but the essential components are adequate rehydration, benzodiazepines (the most popular being chlordiazepoxide) in a gradually reducing fashion and thiamine replacement. The latter is usually best given in intravenous ampoules of Pabrinex to then be replaced by oral thiamine.

Summary

When there are lots of patients to see things can get pretty disorganised. With every acute patient you see, ask yourself the following questions and make sure they're all answered one way or the other before moving on to the next patient.

1 Have I instituted basic resuscitation?

2 How sick is this patient? Do I need to involve senior help now or even escalate to the intensivists?

3 Do I have a diagnosis?

4 Does this patient need to go to theatre urgently?

5 Have I ordered all the appropriate tests at this stage?

6 Have I completed all the relevant paperwork, e.g. clerking, drug chart, etc?

Trauma

Managing patients with trauma can be extremely daunting for the newcomer. The range of injury constellations is endless – where on earth do you begin? Fortunately, an excellent system has been developed to bring order to the chaos that can ensue in a major trauma case and it is, of course, the **Advanced Trauma Life Support** (ATLS) system, the international standard for managing trauma. It cannot possibly be the aim of this book to replace such an invaluable course (see page 118), but it will give a very brief overview to get you started, in case you've not yet had the opportunity to go on the course and you're doing your first surgical on call, where you may be called to a trauma.

You're in a provincial hospital. You're holding the on-call surgical bleep. For argument's sake let's assume you are the only one on for surgery. You're it. It's 3 am and your bleeper goes off – '*Trauma team report to A&E immediately*'. Expletive to self. You hurry on down to A&E where there is an A&E staff nurse, an A&E doctor, an orthopaedic doctor, and a junior anaesthetist all, alarmingly, more junior and scared than you.

The patient is being rolled through the door. He is, you are told, in his mid-20s and was the driver of a car that collided with a lamppost. Inner expletive to self. What are you going to do?

On arriving in the A&E resus department, there's usually a few minutes warning time from the ambulance crew so the team can assemble.

1 **Introduce yourself** and find out who else is there, by name and role.

2 Don an **X-ray gown** and **gloves**.

3 Establish the **details of the case** coming in.

4 **Establish roles**: who is going to lead the trauma call, the **team leader**? Will it be you? If so, make sure you know everyone's names and give them roles. As a minimum: (i) Airway management (the anaesthetist); (ii) primary survey (anyone, ideally ATLS trained); (iii) lines and other things.

5 **Prepare** – get IV cannulae set up, a bag of Hartmann's solution ready to roll and blood bottles on standby (the A&E nurse will usually have already sorted all this out – they're excellent at this sort of thing).

The patient arrives. Take a **clear handover** from the ambulance crew, this is usually done as the patient is being transferred on to the bed. Now to get started on the main substance of the ATLS guidelines which broadly consist of:

Primary survey
↓
Adjuncts to the primary survey
↓
Secondary survey
↓
Adjuncts to the secondary survey
↓
Post-resus monitoring
↓
Definitive care

Synchronous resuscitation

In reality this doesn't tend to occur in quite such a rigid, linear progression. There may be much overlap depending on the case and the personnel available, but the A, B, C, D and E of ATLS are unshakeably the most important life savers. Furthermore, the treatment is being given as the assessment is being made.

Primary survey

Airway management with cervical spine protection

Check the airway for **patency**. If the patient can talk normally, the airway is patent, for now. So ask them a question. If they can't talk, it may be from airway obstruction or reduced levels of consciousness (the airway is particularly at risk if the Glasgow Coma Scale (GCS) score is less than 8). Assess for facial or anterior neck injuries and listen for stridor. If present attempt a **chin-lift** or **jaw-thrust** manoeuvre and consider inserting an airway adjunct such as an oropharyngeal tube (Guedel airway). During all of this, make sure that the patient's neck is completely immobilised in a cervical collar between some form of bolsters, with the head taped to the trolley (or held in line by the anaesthetist). If the airway is sufficiently threatened it may even be appropriate to prepare for formal endotracheal intubation. Proceed to B when you've done as much as you can to secure A.

Breathing and ventilation

With the airway secure, proceed with the assessment of the patient's ability to ventilate their lungs properly. **Palpate the trachea** to ensure it is in the midline (if deviated this indicates a tension pneumothorax). **Inspect** the exposed chest for symmetrical expansion on inspiration, **palpate** for injuries and **auscultate** for air entry. What are the oxygen saturations on the **pulse oximeter** and what is the **respiratory rate**? The major things in B that you're looking for on the primary survey are:

- **tension pneumothorax** → without further ado, perform needle decompression with a large-bore cannula in the midclavicular line through second rib space
- **flail chest with pulmonary contusion** → may lead to profound hypoxia, and will require high-flow oxygen and may even need a period of formal intubation
- **open pneumothorax** → apply an occlusive dressing over the site of injury, taped down on three sides, with one side open. This way, when the patient breathes in, the dressing is sucked onto the skin closing the defect. When they breathe out, the air in the pleural cavity partially blows the dressing off the skin, allowing the air to escape. This should prevent the development of a tension pneumothorax for the time being and allow you to continue the assessment, but they'll obviously also need a formal chest drain
- **massive haemothorax** → aside from the circulatory effects of all the blood loss, which will require circulatory support, you will have to insert a large-bore chest drain to take the pressure off the lungs.

Circulation with haemorrhage control

Hypotension in the context of trauma is caused by haemorrhage until proven otherwise. Assess the pulse, the blood pressure, the skin colour and the level of consciousness (see Table 2.3 in Chapter 2). Attacking this problem is double pronged and consists of replacing the lost fluid (blood) and turning the tap off by stopping the bleeding. Insert **large-bore intravenous cannulae** into each antecubital fossa and give 1 litre of warmed Hartmann's solution. If there is obvious external bleeding, **press on it firmly**. However, there may be **occult bleeding** in the chest, abdomen, retroperitoneum, pelvis or the long bones (a femoral shaft fracture for instance) – if you suspect occult haemorrhage these will all need assessment by examination and/or imaging, and shaft fractures must be splinted to reduce blood loss. **Cross-match blood** urgently but use type O negative if the situation is critical.

Disability: neurological status

Assess the **GCS**, the **pupillary size** and **reaction**, the presence of any **lateralising signs** and any **spinal cord injury level**. At this stage this does not include such fancies as proprioception and temperature sense. You just need to gauge the presence or absence of significant neurological injury. Where the GCS is below 8, usually the patient will require substantial airway support, including intubation.

Exposure/Environmental control: completely undress the patient but prevent hypothermia

The resus room is no place for modesty – the clothes need to come off, and if this means cutting them off, so be it. Any obvious injuries should then make themselves known by basic inspection. Ensure the body is covered up again as soon as possible – you may be getting hot and sweaty with all the excitement, but hypothermia is a real risk for these patients.

In practice, all of the above can often be completed very quickly. If things don't seem to be progressing as they should or there seems to be some form of deterioration, always return to the start, checking that in sequence, A, B and C haven't changed.

Once you're confident you've secured the primary survey, there are various **adjuncts** to consider and their use depends, of course, on the case. You're not going to insert a urinary catheter if the primary survey has revealed no abnormality and it looks like all that's wrong with the patient is a fractured ankle.

1 **Cardiac monitoring**.

2 **Urinary catheter**, providing you've excluded a urethral injury (blood at the meatus, perineal ecchymosis, scrotal bruising, 'high-riding' prostate on DRE or pelvic fracture).

3 **Nasogastric catheter** to reduce stomach distension and aspiration risk.

5 **Arterial blood gas** assessment.

6 **Imaging**. The current advice is that at this stage a portable chest X-ray and pelvic X-ray should suffice, and if available a bedside focused assessment sonography in trauma (FAST) scan performed to look for occult chest and abdominal bleeding.

It may be obvious at this stage, if you are in a small provincial hospital, that the patient's injuries are beyond your collective capabilities. Consider the need for transfer now to another unit; simply stabilising the patient may be all that is appropriate, or you may need to call in specialists from other hospitals, or from their beds, depending on your local policies. Otherwise get on with the next step, the secondary survey.

The secondary survey

This consists of a focused history and a top-to-toe examination to find every little detail of the injury. On the history focus first on the most important questions, the AMPLE history:

- **A** – allergies
- **M** – medications
- **P** – past illnesses/pregnant?
- **L** – last meal
- **E** – events leading up to the injury (what happened?)

Table 4.1 Glasgow Coma Scale

	1	2	3	4	5	6
Eyes	Does not open eyes	Opens eyes in response to painful stimuli	Opens eyes in response to voice	Opens eyes spontaneously	N/A	N/A
Verbal	Makes no sound	Makes incomprehensible sounds	Utters inappropriate words	Confused, disoriented	Oriented, converses normally	N/A
Motor	Makes no movements	Extension to painful stimuli (decerebrate response)	Abnormal flexion to painful stimuli (decorticate response)	Flexion/ withdrawal to painful stimuli	Localizes painful stimuli	Obeys commands

From Teasdale, G. and Jennett, B. 1974. ASSESSMENT OF COMA AND IMPAIRED CONSCIOUSNESS. The Lancet, Vol 304, Issue 7872, p. 81–84 reprinted with permission.

Proceed with the **full examination of every system** only when you know the patient is stable with the ABCs, and if anything changes don't hesitate to recommence the primary survey. The patient needs to be **removed from the long spinal board** that he is on as soon as possible. The spinal board is for safe transfer only – it is no longer needed now that the patient is on a hospital trolley. It is best removed by sliding it out when performing a log roll to examine the back. Not only is the spinal board now unnecessary and uncomfortable, but it takes a frighteningly short amount of time to develop decubitus ulcers.

It's often helpful to start literally at the top of the head and work down to the toes, this can usually be at a more leisurely pace than the primary survey. This is the time also to more carefully assess the cervical spine for injury and see whether you can remove the cervical spine protection measures you have in place.

It's often during this time once the acute drama is over that everyone seems to disappear. This can be a very dangerous time for the patient and it is crucial that continuous monitoring occurs as this can be the time for deterioration as a result of previously undetected problems.

You can then proceed with any adjuncts to the secondary survey such as X-rays of suspected fractures.

Definitive care

By now you will have a diagnosis, i.e. what's been injured and to what extent this has compromised the patient. At this stage it should be clearer who will be taking over this patient – if a head CT has shown an extradural haematoma and this is the patient's isolated injury, obviously they need to be transferred to a neurosurgical centre, assuming you don't have neurosurgery on site. If they have a major abdominal injury, they will be going for a laparotomy in theatre and so forth.

Summary of trauma

Nothing can replace going on the ATLS course and you should do this as soon as you can because there is so much more to managing trauma than just what's described here. If you are still too junior to attend as a full student, it is possible to go on a course as a medical student as an observer. Ask your local ATLS course organisers. A list of where the course is available can be found on the Royal College of Surgeons website.

References

American College of Surgeons Committee on Trauma (2008) *Advanced Trauma Life Support for Doctors. ATLS Student Course Manual* (8e). Chicago: American College of Surgeons.

Shem S (1998) *The House of God*. London: Black Swan.

Chapter 5
THE FOUNDATION YEARS

Shelly Griffiths and Helen Dent

Overview, 89
Recruitment to foundation training, 90
Aims of foundation training, 94
Courses, 95
Examinations, 98
Progression, 98
References, 99

Overview

All doctors qualifying and commencing work in the UK will go through foundation training. The foundation programme is designed to train newly qualified doctors to practise safely and effectively, and covers the first two years of work (in the old system: pre-registration house officers and year one senior house officers). Doctors in the foundation programme will also fill a service need in their allocated trust (meaning you work while you train). Foundation training will include medical, surgical and specialty rotations, and you must complete it satisfactorily before commencing further surgical training.

Being a foundation doctor requires good organisational skills above all else, particularly in foundation year one (FY1) when most of your tasks will be administrative. While this is frustrating, remember that all of your seniors have been there too. This is the year where you will learn how a hospital actually runs, and how to manage the system to your advantage. This is also the time to make sure your basic skills, such as venepuncture and cannulation, are up to scratch. When possible (mainly when you're on call) make the most of opportunities to see acute presentations in both surgery and medicine. The more you see as an FY1, when little is expected of you medically, the more confident you will be going into foundation year two (FY2).

Equally, you'll need to try and create opportunities to get into theatre as well. This is difficult, as you are the first port of call for nursing staff when there are any jobs to be done for the ward patients (urgent or otherwise), and you'll find that during FY1 your bleep goes off almost incessantly. If possible, find a like-minded colleague and offer to hold their bleep while they're in theatre if they'll do the same for you. Even better, find a colleague who would rather be anywhere other than in theatre and get them to hold your bleep while you attend their firm's theatre sessions. If

The Hands-on Guide to Surgical Training, First Edition. Matthew Stephenson.

you do get into theatre as an FY1, remember that your ward duties are still a priority. Your colleagues will not thank you if they end up covering your workload and you will suffer in the long term if nursing staff think you're unreliable. Furthermore, if you know nothing about the progress of the ward patients your consultant will not be impressed.

There is a big change when you get into FY2. In most of your jobs you will now have an FY1 doctor to do the sorts of job you were responsible for previously. Some specialties in certain trusts, particularly orthopaedics and urology, don't have FY1 doctors, so you will find in these your administrative tasks persist. However, for the most part, ward jobs will be somebody else's responsibility and you will be expected in clinic and theatre after the ward round. Don't forget what it was like to be an FY1 though – make sure you're available if and when you're needed on the ward and offer to help when it's busy. It's a good idea to do some more medicine (there are in fact very few FY2 rotations that don't include a medical job), particularly intensive care, as this will give you a greater understanding of postoperative care and more confidence in both the practical skills and theoretical knowledge needed when surgical patients become unwell.

Recruitment to foundation training

Process

Recruitment to foundation training starts in October the preceding year and most trainees apply for generic foundation training. The academic foundation programme will be dealt with separately. For most, applications will be made during your final year at medical school. If this is not the case you need to confirm your eligibility for application with the UKFPO eligibility office. If you graduated more than two years before your application, you will need to sit the clinical assessment, which is an Objective Structured Clinical Examination (OSCE) organised by the University of Manchester (costing £800 in 2011).

The application form is split into two main sections, with 100 marks available. The first deals with performance at medical school, with a maximum of 40 points up for grabs, dependent on which quartile you're ranked in at medical school:

- first quartile (0–25th centile) 40
- second quartile (26th–50th centile) 38
- third quartile (51st–75th centile) 36
- fourth quartile (76th–100th centile) 34

As is apparent, there is very little difference between the candidate ranked top of the year and the candidates towards the bottom. The second part of the application form is much more heavily weighted, with 60 points available. There are a number of questions in this section that are designed to assess your strengths and suitability for foundation training, and will ask you, for example, to describe a situation where you have worked in a team, a significant clinical encounter you have had or a significant achievement either within or outside of medicine. It's sensible to look up the person specification for foundation training and ensure your answers highlight these skills. Your overall score for the application form determines your rank, and foundation placements are offered accordingly.

Competition

Most students who pass their medical school finals will be successful in getting on to a foundation training programme. Applicants will rank all 21 foundation schools, which each cover a particular area of the country, in order of preference at the time of submitting their application. While you may have personal reasons for applying to particular geographical locations, it's important to look at competition ratios for each foundation school, as certain ones, particularly in north London, are highly competitive. If you do have a need to be in a particular area of the country, you can apply for special circumstances to be considered. You still need to complete the application form though, as your score will be used to determine which rotation you do. In the first round of offers, all jobs in each foundation school will be offered to candidates with the highest scores that ranked that school first. Only if there are unfilled rotations in that school are jobs offered to candidates who ranked that school as a lesser option. This means that candidates who are unsuccessful in applying to their first choice school often end up with a much lower choice, even if they have done relatively well (just not well enough) on their application form. You can appeal if you feel that correct procedures weren't followed in the assessment of your application – but not just if you disagree with the score you've been allocated. If you decline your offer you are effectively withdrawing from the process, and you won't be offered any other job.

Table 5.1 Competition ratios for 2010 by foundation school

Foundation school	Vacancies	Applicants choosing FS as first preference	Competition ratio (%)
Coventry and Warwickshire FS	84	85	101
East Anglian FS	288	245	85
Keele (Staffordshire) FS	102	39	38
Leicestershire, Northamptonshire and Rutland FS	143	144	101

(Continued)

Table 5.1 (*Continued*)

Foundation school	Vacancies	Applicants choosing FS as first preference	Competition ratio (%)
Mersey FS	290	259	89
North Central Thames FS	313	451	144
North East Thames FS	312	299	96
North West Thames FS	267	506	190
North Western FS	532	499	94
Northern FS	390	288	74
Northern Ireland FS	252	252	100
Oxford FS	225	261	116
Peninsula FS	198	160	81
Scotland FS	747	684	92
Severn FS	270	270	100
South Thames FS	814	1032	127
Trent FS	292	222	76
Wales FS	324	296	91
Wessex FS	294	239	81
West Midlands, North, Central and South FS	408	436	107
Yorkshire and the Humber FS	600	483	81

On being allocated to a foundation school, successful applicants then have to rank all jobs within that school in order of preference. In South Thames Foundation School, there is a further split into separate areas, with candidates ranking just the jobs in one of those areas, due to the number of rotations within the deanery. Most FY1 placements will consist of three four-month placements, including medicine, surgery and a specialty. This is variable, though, and the year may consist of any combination of two-, three-, four- or six-month rotations.

Foundation year one jobs are linked to FY2 jobs. The exact job the following year may be specified, or the trust to be worked in indicated. In a few cases the second foundation year will not be confirmed until after the application process. Obviously all jobs are subject to possible changes, but you must consider both years when making your choices.

All applicants must think about what jobs they do and where they do them to optimise applications for surgical training. Unless you're aware of a department's training record (normally from having spent time there as a student or having spoken to previous trainees) it's difficult to choose wisely. Time spent in surgical departments should be maximised, particularly in FY2, as this is the year when the ward jobs are not your only responsibility anymore. Remember, though, that medical knowledge is important and jobs in other departments are vital for proper training.

The academic foundation programme

There are about 450 academic foundation programme places available each year. These are intended for those with a strong interest in research or education, and competition is fierce. Recruitment begins in June more than a year before the training programme starts and is also a national process, with candidates choosing three 'units of application' (geographical areas) from the 17 that the UK is divided into for this. The first application form is a generic overview of personal details, qualifications, etc., and is identical to the first section of the main foundation programme application. After the first application is completed, candidates then have to complete local application forms for each area. Interviews for short-listed candidates normally take place between June and September, with offers out in mid-September (before the main foundation programme recruitment begins), so if you don't get into the academic programme you can easily slot into that application process. If this happens to you, you will use the same log on details for this application and won't have to enter all the information from your first form again.

The academic foundation programme is identical to the main programme in FY1. During FY2, which will be in the same trust as FY1 jobs, one of the four-month placements will be in research. The project depends on what that department is researching at the time. For more details we would advise speaking directly to the foundation school or hospital. This can be a useful thing to do, especially if you're interested in a career in academic surgery. However, remember that you will be non-clinical for these four months (and unbanded) and you will have little choice over the project you become involved in.

Aims of foundation training

If you're committed to a surgical career, you must start preparation for core training as early as possible. Remember, though, that core foundation competencies must be achieved in order for successful completion of foundation training. Look at the person specification for core training early on and make sure you meet all essential characteristics. Then work on making sure you meet as many of the desirable characteristics as possible.

During foundation training, you're able to undertake a taster week in a specialty of your choice. You can take up to five days to do this, and while it's advertised as a perk of FY2, most trusts will let you do this late in FY1 (although this eats into your total of five days allowed for the whole of foundation training). This can be done in any hospital, providing a local consultant agrees to have you. This is a good opportunity to show your interest to people in that department and get involved in departmental projects that you can continue with after the week is over. It can be done at any point in foundation training, but it's useful to do it before interviews in January of FY2, as it's a good way of showing your interest in surgery in general or one of the surgical subspecialties. If you do have an interest in a more unusual subspecialty, such as hepatopancreaticobiliary surgery for example, this is a great opportunity to get some exposure to something you wouldn't otherwise see. Some trainees have been allowed to do a career-specific course (such as a teaching course for those interested in medical education) during a part of this week, but this is at the discretion of your trust and the foundation school.

There is no set list of which surgical procedures you should be able to perform by the end of foundation training. A lot of consultants involved in the foundation programme will tell you that during foundation training you are meant to be learning how to be a good doctor rather than how to be a surgeon. However, few of them are surgically minded. In reality, by the end of foundation training you should feel comfortable performing the following procedures.

1 Suturing – including subcuticular, interrupted and mattress sutures for skin, and layered internal closures.
2 Simple skin excisions, e.g. lipoma, sebaceous cyst.
3 Incision and drainage of abscesses.

Of course, depending on which rotations you do, how keen you are and how supportive your seniors are, you may be competent to do a lot more than this.

How to get into core training is discussed further in Chapter 6. However, there are a number of things you can do during foundation training to try and get ahead:

1 Start a **logbook** of surgical procedures you assist with or perform as early as possible. There are a number of online systems you can do this through, such as elogbook.org. The ISCP specific logbook was discontinued in August 2011.
2 Complete at least one **audit** project relevant to surgical training and present it at least locally.

3 Try and write up a **case report** – consultants often have interesting cases just waiting for somebody to volunteer to write them up.

4 Involve yourself in **teaching** if possible – set up a journal club or offer to facilitate teaching that is already up and running. Remember to get evaluation forms filled in for whatever you do – as far as the portfolio is concerned, you need proof of what you say you're doing.

5 Get involved in teaching medical students – it's a great time to **organise OSCE teaching sessions** and a mock exam, as you yourself will have just been through the process and know what's needed to get through, especially if the local students attend the same medical school as you did.

6 Check out the list of things medical students should do in the *So you want to be a surgeon?* section and try and catch up with these if you haven't already.

Courses

The Royal College of Surgeons (RCS) recommends a number of courses to be completed during foundation training.

STEP foundation (Surgeons in Training Education Programme)

What?	A distance learning programme, covering ethics, law, postoperative management, management of acutely unwell surgical patients and some practical skills. The website includes case discussions, questions and recommended reading. The day events cover the portfolio and interview skills
How long?	Distance learning over a recommended 20 months (web access is included for a maximum of 24 months) and attending two day courses during this time
When?	Distance learning – as and when. See the Royal College website for details of the day events
Where?	Home, with the day events at the Royal College
Why?	When you're doing non-surgical jobs in the foundation programme, it'll help to keep up your surgical learning throughout
Assessment	None
How much?	£450

Systematic Training in Acute Illness Recognition and Treatment for Surgery (START Surgery)

What?	A one-day lecture course aimed at advancing skills in the care of critically ill surgical patients. A foundation for the Care of the Critically Ill Surgical Patient (CCrISP) course aimed at core trainees
How long?	One day
When?	See the Royal College website for details
Where?	Royal College of Surgeons
Why?	The sooner you learn to manage complicated, sick surgical patients safely, the better. Also, looks good when applying for core training that you're already doing surgically focused courses
Assessment	None
How much?	£150 (£130 if you've enrolled onto the STEP foundation course)

Clinical Anatomy of Practical Procedures

What?	A two-day interactive course reviewing prosections relevant to a range of basic procedures, such as cannulation, to more advanced procedures such as cricothyroidotomy
How long?	Two days
When?	See the Royal College website for details
Where?	Royal College of Surgeons
Why?	Useful preparation for the real thing
Assessment	None

There are also other courses available that trainees may be interested in.

So You Want to be an Orthopaedic Surgeon?

What?	A careers advice day
How long?	One day
When?	See the Royal College website for details
Where?	Royal College of Surgeons
Why?	If you're interested in a career in orthopaedics this course could be used as an example of commitment to specialty at interview
Assessment	None

Clinical Skills in Examining Orthopaedic Patients

What?	An extension of 'So You Want to…', looking at the skills necessary for a foundation doctor interested in orthopaedics
How long?	One day
When?	See the Royal College website for details
Where?	Royal College of Surgeons
Why?	As 'So You Want to…'
Assessment	None

These last three courses are run intermittently as interest is variable, so dates and prices are not available. Trainees who are interested in them are asked to register on the RCS website.

There are a number of other courses that the Royal College recommends taking during core training. Some of these, such as Basic Surgical Skills, CCrISP and Advanced Trauma Life Support (ATLS), can be taken during foundation training. It will certainly do an application to core training no harm to have completed these well in advance, but they are detailed in Chapter 6 because of this recommendation.

While you're not entitled to any study leave during FY1, some trusts will let you take single days for exams and such-like. Be aware, though, that you may end up having to use annual leave. During FY2 you have an allowance of 30 days – most of this is taken up with mandatory trust teaching. Find out what your trust offers early on, and plan well in advance.

There are also a few e-learning modules that you can complete. These can be accessed through www.e-lfh.org.uk, the official site for the foundation programme. Some of these are mandatory, such as Safeguarding Children and Young People. When you've completed a module you will be given a certificate that you can print off and place in your portfolio as evidence of continued professional development. Other websites, such as Doctors.net.uk and BMJ Learning, also have modules that you can complete and which you also get a certificate for. These modules rarely take more than an hour or so and are a good way to fill some free time if you are in a reasonably quiet job.

Examinations

The Royal College recommends membership exams to be taken during core training. However, most trainees will find Part A Membership of the Royal College of Surgeons (MRCS) easily attainable within foundation training. Full information about Membership of the Royal College of Surgeons can be found in Chapter 6.

Progression

There are a number of hoops to jump through as you progress through foundation training. Some of them are genuinely beneficial to you, others are a necessary evil. Either way, it's best to be organised and get everything done in a timely fashion. Nobody will appreciate you running around in the last few weeks of the year pestering people to sign you off for a cannula they may have watched you do six months previously. There is a long list of competencies that need to be achieved, covering attitude, knowledge and skills. These are monitored through a range of assessments, which you will access through your online ePortfolio.

- **Mini clinical evaluation exercise (Mini-CEX)**: you must do at least six of these each year. It's an assessment of an interaction with a patient, such as history taking or management.
- **Case-based discussion (CBD)**: these are more formal reviews of a case in which you had a particular involvement, and should be done with a registrar or consultant. You should again do at least six of these each year.
- **Team assessment of behaviour (TAB)**: this is a form of multisource feedback, where you need to get a number of different colleagues from a range of medical and allied professions to assess your ability at work. You must have at least one satisfactory TAB each year.
- **Procedural logbook**: this has been designed to allow you to provide evidence of competency in a number of basic procedures that are on the GMC list of core skills. You should be able to perform and teach these by the end of foundation training. Skills include venepuncture, cannulation and catheterisation, and you must get each skill

signed off by either a more senior doctor or another health professional.

- **Direct observation of procedural skills (DOPS)**: this is to record practical procedures that do not fall into the remit of the logbook. You should aim to do three of these each year, though they are not mandatory since the introduction of the procedural logbook.
- **Developing the clinical teacher assessment**: this is a review of a teaching session you have given, for example a presentation at a journal club. You must do at least one assessment each year.

These assessments are accessed through the NHS ePortfolio website (www.nhseportfolios.org), through which you also have to complete induction meetings and end of placement reviews with your consultant. As a foundation trainee, registrars and consultants can complete CBDs for you. All grades can complete mini-CEX and DOPS assessments.

In order to get 'signed off' (i.e. successfully complete foundation training) you will need to have completed each year without taking too much additional time off (including sick and compassionate leave), completed the necessary number of assessments as detailed above and attended a minimum of teaching sessions (normally 70%, excluding sessions you couldn't attend due to annual leave or on-call commitments). In each year, the trust will then sign a 'Foundation Achievement of Competency Document', which will be forwarded to the foundation school, who will also sign and keep a copy, returning a copy to you for your records. This is the FACD5.1 (Foundation Achievement of Competency Document) for FY1 and FACD5.2 for FY2. Most trainees will need to present this at interview for further training.

References

www.foundationprogramme.nhs.uk
www.mmc.nhs.uk
www.nhseportfolios.org
www.surgeryrecruitment.nhs.uk

Chapter 6
THE CORE TRAINING YEARS

Shelly Griffiths, Helen Dent and Matt Stephenson

Overview, 100
Recruitment to core training, 101
Academic clinical fellowships, 106
Aims of the core training years, 107
syllabus, 110
Membership of the Royal College of Surgeons (MRCS), 111
Courses, 117
Annual Review of Competence Progression (ARCP), 120
References, 121

Overview

The core training years consist of CT1, CT2 plus or minus CT3 (also called CT2+, see later) and follow on directly from foundation year 2. When the time comes in FY2 to apply for core training you should have decided which branch of medicine to move into and if you're reading this book presumably you'll be considering surgery! The overall options though include surgery, medicine, paediatrics, ACCS (acute common care stem), psychiatry, radiology, general practice and other smaller specialties.

Once you've decided to pursue a surgical career, you must decide if oral and maxillofacial surgery (OMFS) or neurosurgery (and if you're in Scotland, trauma and orthopaedics) is for you, as these must be applied for separately at this point (see Chapter 11 or 14 respectively). If not, then the other subspecialties are combined into a two-year rotation termed core surgical training, which will be themed towards one of the subspecialties.

In general, CT1 is more generic, covering three four-month posts in surgery and CT2 is more specialised covering two six-month posts. Some core programmes are more generic as a whole and some are more themed throughout for those who already know which subspecialty they wish to pursue. Rotation allocation varies between deaneries. In some, your CT2 year will be determined by a matching process, which may involve an interview or a review of your performance during CT1. In others, the posts for the full two years will be decided before starting CT1. CT3 is currently an optional year and again the process varies between

The Hands-on Guide to Surgical Training, First Edition. Matthew Stephenson.

deaneries, with some actively encouraging this year and others keeping it as a reserve for those trainees who are not successful in progressing to higher training after completion of core training. It's likely to become more common to take CT3 in the future, largely due to the working time restrictions meaning trainees do not have sufficient experience to progress to registrar level after CT2.

The priority for core trainees is obviously to increase experience and confidence in being a surgical doctor. The higher training years are looming, when you will often be the most senior doctor in hospital, so now is the time to prepare yourself for that. Most people head for theatre first to get as much cutting experience as possible, but don't miss out clinics, multidisciplinary team meetings (MDTs) and departmental meetings just to get scrubbed – you will regret it later. Most core trainees won't have a full timetable but will often have an FY1 to do the ward work, so it's time to leave the FY1 to look after the patients and plan your days carefully. It's too easy to get stuck on the wards and wonder where the time went.

One of the big difficulties for core trainees is being allowed to operate. It seems that each day in theatre lands you with a different supervisor, who will inevitably say 'Let me show you, you can do the next one' even if it's the fifth one you've seen. Find out which days are quiet for your firm and see if there are any surgeons who have a regular list that day who do not have trainees with them. That way you could join them in theatre every week, get to know them and they get to know you. That's the way you'll get to operate. In the near future it's unlikely a surgical trainee will get enough cutting time without putting in some of their own free time, so make it a habit to walk past the CEPOD theatre each day to see what's booked and let it be known you are keen to help out in theatre so people will call you when an extra pair of hands is needed.

If you don't have FY1s to cover the wards it's still possible to arrange extra theatre time. Agree with your colleagues to hold each other's bleeps in turn so you can attend theatre and clinic without interruption.

Some posts give the core trainees a lot of administrative responsibility – if they do, make it work to your benefit and include aspects like 'Booking theatre lists' and 'Arranging MDTs' in your portfolio as examples of managerial roles. Other posts don't give any responsibility so volunteer for these things and make use of your time. Use free sessions for research, audit or teaching. There is never any need to sit in the mess!

Recruitment to core training

Competition

It can be useful to look at competition ratios from years gone by to help decide the subject and area you wish to apply for, although of course it's no guarantee of what's to come. To put surgery into perspective, Table 6.1 shows how much more competitive surgery is compared with the other career options. In 2011, the overall competition ratio for core surgical training was 4.2:1 (and 11.2:1 for neurosurgery ST1). Competition ratios are not available by theme of the rotation.

Table 6.1 Competition ratios by speciality, 2010 (England only)

Subject	Number of posts	Number of applicants	Applicants per post
Core surgical training	594	4,794	9.7
Core medical training	1,171	2,455	2.1
General Practice Vocational Training Scheme (VTS)	2,783	4,850	1.7
Obstetrics and gynaecology	249	1,252	5.0
Paediatrics	340	1,386	4.0
Psychiatry	383	1,066	2.8
Clinical radiology	179	1,251	7.0

Process

Recruitment to core surgical training up until 2010 was deanery based – you would apply to as many deaneries as you wanted, up to 14 in some cases (see Table 6.3).

In 2011 this changed (see Table 6.2), in common with all of the surgical subspecialties, to national recruitment, in this case administered by the Kent, Surrey and Sussex deanery. Applications were open for two weeks in early December. The application form in 2011 was very basic, consisting of drop-down boxes to rate the level achieved in terms of audit, presentations and publications. It's likely that this will continue as all candidates are guaranteed interviews in the two deaneries they rank highest, meaning there is little point in an in-depth application form. Candidates can rank as many deaneries as they would consider working at, though in reality as most deaneries are oversubscribed you are unlikely to be considered in deaneries apart from those two you rank highest.

Interviews then followed in January and February and comprised three 10-minute stations.

- The **clinical scenario** station – the most heavily weighted station comprising a scenario to read immediately before interview and another during it. Examples in 2011 included a paediatric trauma case, reaction to local anaesthetic and high stoma output.
- The **management** station – ethics, judgement and management of time. Examples in 2011 included methods to meet training needs considering European Working Time Directive

Table 6.2 The figures for applications to the 2011 round of recruitment by deanery

Deanery	Post numbers	Ranked first by candidates invited to interview	Ranked second by candidates invited to interview	Total number of candidates invited to interview	Competition ratio
East of England	49	71	127	198	4:1
East Midlands North	22	28	49	77	3.5:1
East Midlands South	18	15	33	48	2.7:1
Kent, Surrey and Sussex	41	53	213	266	6.5:1
London	98	487	135	622	6.3:1
Mersey	32	40	54	94	2.9:1
Northern	40	89	31	120	3:1

(*Continued*)

Table 6.2 *(Continued)*

Deanery	Post numbers	Ranked first by candidates invited to interview	Ranked second by candidates invited to interview	Total number of candidates invited to interview	Competition ratio
North Western	59	107	160	267	4.5:1
Oxford	19	41	72	113	5.9:1
Severn	31	61	85	146	4.7:1
South West Peninsula	34	15	25	40	1.2:1
Wales	30	49	30	79	2.6:1
Wessex	29	29	39	68	2.3:1
West Midlands	67	105	77	182	2.7:1
Yorkshire and the Humber	77	78	104	182	2.4:1

Table 6.3 Number of applications made to core surgical training in 2010

Number of applications	Applicants	%
1	344	27.50
2	183	14.63
3	200	15.99
4	159	12.71
5	120	9.59
6	73	5.84
7	39	3.12
8	29	2.32
9	19	1.52
10	18	1.44
11	19	1.52
12	18	1.44
13	13	1.04
14	17	1.36
Total	**1251**	**100**

(EWTD) restrictions and dealing with misdiagnosis.

- The **portfolio** station – the portfolio prompts discussion around achievements and career development and will look at your motivation for pursuing a surgical career.

Each candidate is then awarded a score out of a maximum of 60 points.

There are four possible outcomes following interview.

1 Being deemed **successful** and **offered** a job.

2 Being considered successful at interview but **failing to achieve a high enough score** to be offered a job in the initial round of offers. These candidates are **eligible to receive offers** if any jobs were rejected after the first round of offers.

3 Being considered successful at interview but **failing to achieve a high enough score** to be offered a job in that deanery, and being placed on the **reserve list** for other deaneries.

4 Being considered **unappointable** at any deanery due to an overall low score at interview, or receiving less than 50% in any one station.

In 2011, offers were made at the end of February. Further iterations of offers came out quickly, as some jobs were rejected, with several rounds occurring each week. Those candidates receiving an offer then had three options: to accept, decline or hold that offer. A decision had to be made within 48 hours. Offers could be held until the national cut-off date at the end of March, to allow offers from other specialties; however, if a candidate was holding an offer they would not receive any further offers from the surgical national recruitment programme. It's only possible to hold one offer across all specialties. There is some talk at the moment of candidates in the future being able to 'upgrade' offers if a job they ranked higher than the job they have been offered becomes available further down the line. This system is not currently in place though, and once a candidate has accepted a job they are bound to take it.

Most posts in 2011 were filled with applicants who had been interviewed at that deanery. However, there were a few jobs available in certain deaneries with low subscription rates that were not filled following all appointable candidates in that deanery being offered a job. A process of national clearing began in April, whereby all eligible candidates were invited to rank the remaining deaneries that still had posts available. Job offers were then made based on the highest score each candidate received at interview. Think carefully before ranking the deaneries, as you are wasting time if you rank a deanery that you would not agree to work in.

It's essential to prepare early for applications to core surgical training to ensure you fulfil all the eligibility criteria on the person specification and as many of the desired criteria as possible. To standardise recruitment and make it a fair process, recruitment has become somewhat tick-box. However, this means it's very clear what's required and how to gain a high score before even attending the interview. Plan ahead to ensure exams are passed and courses attended in plenty of time for the application process.

You will also need to demonstrate that you have completed all the foundation competences, usually with the form FACD 5.1 (Foundation Achievement of Competency Document), to indicate successful completion of FY1 with an agreement to provide FACD 5.2 on completion of FY2 later that year

Academic clinical fellowships

The alternative to core surgical training is to do an academic clinical fellowship. Like the academic foundation programme, these are aimed at trainees with a particular interest in research. They are targeted at subspecialties, such as paediatric or colorectal surgery, and include nine months dedicated to research, during which time it's expected that you would gain funding in order to complete a PhD. This is completed during an Out of Programme Experience period (OOPE), but can include time spent on call or in clinics if required.

Recruitment begins earlier than for core training, but outcomes are not known when core training recruitment begins, meaning unless you're extremely confident you should apply for core training as well. The application form is much more formal, as true short-listing does occur. In 2011, the following questions were asked of candidates.

- Give details of outstanding achievements outside the field of medicine gained in parallel.
- Give details of presentations and publications:
  - presentations at a regional/national level
  - presentations at a local level
  - publications in peer-review journals
  - other publications (e.g. conference abstracts).

- Teaching and audit:
  - what experience do you have of delivering teaching?
  - what experience of clinical audit do you have?
- Describe how you meet the person specification for the programme you are applying for, including particular skills and attributes that make you suitable for a career in this specialty.
- Provide evidence of activities and achievements that demonstrate your commitment to a career in this specialty and how they have led to the development of skills relevant to a career in this specialty.
- Research experience and academic career plans:
  - give details of all research projects you have undertaken, including methods used
  - describe in detail a research project you have been involved in
  - explain why you want this particular academic clinical fellowship, indicating your medium- and long-term career goals in relation to an academic career in this specialty area.

If an academic career interests you, you need to make sure you have something to write for each of the above questions. Short-listing takes place in December and interviews are held in early January. The clinical training should match that received by the core trainees, and the aims and assessments are largely identical, except for the research component.

Aims of the core training years

The overarching aim of the core training years is to instil trainees with basic surgical knowledge and ensure they are competent and confident in the management of common surgical conditions. By the end of core training, in general, trainees need to be comfortable working in theatre and performing certain index procedures, assessing acute surgical patients in A&E, seeing patients in clinic with supervision and managing common problems on the ward. There are far more specific competences to achieve though, the details of which are on the Intercollegiate Surgical Curriculum Programme (ISCP) website and are assessed particularly through workplace-based assessments.

You cannot complete core training without passing your Membership of the Royal College of Surgeons (MRCS) exams, and this must be completed in order to progress to ST3; there are also a number of courses that must be attended. From CT1 onwards you will be expected to pay an annual fee (currently £125) to the Joint Committee on Surgical Training (JCST) and this enables you to use the ISCP website, which helps coordinate your learning portfolio.

As well as gaining clinical experience, the time should be spent beefing up your portfolio in preparation for ST3 applications. The easiest way to do this is to look at the ST3 person specifications (see Chapter 7) early in your core training and ensure you have something to put in each section. The basics are unlikely to change each year and include things such as publications, presentations, teaching and demonstration of commitment to specialty.

There are some specific areas to focus on during your core training years to optimise your progression through core training and future success at ST3.

Audit

Most trainees will have done one or two audits during their foundation years, but it's important to continue participating in audits, leading one if you can and really trying to close the loop on one if possible. Most hospitals have an audit department that can help with pulling notes and with some of the leg work, but this can often take a while. Ask your consultant during your initial meeting what projects they're interested in performing and maybe even start two or three so time is not wasted waiting for notes to arrive. One recent ST3 application form asked for audits performed during the past four years only, so an audit done in the FY1 year will be getting close to the cut-off point. When doing an audit later in training, take advantage of the fact you have juniors working for you, and supervise an FY1 in collecting the data, focusing your own efforts on the interpretation and presentation of results. Often, the application form will ask you to detail four or five audits, so don't just leave it at one. It also helps to have presented the audits to directorate meetings.

Research

Application forms and person specifications ask for involvement in research, and understanding of the process of research. In reality it's necessary to have at least one publication under your belt by the time of application for ST3, but the more the better. Don't forget that as well as big research projects, letters to journals, case studies and abstracts published after conferences can be included in applications too.

Teaching

To be awarded the points on an application form for 'teaching' it's not enough to just talk to the medical students on the ward round. Teaching achievements range from bedside teaching to tutorial teaching, tutoring in a series of sessions, lecturing and developing courses. If you don't have scheduled teaching sessions in your hospital (or even if you do) you could arrange a time each week to meet with other trainees and recruit registrars and consultants to each talk about a topic. Teaching also includes assessing work and designing and marking exams. Try to keep a record of any teaching you do, and ask for feedback from the students. You can write a feedback form to hand out after sessions that you can summarise and keep in your portfolio. Don't forget to also keep a record of teaching you attend.

Courses

The Courses section of this chapter has more details on the specific courses available. It's a requirement for some applications to ST3 (check the individual person specifications for each subspecialty) to attend Advanced Trauma Life Support (ATLS), Care of the Critically Ill Surgical Patient (CCrISP) and Basic

Surgical Skills (BSS), but be warned that some courses (particularly ATLS) have a long waiting list, so it pays to be organised. Bonus points are available for achieving 'recommendation for faculty', so don't just turn up and expect that to be enough. If you perform well enough, the course tutors will register you as someone who may be suitable to teach on the course, which shows you've done particularly well and can be mentioned in application forms and provides a talking point in interviews.

Logbooks

It's essential to keep a surgical logbook. There are a variety of different methods of doing this, for example www.elogbook.org. An alternative is the Orthopaedic Curriculum & Assessment Project (OCAP) logbook for orthopaedic trainees. The best way is to go online after each theatre session to log the operations; but at the very least it should be updated regularly. Do not rely on hospital records, because, as the junior surgeon, you will often not be logged by name.

Workplace-based assessments

CBD (case-based discussion): this assesses clinical judgement and management planning skills. The assessment compares the trainee with the average person at that level of training and should be performed by your assigned educational supervisor (AES) or clinical supervisor.

DOPS (direct observation of procedural skills): assessing practical procedures against the level of an average trainee. There is a set list of procedures available from the ISCP website that includes subjects such as 'Banding of haemorrhoids', 'Injection of local anaesthetic' and 'Open and close midline laparotomy'. These can be assessed by more senior doctors.

PBA (procedure-based assessment): this is an assessment of full surgical procedures such as appendicectomy or hernia repair, for example. These are assessed compared with someone performing at the level of Certificate of Completion of Training (CCT), so even an ST3 trainee, for example, would not be expected to achieve the highest mark. Since they are marked at CCT level, they can only be assessed by people at CCT level themselves. These may or may not be required at core trainee level, but will become more important in higher specialty training. Even if not a requirement, there is no reason why a core trainee may not start using the PBA assessments.

Mini-CEX (clinical examination): assesses patient interaction, including history taking, examination and communication. These can be completed by senior doctors.

Mini-PAT (peer assessment tool): this is a form of 360 degree assessment. Several of these should be performed over the whole period of training, specifically in years CT1, ST4 and ST7. However, it will look good anyway if one is completed every year and it doesn't take too long. Raters should be selected on ISCP, and they will then receive an email invited them to share their opinions on your behaviour. Choose your raters carefully!

Syllabus

The purpose of a curriculum is to ensure that trainees get a standard level of training with similar content irrespective of their deanery or hospital. It also aims to keep the training similar across the different specialties. The curriculum is for higher trainees as well as core and is designed to take trainees to CCT level.

The surgical curriculum consists of four parts:

- syllabus – what trainees should know and be able to do
- teaching and learning – how trainees cover the content of the syllabus
- assessment – how to measure the progress of trainees
- training systems and resources – how the programme is organised.

The syllabus has been standardised and is published on the ISCP website. The current version was updated in August 2010 and is the curriculum that should be followed.

There are various aspects, including (for example):

- theoretical knowledge
- practical and operative skills
- clinical judgement
- professional and leadership skills
- the responsibilities of being an NHS employee.

The Curriculum Framework page of the ISCP website gives a list of recommended reading and suitable textbooks for the trainee to use.

The curriculum is competence based rather than being based on time spent in training and so is flexible as to when certain levels are reached. Core (early years) training focuses on common competencies that are standard across all the subspecialties, with only a few specialty-specific competencies.

Early year training aims to ensure trainees achieve the competencies required to enter ST3 training. These competencies include:

- managing patients who present with a variety of elective and emergency conditions. Both listed in the Core and Speciality syllabus sections.
- professional competencies derived from the Good Medical Practice publication (GMC).

There are 10 modules, as foloows.

1 Basic science knowledge relevant to surgical practice, including anatomy, physiology, pharmacology, pathology, microbiology and radiology.

2 Common surgical conditions. To be able to investigate and manage common surgical conditions.

3 Basic surgical skills, including handling surgical instruments and tissues, tying knots and good assisting.

4 The principles of assessment and management of the surgical patient, including history, assessment, basic consent.

5 Perioperative care of the surgical patient, including fluid management, use of blood products and nutritional management.

6 Assessment and early treatment of the patient with trauma, including head injury, chest trauma and abdominal trauma.

7 Surgical care of the paediatric patient, including the surgical conditions and issues of child protection.

8 Management of the dying patient, including consent issues, palliative care and DNAR orders.

9 Organ and tissue transplantation, including brain stem death.

10 Professional behaviour and leadership skills, including good clinical care, teaching, managing people and ethical issues in surgery.

Within the syllabus itself, each module contains a list of topics to be covered. Each clinical topic is presented with a standard required by the completion of CT2. These standards are numbered 1–4.

Clinical standards:

1 has observed

2 can do with assistance

3 can do whole but may need assistance

4 competent to do without assistance, including complications.

The syllabus is useful to guide revision for the MRCS exams and knowing what clinical exposure you should be getting. It's important to show in your Annual Review of Competence Progression (ARCP) that you have been following the syllabus and have progressed in your knowledge of each of the topics.

Membership of the Royal College of Surgeons (MRCS)

Probably the most significant milestone in your early career is achieving membership of the Royal College of Surgeons by passing the MRCS exams. It not only changes your title from Dr to Mr or Miss (or Mrs), it is a necessary step for career progression to higher surgical training and is a recognisable benchmark for your colleagues to measure you by.

A few years ago the advice given to trainees was to not take MRCS too early – wait until you've done a few senior house officer (SHO) jobs – 'passing the vascular station will be difficult if you have never done a vascular job' – was the official advice. Times have changed and with the accelerated pace due to MMC, generally the unofficial advice is to start taking the exams as early as you can. However, the Royal College of Surgeons suggests that Part A be taken in CT1 and Part B in CT2, and that doctors in their foundation years are very unlikely to pass Part B. Given that there is a limit on the number of times you're allowed to fail Part B, you would be unwise to take it too early. The counter argument is that in order to apply for ST3, you need to have passed both parts by the time applications close, usually in February/March of your CT2 year.

You need to be careful that MRCS should not be seen merely as a hoop to jump through. It should be seen as an opportunity to study properly for the first time since medical school.

Figure 6.1 shows a number of points. Knowledge and ability gradually rise during medical school with a blip towards finals. After qualifying, your practical skills improve – you can put a cannula in blindfolded – but because you're now earning money, there are more interesting things to do with your evenings than read the *British Journal of Surgery*. Eventually we realise

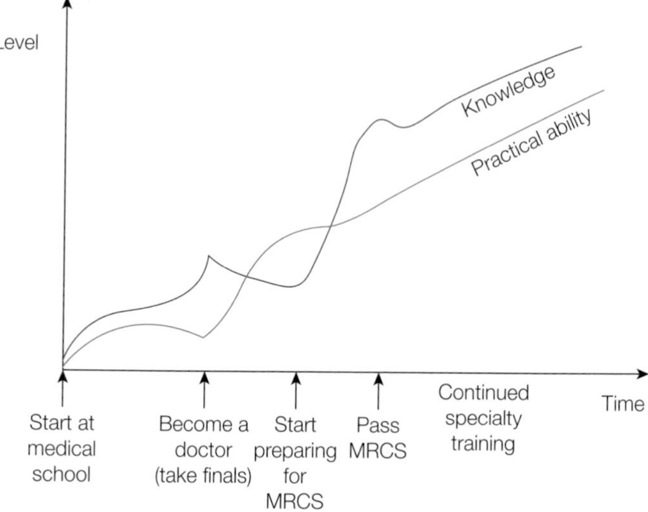

Figure 6.1 A schematic representation of the development of knowledge and practical ability.

our knowledge is waning, the facts we learnt at finals, which we were never entirely sure were accurate anyway, are becoming a vague memory. Is Crohn's more common than ulcerative colitis? What are the branches of the brachial plexus? When you start preparing for MRCS you are preparing to put half-baked medical student concepts that got you through finals to bed. Now is the time for the **absolute acquisition of knowledge**. A thorough commitment to the forever part of your memory of the epidemiology of inflammatory bowel disease, the steps of an inguinal hernia repair and the clinical application of Starling's curve.

MRCS is not a time for cramming the week before the exam. People have probably passed before by doing so, but you are denying yourself the opportunity for MRCS to mean so much more than the letters before and after your name.

So start early, six months before perhaps. Prepare properly. If you're going to use revision guides, use them as final revision guides, not the main substance of your study. To learn the basic surgical sciences go to some established textbooks. To learn physiology use a proper physiology textbook like Ganong. To learn anatomy read the poetic words of Last with the beautiful atlas of Grant's in front of you. To learn pathology study Underwood or some similar tome. You will never regret preparing properly for your MRCS exams, and you can tell the difference between the surgical registrar who did, and the one who didn't.

Popular books that cover the whole syllabus include *Essential Revision Notes for Intercollegiate MRCS*, which comes in two volumes, with a third addition to the collection looking at communication skills for Part B. DrExam also publishes an Objective Structured Clinical Examination (OSCE) guide that includes a lot of the theoretical knowledge that you can be quizzed on. Pastest and OnExamination also have online question banks that are a really useful way of testing your knowledge in preparation for Part A. To prepare for any operative questions and indeed just to learn how to operate, *How to Operate* is a DVD and book box set, which has 40+ operations to watch on the DVD and read about in the book.

What is MRCS?

MRCS is the shorthand way of saying Intercollegiate MRCS examination. Intercollegiate because since 2004 the three Royal Colleges in the UK: RCS of England, RCS of Edinburgh and RCPS of Glasgow have been doing the same one (yes, there are two in Scotland; in Glasgow it's called the Royal College of Physicians and Surgeons of Glasgow).

Where should you do it?

You can apply to take the exam at any of the three colleges, but only one at a time. It used to be possible to apply for the exam in London and Edinburgh and use the other as a back-up in case you failed the first. If you do this now you just forfeit the fee.

In short it doesn't really matter which one you take it at, although many people will feel a strong attachment to one particular college, and that matters to some extent because the college in which you apply for Part B of the exam is the one that you will belong to lifelong. The exam is the same in all colleges.

Which MRCS?

Because MRCS has been transformed in recent years along with a new curriculum, some trainees will be taking an older version of it, which has pretty much died out. If you've not taken any part of MRCS before you will be taking what are called the September 2008 guidelines.

Eligibility

Candidates must possess a:

- primary medical qualification that is acceptable to the UK GMC for full or provisional registration *or*
- primary medical qualification that is acceptable to the Medical Council in Ireland for full or temporary registration *or*
- for overseas candidates, a primary medical qualification acceptable to the Councils of the colleges. To see the acceptabilities of each country see the international Medical Education Directory on http://avicenna.ku.dk/database/medicine.

And that basically is it, with a few small print exceptions regarding re-attempts following a previous failure. You can theoretically take your MRCS in foundation year 1, never having done a surgical job, but it would be very unwise.

What can you do with it?

MRCS is mandatory for progression to ST3 (or ST4 in neurosurgery). ENT trainees also require the Diploma in Otorhinlaryngology – Head and Neck Surgery to progress to ST3 (for full details see Chapter 12).

Costs

Postgraduate examinations are not cheap in any specialty. The costs at the time of going to press were:

Part A	£460
Part B	£835
Total	**£1,295**

Even after you've passed you will of course still have to pay the annual subscription to the Royal College of Surgeons of £285. If you don't pay it, technically you aren't allowed to use the letters MRCS after your name as these formally denote current membership of the college, not of passing the exam, as the College will remind you if you're late for your annual payments.

Usual dates

Diets, better known as exam sittings, are held three times a year in each college. Part A is held in January, September and April; Part B is held in October, February and May.

Structure of the exam

Part A Multiple-choice questions (MCQs)

MRCS has undergone some radical changes over recent years but the dust is beginning to settle and the system is looking more consistent from year to year; however, check www.intercollegiatemrcs.org.uk for precise, up-to-date information when you're planning to take it.

This comprises two separate MCQ papers, each two hours long, sat on the same day at one of the Royal Colleges. So four hours of written papers assessing your core knowledge of applied basic sciences in all nine surgical specialties.

- Paper 1 – Applied basic sciences (single best answers)
- Paper 2 – Principles of surgery in general (extended matching items)

To pass, you must achieve an undisclosed minimum score both in the combined total of the two papers and also on each individual paper. So you can't ace the second and flunk the first and still pass Part A.

Part B Objective Structured Clinical Examination (OSCE)

This consists of 18 stations, each lasting nine minutes. Broadly, you will be examined on four areas.

1. Anatomy and surgical pathology.
2. Applied surgical science and critical care.
3. Communications skills in giving and receiving information and also history taking.
4. Clinical and procedural skills.

When you apply for MRCS you are asked to choose three different 'specialty context areas' out of a choice of four:

- trunk and thorax
- head and neck

- limbs and spine
- neuroscience.

Twelve of the stations will have a general context and the remaining six will be given a slant towards your chosen area, with your first choice given three stations, your second choice given two stations and your third choice given one station. There are four broad content areas the examiners are looking for:

- clinical knowledge and its application
- clinical and technical skill
- communication
- professionalism.

You will be scored on each of these domains for each station (with a maximum mark per station of 20).

Pass rates

Tables 6.4 and 6.5 shows the pass rates for Part A and Part B of MRCS; these figures didn't used to be available but the system has now become more transparent. Part A is in the region of 62% and Part B 60%. Anyone telling you the pass rates have gone up massively compared with 'their day' should remember that even if that's the case (and it can't be proved), the fact is that you only get one chance per diet as opposed to olden times when you could put in for all three colleges in each diet in case you failed one, which was expensive but gave you a pretty good chance per diet of winning at least once.

If you've never failed an exam in your life, unfortunately you just might be

Table 6.4 Pass rates for Part A over three diets

	Total number sat	Passing % (and number)	Failing % (and number)	Pass mark (%)
September 2008	636	63.2 (402)	36.8 (234)	64.7
January 2009	664	60.4 (401)	39.6 (263)	66.9
April 2009	566	61.5 (348)	38.5 (218)	65.6

Table 6.5 Pass rates for Part B over three diets

	Total number sat	Passing % (and number)	Failing % (and number)	Pass mark (%)
October 2008	155	63.9 (99)	36.1 (56)	69.5
February 2009	278	54.7 (152)	45.3 (126)	68.0
May 2009	432	60.4 (261)	39.6 (171)	67.6

in for an unpleasant surprise. Pass rates (as above) are far lower than those you'll have experienced before in undergraduate exams and that's among other candidates who have also never failed anything in their life. Don't feel too bad, some of the best surgeons have failed at least part of MRCS once, twice or even three times. Dust yourself off, take a holiday, and come back and focus on your weaknesses and get to work on fixing them.

The MRCS exam – an examiner's perspective

Sam Andrews is an MRCS examiner and the author of *MRCS Core Modules: Essential Revision Notes*

The OSCE part of the MRCS examination has been phased in over the past three years to replace the traditional viva and clinical sections of the exam, which have now been completely replaced for the MRCS UK exam. However, at the time of going to press the traditional clinical and viva format is still used by the Irish college, and for the MRCS examinations in overseas centres, currently Kolkata, Colombo and Cairo.

It is no secret that many examiners dislike the OSCE format. Although perceived to be fairer, standardised and more reproducible, it does not allow candidates with exceptional knowledge or skills to stand out, and is undoubtedly more onerous to examine in. Nevertheless the new format is here to stay and candidates should prepare accordingly.

Believe it or not, the examiners want you to pass. It is far easier and more fun to examine a good or exceptional candidate than it is to examine a poor or borderline one.

Some general rules

DO – dress smartly. A tie is not necessary but a smart shirt and trousers, or blouse and skirt is ideal. Candidates are expected to be 'bare below the elbows' and many carry their own alcoholic hand gel, although this is available in the exam.

DO – look and act professionally. The exam is supposed to reflect the way you would treat patients and colleagues in the real clinical situation.

DO – answer the question asked. Avoid waffle, repetition and confabulation. If you do not know the answer, do not guess or make it up. The examiner has the correct answer on a card in front of him, so he will know! It is better to admit to not knowing the answer and move on.

DO – talk slowly and clearly. Remember you may be the twentieth candidate the examiner has seen in the same station that afternoon. Imagine he has had a heavy lunch with fine wine and port (at the candidate's expense) and he may be feeling soporific. Use plenty of eye contact to try to keep the examiner interested (or awake).

(*Continued*)

The marking of the MRCS OSCE is complex. Each station is marked separately for domains and broad content areas. The four broad content areas are clinical and technical skills, anatomy and surgical pathology, surgical physiology and critical care, and communication skills. The domains are marked for clinical knowledge, clinical and technical skill, communication and professionalism (including judgement, organisation and planning). Obviously different stations have different weighting for each domain and broad content area.

It is probably unhelpful to worry too much about the marking scheme. Candidates who prepare and revise carefully, act professionally and communicate clearly will be rewarded with a pass!

Finally – GOOD LUCK.

Sam Andrews

Courses

The big three courses to get under your belt are Basic Surgical Skills, Advanced Trauma Life Support (ATLS) and Care of the Critically Ill Surgical Patient (CCrISP). The majority of people you're competing with for jobs will have done all three at the very least (even in subspecialties that don't require all three) and don't forget about more general courses such as Advanced Life Support (ALS). There are also some specialty-specific courses to think about in the core training years and these are discussed in Chapters 8–16.

Basic Surgical Skills (BSS)

What?	You are taught and then practise various basic surgical techniques. It covers open surgery, trauma and orthopaedics, and minimal access surgery. Lots of hands on practise and individual tuition.
How long?	2.5 days
When?	Aimed principally at CT1s but the range is FY2–CT2. It's essential to do this course fairly early on so that you can properly assist in theatre and later it becomes less useful as you will have picked up the skills already, and you may have got into some bad habits
Where?	The course is run at the Royal Colleges but these courses get booked up very quickly and are more expensive. Check the Royal College of Surgeons website for all the peripheral centres running the course

Why?	It's mandatory and it's very helpful for acquiring the basic skills essential for competent operating. You get a DVD, a handbook and a certificate at the end
Assessment	No exam, continued observation and informal assessment throughout the course
How much?	£740

Advanced Trauma Life Support (ATLS)

What?	International course originating in the US. Will teach you a simple approach to the management of trauma patients. Interactive tutorials, skills teaching and simulated scenarios (called moulages). If you perform particularly well you may be recommended to become an ATLS instructor (even if junior) which can look good on the CV
How long?	Three days
When?	Recommended CT1–2 but can be from FY2
Where?	The course is run at many centres across the UK, indeed the world
Why?	It's mandatory and essential for safely managing trauma patients. You get a course manual and a certificate
Assessment	Pre-course MCQ, continual assessment by faculty throughout three days and final written MCQ and assessed simulated patient management scenario
How much?	£550

Care of the Critically Ill Surgical Patient (CCrISP)

What?	Run by the Royal College of Surgeons. Advances practical and theoretical skills for the management of critically ill surgical patients through small group tutorials, lectures and practical sessions
How long?	2.5 days
When?	Recommended CT2, but CT1 can apply if sufficient experience. The course organisers advise having done at least six months of general surgery
Where?	The course is run at many centres across the UK including the Royal Colleges
Why?	It's very useful for safely managing very sick patients. While it's not mandatory, you'd be very foolish not to do it, both for your own experience and for your CV. You get a course manual and a certificate
Assessment	Ongoing assessment throughout the course
How much?	£550

STEP courses

The Royal College of Surgeons for many years now has been running a distance learning course for surgical trainees called STEP, Surgeons in Training Education Programme. This has been modified to fit recent changes in the surgical curriculum. There is now a STEP Foundation and a STEP Core

What?	Mainly a distance learning course aimed at CT1–2 trainees for preparation for MRCS. It's flexible so can be tailored to fit with the clinical placements you're doing. Some deaneries supply the STEP programme as part of the core training, so check with the deanery and your hospital before paying up

How long?	The College suggest that with 15 hours a week work this can be completed over 20 months. Within this time there will be two STEP Core events at the college to attend. There are four modules including: **1** The human body in health (anatomy and physiology) **2** The human body in disease (pathology, microbiology and radiology) **3** Surgical skills and procedures (basic surgical skills, the surgical Patient and perioperative care) **4** Special topics (including topics such as nutrition, trauma and child protection)
When?	See How long?
Where?	Distance learning with occasional college events
Why?	Supports continued learning and preparation for MRCS. Side benefits include subscription to *Surgery* journal, discounts on MRCS revision courses and access to other surgical websites for learning
Assessment	Participation in this programme also permits access to the eSTEP Core website which has a forum for discussions, and MCQs and clinical cases for learning and revision
How much?	£550 (£500 for those who enrolled in STEP Foundation). Older versions of the STEP course can be obtained from colleagues who have completed it or from sites such as eBay at a much reduced price, but bear in mind that the format has changed significantly over the years and you would not have access to the online resources

Annual Review of Competence Progression (ARCP)

To pass the core surgical training years you must pass an ARCP each year. This looks at a variety of activities, including attendance at teaching days, progress with exams, research and audit activity, and the contents of your logbook. Make sure you keep track of all of your activities on the ISCP website under the Evidence section. This allows the assessors at your ARCP to see what activities you have completed during the year.

A big focus, however, is on the completion of workplace-based assessments

(WBAs). These take several forms, including DOPS, mini-CEX, CBDs, PBAs and mini-PATs. It's important to check the requirements of your local deanery as there is variation between the core years, different deaneries and changes each year, but they will usually consist of a minimum requirement of a certain number of each type of assessment. As an example, one deanery asks for (minimum per year):

- 12 CBD
- 12 DOPS
- 12 mini-CEX.

There will be an interim review (usually in January/February) at which point half of the assessments should be completed, along with some content in the Evidence section. The final assessment of the year is the ARCP, which happens quite far in advance of the actual end of the year, so bear that in mind when keeping an eye on the assessments that you have completed.

You must pass the MRCS before your final ARCP in order to progress.

References

A Reference Guide for Post Graduate Specialty Training in the UK. The Gold Guide Core Training Supplement (3e) (2009). London: MMC.

Applicant Guide (2010) Core Surgery National Recruitment Office, Kent, Surrey and Sussex Deanery.

Intercollegiate Committee for Basic Surgical Examinations (2009) *2008/9 Annual Report. The Membership Examination of the Surgical Royal Colleges of Great Britain MRCS Part A and B (OSCE)*. London: ICBSE.

National Recruitment Bulletin (2011) Core Surgery National Recruitment Office, Kent, Surrey and Sussex Deanery.

www.elogbook.org

www.intercollegiatemrcs.org.uk/

www.iscp.ac.uk

www.jcst.org

www.mmc.nhs.uk/

www.rcseng.ac.uk

www.surgeryrecruitment.nhs.uk/kent-surrey-sussex-deanery

NON-CLINICAL

Chapter 7
THE SPECIALTY TRAINING YEARS

Matt Stephenson

Choosing a specialty, 122
Overview of specialty training, 122
Recruitment, 124
Aims of the specialty training years, 136
Out of Programme, 136
Courses, 137
Annual Review of Competence Progression, 137
Postgraduate degrees, 138
Fellowship of the Royal College of Surgeons, 138
References, 139

Choosing a specialty

Deciding which subspecialty to choose can be immensely difficult if you aren't completely head over heels in love with one particular one. One of the main reasons for this is that it can be very difficult to judge what your likely chances are of career progression. Over time, the surgical subspecialties grow and shrink. The number of jobs available, the number of people required to provide the service and the popularity of the specialty changes each year. It's difficult to predict which specialties will become more or less popular, but the Centre for Workforce Intelligence (CfWI) aims to recommend how recruitment should change.

Table 7.1 shows the current situation and is somewhat surprising given how cardiothoracics has for years now been considered by some a dying art. Clearly this is untrue, but it demonstrates how workforce demand varies with time.

Reports of each of the subspecialties can be found on the CfWI website. It can't be emphasised enough though just how much this changes over time. It should not be used solely to guide your choice of specialty. Within reason, if you're dead set on neurosurgery, for example, then you should go for it. There will always be a need for more neurosurgeons, the catch is, they may not all be consultants.

Overview of specialty training

Of course there are huge differences between the surgical specialties in terms of specifics of specialty training and these are covered in Chapters 8–16, but there are also some consistent points which

The Hands-on Guide to Surgical Training, First Edition. Matthew Stephenson.

Table 7.1 Future projections for specialty recruitment, in England

Grow	Reduce	Stay the same
Cardiothoracics	General surgery Trauma and orthopaedic Otorhinolaryngology (ENT) Neurosurgery	Urology Oral and maxillofacial surgery Plastics

NB Do not read too much into this table, the situation is changing all the time and is notoriously difficult to predict.

will be looked at here. In addition to the following nine surgical specialties, it is highly likely that by around 2013 this list will go up to 10, as vascular surgery plans to split off from general surgery to form its own career structure – see the vascular section of Chapter 8.

Technically all doctors are 'junior doctors' until they have completed their training and achieved Certificates of Completion of Training or equivalent. However, among that broad spectrum there is the division between the registrar grade (or 'middle grade' to encompass non-training grades like clinical fellows that are more senior than core trainees) and those more junior to it. Specialist registrars (SpR) were the name for this breed post-Calmanisation (see Chapter 20), but since Modernising Medical Careers (MMC) the name has changed to specialty registrars (StR) (spot the all-important difference of -ist and -ty). The only implication this has in real terms is in run-through posts where there are no core training stages, so in neurosurgery you technically become a 'registrar' (ST1) after FY2, albeit a specialty one and not a specialist one, and to all intents and purposes you are doing the job of an old-style SHO. Such tiresome semantics! The bottom line is that specialty training (or higher surgical training [HST]) begins at ST3 in all specialties (except neurosurgery) just like the old-style year 1 specialist registrar, and at this stage you become a registrar and suddenly the world starts to look rather different.

The step from core training to specialty training can feel like more of a giant leap. You will, overnight, be expected to be able to do far more and with less supervision, your responsibilities grow and your learning opportunities increase. Getting an ST3 job (or ST1 in neuro) with run-through training means that you are in secure employment being trained for the next six years, subject to satisfactory progression as judged by your Annual Review of Competence Progression (ARCPs; see later). You will have heard of the phrase 'getting a number'. This refers to a national training number (NTN), which is awarded to you on successfully getting an ST3 job. It is considered a golden ticket because of the security of getting you all the way to completion of training.

Of course, not everyone is lucky enough to get a 'number' and instead get stand-alone jobs that may or may not count towards training. Training jobs are in the form of either fixed-term specialty training appointments (FTSTAs) or locum appointments for training (LATs), the latter being more of an ad hoc appointment, usually for one year. These can be extremely valuable for learning whether or not that particular specialty is right for you, but there is at least anecdotal evidence that some people get stuck in a rut doing these fixed-term jobs over and over again, which may disadvantage you from getting an ST3 run-through post. Non-training jobs such as LAS (locum appointment for service) or trust grade doctors have no deanery support to help with training and are largely dependent on the whim of the trust and consultant you are working for. In practice, of course, we all know doctors working in LAS posts getting just as much if not more training than those in ST training posts. The distinction between a training and a non-training job is often purely only a technical paper distinction, but an important one for career progression.

The Gold Guide is the official 112-page guidance document for specialty trainees and is updated annually. It covers a whole range of issues relevant to these years from interdeanery transfers to relocation expenses, so is worth a look. It's available from the MMC website (www.mmc.nhs.uk/specialty_training/specialty_training_2011_final/gold_guide.aspx).

Recruitment

Competition

Getting an ST3 run-through post is extremely competitive. In 2010, there were 621 posts in CT1 and another batch of 190 free-standing CT2 posts dished out, but only 288 ST3 appointments that year (these figures exclude oral and maxillofacial surgery [OMFS] and neurosurgery but the equivalent positions are similar). Assuming numbers through the system stay reasonably stable overall (which they do), this equates to roughly 36% of core trainees to higher surgical trainees; in 2007 the figure was 35%. That doesn't even equate to the competition ratios as it doesn't include other doctors in other grades applying for ST3 posts. There was talk during the introduction of MMC of a 'lost tribe' of SHOs unable to progress to higher surgical training. Not much has changed, the progression from CT2 to ST3 is just the same as the old senior house officer (SHO) to specialist registrar bottleneck. The system is intrinsically pyramid shaped with more doctors in the junior grades, fewer in the registrar grades and even fewer in the consultant grades (when you take into account length of time in grade). As you'll read in Chapter 12, for instance, there are currently 337 ENT specialist/specialty registrars and only 565 ENT consultants (bearing in mind the registrar years are only supposed to last around six years and a consultant surgical career can be from 20 to 30 years – that's a long time to wait for someone to retire). This pyramid is unlikely to change any time soon and will if anything become more marked as hospitals will need plenty of juniors to man the European Working Time Directive (EWTD) compliant rotas. It is also considered to encourage healthy competition. However, under pressure to reduce this high attrition ratio of core training posts to specialty training posts,

Table 7.2 Ratio of CT posts to ST posts in given specialties, 2010

Specialty	Total number of themed CT posts	Number of ST3 opportunities	Ratio of CT:ST
General surgery	270	93	2.9 : 1
Trauma and orthopaedics	260	90	2.9 : 1
Plastic surgery	64	9	7 : 1
Paediatric surgery	22	6	3.7 : 1
Urology	58	41	1.4 : 1
ENT	72	27	2.7 : 1
Cardiothoracic	10	22	0.45 : 1

it's quite possible that we may face a reduction in the number of core training posts, not a rise in the number of specialty training posts. This could mean doctors having to move into service grade posts even earlier in their careers.

Competition ratios of course vary depending on the specialty and from year to year. The figures for the ratio of CT posts to ST posts in 2010 are shown in Table 7.2.

This doesn't tell the whole story however. For example, don't go thinking that if you were a cardiothoracic core trainee that year you'd be begged to take up an ST3 post – there are many others in other grades applying for these jobs.

In fact, in 2011 across the board there were three times as many non-core trainees (i.e. service posts) as core trainees applying for specialty training. In 2011, statistically speaking core trainees had a higher chance of landing an ST3 post than someone coming from a service job; however, this only amounted to 24% of core trainees getting an ST3 job and some of these had done a CT3 year as well. However, significantly, the majority of ST3 numbers in fact went to those in service posts. This is important to remember if you've wandered off the formal training pathway: all is not lost (although the proportion of core trainees getting ST3 jobs was still higher than the proportion of non-core trainees).

Table 7.3 looks really rather complicated but has been presented in its entirety to make two, hopefully slightly optimistic, points in the face of all this gloom. There is often a difference between the frequently advertised competition ratios and the truth. For instance, imagine some make believe country where there are five medical schools each with 100 places. If 1,000 sixth

Table 7.3 The 2008 competition ratios

Specialty	Number of applications	Number of applicants	Number of posts	Ratio of posts to applications	Ratio of posts to applicants
General surgery	1463	930	80	19	12
Trauma and orthopaedics	757	460	50	15	9
Neurosurgery (ST1)	150	150	30	5	5
Cardiothoracic surgery	115	90	5	23	18
Urology	206	160	14	15	11
ENT	267	180	19	14	9
OMFS	219	75	17	13	6
Plastic surgery	210	170	9	23	19
Paediatric surgery	40	40	1	40	40

formers apply for a particular medical school, the competition ratio will be 10 : 1 – sounds gloomy. However, those same medical students will all be applying to the other four medical schools, so as long as the sixth former doesn't mind going to a medical school that isn't their first choice, this makes the true competition ratio of sixth former to medical student 2 : 1 – not so bad. The same has been the case with ST3 applications to surgery until they all started organising national recruitment. The number of applicants is not necessarily the same as the number of applications, as one applicant could make more than one application. In other words, the headline competition ratios often banded around are not necessarily always as bad as they seem.

The second point is that particularly with the smaller specialties, the number of posts may vary considerably from one year to the next depending on the number of senior trainees leaving the other end of the training system. For example, while there was only one ST3 post in paediatric surgery in 2008, in 2011 there were six.

The process

It's difficult to be too specific about the process of applying to specialty training. There has been so much flux in recruitment in recent years that not much has stayed the same year on year since the Medical Training Application Service (MTAS) debacle of 2007. What has become more consistent, however, is that applications to specialty training are now once a year at about the same time, and instead of applying to separate deaneries you apply to one deanery that manages recruitment for the whole country. The deaneries responsible for this task in 2011 are listed in Table 7.4. It's unclear currently whether this will stay the same long term.

The first stage of recruitment, Round 1, starts in early December to fill jobs the following August. However, this is for more junior posts such as core training rotations. Round 2 starts in early February and this is where ST3 posts are advertised (later than the first round as this helps them work out how many posts will be available) and ST3 jobs generally start in October, not August (giving a rare opportunity to take a two-month career break between the end of your core training job finishing in August and the start in October).

Well before this you should make sure that you fit the eligibility criteria for appointment, which you can find in the person specifications on the www.mmc.nhs.uk website. An example of the person specifications is shown below and these are pretty consistent across the specialties; however, there are some important differences between the different specialties in terms of the 'Eligibility' and 'Career progression' sections. For instance, in cardiothoracic surgery you're ineligible if you've already taken the Fellowship of the Royal College of Surgeons (FRCS) exit exam, in other words if you're too experienced already. You then need to keep your eyes peeled for the advertisement of any jobs. Such vacancies tend to remain open for four weeks – if you're late in applying, your application will be immediately rejected so don't leave it until the last minute. All applications these days are electronically submitted. You will be asked to rank the deaneries in order of

Table 7.4 The lead deaneries for national selection for each specialty

Specialty	**Deanery**	**Website**
General surgery	London	www.londondeanery.ac.uk
Trauma and orthopaedics	Yorkshire and the Humber	www.yorksandhumberdeanery.nhs.uk
Neurosurgery	Yorkshire and the Humber	www.yorksandhumberdeanery.nhs.uk
Cardiothoracic surgery	Wessex	www.wessexdeanery.nhs.uk
Urology	Yorkshire and the Humber	www.yorksandhumberdeanery.nhs.uk
ENT	Yorkshire and the Humber	www.yorksandhumberdeanery.nhs.uk
OMFS	Severn	www.severndeanery.nhs.uk
Plastic surgery	London	www.londondeanery.ac.uk
Paediatric surgery	Yorkshire and the Humber	www.yorksandhumberdeanery.nhs.uk

Source: www.mmc.nhs.uk

preference. Also bear in mind that the person reading your form will not be able to see your personal details – this is particularly relevant in the very small specialties.

All applications will go through a process of long listing, which means all applicants that fit the eligibility criteria. These will then be short-listed using a scoring system that should be made transparent to you by the relevant deanery. However, in 2011 all applicants to ST3 general surgery, for example, were interviewed; there was no short-listing. You'll then hear from the relevant deanery whether or not you've been short-listed and will be sent an invitation for interview.

There are a number of things you're likely to be asked to take with you, such as:

- original proof of identity (e.g. passport or other photo ID)
- original and photocopy of your GMC certificate
- original and photocopies of all qualifications listed on your application form (translated if necessary)
- verified evidence of competences cited on your application form – your professional portfolio

- evidence of educationally approved posts cited on your application form
- evidence of nationality/immigration status
- evidence of skills in written and spoken English.

Interviews have typically lasted 60 minutes and often comprised three separate stations, but you will need to check up-to-date information about your round of recruitment.

If you're offered a post you should be allowed at least 48 hours to accept or reject it, and if you accept it you must withdraw from the application process altogether. However, now that recruitment is coordinated nationally, you should know for sure that nothing better will be coming your way as you're not waiting for any other deaneries to get back to you. The exception of course would be if you've applied to do more than one surgical specialty, but if you're doing this you may struggle to show how you've demonstrated your commitment to one particular specialty.

Regional variations

National selection to the following specialties encompasses England, Wales and Scotland:

- neurosurgery
- urology
- paediatric surgery
- OMFS
- cardiothoracic surgery
- plastic surgery.

Only in paediatric and cardiothoracic surgery does national selection reach Northern Ireland. You are of course entitled to apply for the specialties that recruit regionally in all separate countries if you so desire.

Wales

Information can be obtained from www.mmcwales.org or http://specialty.walesdeanery.org/. The Wales School for Surgery is responsible for the usual nine surgical specialties (and also ophthalmology) at core and specialty levels. There are obviously fewer posts across the board in Wales than England, and those specialties that are not part of national selection are advertised over roughly the same time span as in England. The whole process is broadly similar to England's.

Scotland

NHS Education for Scotland (NES) is responsible for Scottish Medical Training and manages the application and recruitment process; information about recruitment is available from their website: www.scotmt.scot.nhs.uk/. The main notable difference is that trauma and orthopaedics is still run-through in Scotland and not uncoupled, i.e. you apply for ST1 directly from FY2 and that takes you right through to ST8.

The three remaining specialties (ENT, general surgery and orthopaedics) that don't recruit nationally are managed through Scottish Medical Training but run at roughly the same times as in England. Of note, as orthopaedics is run-through from ST1, you need to keep an eye out for Round 1, rather than Round 2.

Table 7.5 2011 Person specification: application to enter specialty training at ST3, general surgery

Entry Criteria	Essential Criteria	When Evaluated
Qualifications	■ MBBS or equivalent medical qualification ■ Successful completion of MRCS or equivalent at time of application	Application form
Eligibility	■ Eligible for full registration with the GMC at time of appointment and hold a current licence to practice.	Application form
	■ Evidence of achievement of **Foundation competences** from a UKFPO affiliated Foundation Programme or equivalent by time of appointment in line with GMC standards/Good Medical Practice including: ■ *Good clinical care* ■ *Maintaining good medical practice* ■ *Good relationships and communication with patients* ■ *Good working relationships with colleagues* ■ *Good teaching and training* ■ *Professional behaviour and probity* ■ *Delivery of good acute clinical care*	Application form Interview/Selection centre
	■ Evidence of achievement of **CT/ST1 competences** in general surgery at time of application & **CT/ST2 competences** in general surgery by time of appointment, supported by evidence from work-based assessments of clinical performance (DOPS, Mini-CEX, CBD, ACAT) and Multisource Feedback or equivalent ■ Eligibility to work in the UK	Application form/ Interview/Selection centre Application form

Fitness To Practise	Is up to date and fit to practice safely	Application form References
Language Skills	All applicants to have demonstrable skills in written and spoken English adequate to enable effective communication about medical topics with patients and colleagues demonstrated by one of the following: ■ *that applicants have undertaken undergraduate medical training in English; or* ■ *have achieved the following scores in the academic International English Language Testing System (IELTS) in a single sitting within 24 months at time of application – Overall 7, Speaking 7, Listening 7, Reading 7, Writing 7.* If applicants believe they have adequate communication skills but do not fit into one of these examples they must provide supporting evidence	Application form Interview/Selection centre
Health	Meets professional health requirements (in line with GMC standards/Good Medical Practice)	Application form Pre-employment health screening
Career Progression	■ Ability to provide a complete employment history ■ Evidence that career progression is consistent with personal circumstances ■ Evidence that present achievement and performance is commensurate with totality of period of training ■ At least **24 months' experience** in surgery (not including Foundation modules) by time of appointment, of which at least **6 months experience** has been in general surgery	Application form Interview/Selection centre

Table 7.5 *(Continued)*

Entry Criteria

	Essential Criteria	When Evaluated
Application Completion	**ALL** sections of application form completed **FULLY** according to written guidelines	Application form

Selection Criteria

	Essential	Desirable	When evaluated
Career Progression	**As above**	■ Completion of **a year's General Surgery experience** at CT/ST level by the time of appointment ■ Less than 4 years experience in General Surgery at CT/ST level (not including foundation modules)	Application form Interview/Selection centre
Courses	Attendance at relevant courses, e.g. ATLS, Basic Surgical Skills or equivalent, CCrISP		Application form Interview/Selection centre

Clinical Skills	**Technical Knowledge & Clinical Expertise:** ■ Capacity to apply sound clinical knowledge & judgment & prioritise clinical need ■ Demonstrates appropriate technical and clinical competence and evidence of the development of diagnostic skills and clinical judgment ■ Validated logbook with summary documentation of surgical exposure to date	**Personal Attributes:** ■ Shows aptitude for practical skills, e.g. hand-eye coordination, dexterity, visuo-spatial awareness	Application form Interview/Selection centre References
Academic/ Research Skills	**Research Skills:** ■ Demonstrates understanding of the basic principles of audit, clinical risk management & evidence-based practice ■ Understanding of basic research principles, methodology & ethics, with a potential to contribute to research **Audit:** Evidence of active participation in audit **Teaching:** Evidence of contributing to teaching & learning of others	■ Evidence of relevant academic & research achievements, e.g. degrees, prizes, awards, distinctions, publications, presentations, other achievements ■ Evidence of participation in risk management and/or clinical/laboratory research	Application form Interview/Selection centre

Table 7.5 *(Continued)*

Selection Criteria	Essential	Desirable	When evaluated
Personal Skills	**Judgement Under Pressure:** ■ Capacity to operate effectively under pressure & remain objective In highly emotive/pressurised situations ■ Awareness of own limitations & when to ask for help **Communication Skills:** ■ Capacity to communicate effectively & sensitively with others ■ Able to discuss treatment options with patients in a way they can understand **Problem Solving:** ■ Capacity to think beyond the obvious, with analytical and flexible mind ■ Capacity to bring a range of approaches to problem solving **Situation Awareness:** ■ Capacity to monitor and anticipate situations that may change rapidly **Decision Making:** ■ Demonstrates effective judgement and decision-making skills **Leadership & Team Involvement:** ■ Capacity to work effectively in a Multi-Disciplinary Team ■ Demonstrate leadership when appropriate ■ Capacity to establish good working relations with others		Application form Interview/Selection centre References

	Organisation & Planning: ■ Capacity to manage time and prioritise workload, balance urgent & important demands, follow instructions ■ Understands importance & impact of information systems		
Probity	**Professional Integrity:** ■ Takes responsibility for own actions ■ Demonstrates respect for the rights of all ■ Demonstrates awareness of ethical principles, safety, confidentiality & consent ■ Awareness of importance of being the patients' Advocate, clinical governance & responsibities of an NHS Employee		Application form Interview/Selection centre References
Commitment To Specialty	**Learning & Development:** ■ Shows realistic insight into general surgery and the personal demands of a commitment to surgery ■ Demonstrates knowledge of the surgical training programme & commitment to own development ■ Shows critical & enquiring approach to knowledge acquisition, commitment to self-directed learning and a reflective/analytical approach to practice	**Extracurricular activities:** ■ Achievements relevant to general surgery, including elective or other experience ■ Attendance at, or participation in, national and international meetings relevant to general surgery	Application form Interview/Selection centre References

Northern Ireland

Full details can be found on the Northern Ireland Medical and Dental Training Agency website, www.nimdta.gov.uk/. In Northern Ireland, the only run-through specialty is neurosurgery, as in England and Wales. Aside from paediatric surgery and cardiothoracic surgery, the other surgical specialties aren't operating a national selection process.

Person specifications

Person specifications are crucial reading well before applying to your chosen specialty training rotation as it will take some preparation to achieve all that they require. Some specifications are specific, such as attending a particular course, others are more general, for instance how are you going to prove that you can 'manage time and prioritise workloads'? There are different person specifications for each subspecialty but the vast majority are the same – the main differences are in the Eligibility and Career progression sections.

Aims of the specialty training years

The aim of specialty training is to take you from core trainee right the way up to preparedness for being a consultant. It takes six years (five years in urology). It may take longer if you don't progress satisfactorily, but it won't be quicker. Many people also take additional years voluntarily in the form of fellowships, which might be at home or abroad and are generally taken towards the end of training. This is usually to learn a highly specialised skill not completely covered during the statutory six years but that will help in your consultant practice.

By your fifth or sixth year of being a registrar, you shouldn't be too far off the full range of abilities of a junior consultant. You should have built up a broad operative repertoire and learnt to make very sensible decisions, but clinical acumen is not all you have to develop. The bottleneck for jobs didn't end at your ST3 interviews, oh no, the competition's just hotting up. In most of the surgical specialties securing a consultant job is a fiercely competitive process (see Chapter 21) so you need to keep on cramming bits into your CV and working on your portfolio. You still need to be doing audits, publishing papers, teaching, attending and presenting at conferences, going to courses, ideally doing a postgraduate degree, albeit part time, and generally trying to set yourself apart from the crowd. All of this will be assessed at least annually at your ARCP. Then towards the end of training you need to do your exit exams (see later). So even though getting a number is a golden ticket, it doesn't mean the hard work has finished, it's only just starting.

Out of Programme

Many trainees take a year, or sometimes more, out of their six years to travel to other units in the UK or internationally. This can provide some extremely helpful experience that you otherwise wouldn't have had on your normal rotation. These time-limited posts, usually in the form of fellowships, need to be agreed with your programme director in advance. There are four types.

- OOPT – Out of Programme for Approved Clinical Training. Vascular surgeons for instance may want to get extra experience of endovascular techniques; colorectal surgeons may want to spend some time in a tertiary referral centre doing advanced laparoscopic surgery. The GMC has to give approval for OOPTs and this therefore counts towards training and towards the CCT.
- OOPE – Out of Programme for Clinical Experience. As for OOPT in terms of the kind of experience, but this doesn't formally count towards training or, therefore, towards the CCT; no GMC approval needed.
- OOPR – Out of Programme for Research. This doesn't tend to count towards training and is usually taken earlier in the specialty training years in the form of a single year or up to three years for a PhD.
- OOPC – Out of Programme for Career Breaks. Obviously taking a year out to prepare for *X Factor* auditions or go travelling around South America needs prior approval and sadly doesn't count towards training.

Start thinking early about the kind of OOP year you might want to do because if you want to go abroad for it, that can take a considerable amount of planning in order to get all the documentation in order so you're allowed to practice abroad.

Courses

There is a huge array of courses available but these are unique to each specialty and are therefore covered in each of the subspecialty chapters.

Annual Review of Competence Progression

Every year you will be summoned in front of a panel of assessors to show them that you have progressed satisfactorily and are on the right trajectory in your training. This is the Annual Review of Competence Progression (ARCP). It used to be called the Record of In-Training Assessment (RITA) for old-style specialist registrars. These days, evidence is king. You need to provide evidence of everything you've done – log books, workplace-based assessments, feedback from your clinical supervisor, etc. If you have already undergone core training you will already be familiar with ARCPs.

Who's on the panel? This varies but it's usually chaired by the chair of the Specialty Training Committee or one of the programme directors. A number of other people may be present, such as consultants interested in training, as well as lay people and employers (i.e. from hospitals).

Find out well in advance exactly what your ARCP panel expects from you, as this varies from deanery to deanery and specialty to specialty, e.g. some are very strict about the number of workplace-based assessments you are expected to fill in. If you know they're expecting you to have done an audit, you'd be foolish not to take the evidence of one along with you. This is where you will be hoping that you've kept your portfolio up to date as you've gone through the year and continually added to it. There should be at least three members on the panel, but there may be many more.

The ARCP process is a two-way street though. It is an opportunity for you to bring up unresolved issues you've had with your training. The panel has two objectives: to consider and approve the adequacy of the evidence provided and, providing this documentation is adequate, make a judgment about your suitability to progress to the next stage of training.

There are a number of outcomes ranging from 'Outcome 1: Satisfactory progress' to 'Outcome 4: Released from training programme', with intermediate grades of remedial effort in between. There are other outcomes for other specific circumstances, such as at the end of training.

Postgraduate degrees

If you haven't already taken out separate time to undertake research or some other postgraduate degree and you're not planning to, a part-time Masters postgraduate degree may be just right for you. There is a wide variety to choose from such as an MSc in surgical practice, an MSc in medical education or an MSc in medical law; some people even do a medical MBA to help present themselves as a consultant who would be able to manage the department (bearing in mind that most surgeons don't like managing this would be music to some interview panels' ears).

These can be costly, however, in the order of £2,000–3,000 per year for two to three years, and most study budgets are only in the region of £800 per annum. Some are purely distance learning and involve lots of written assignments, while others involve up to 20 days of attendance at lectures or seminars (a hefty chunk of your study leave would go on this).

Fellowship of the Royal College of Surgeons (FRCS)

Unlike in medicine, surgical trainees are expected to pass an exit exam ('exit' from training) in the final registrar years, usually ST7–8. What can be confusing is that FRCS used to be the name for the primary Royal College exam undertaken during the SHO years that was replaced by the Membership of the Royal College of Surgeons (MRCS) exam, so some older surgeons may talk about FRCS meaning MRCS. The only difference in the name is that if it's the new, exit exam variety, it has a suffix in brackets denoting the specialty in which you exited.

- Cardiothoracic surgery – (C-Th)
- General surgery – (Gen.Surg)
- Neurosurgery – (Neuro.Surg)
- Oral and maxillofacial surgery – (OMFS)
- Otolarynology – (ORL-HNS)
- Paediatric surgery – (Paed.Surg)
- Plastic surgery – (Plast)
- Trauma and orthopaedic surgery – (Tr and Orth)
- Urology – (Urol)

Getting FRCS (specialty) is an essential step towards acquiring your Certificate of Completion of Training and is colloquially just called the FRCS exam or officially the Intercollegiate Specialty

Examination. Once you've passed it and done all the relevant paperwork, you can apply for Fellowship (not just membership any more) of the Royal College of Surgeons. The format is essentially the same for all surgical specialties, although obviously content will differ.

Unlike MRCS, there are strict entry criteria. You must have a structured reference from three consultants you've worked with who state that you are ready to become a consultant.

There are two sections.

- **Section 1: Written.** Two papers taken on one day consisting of Multiple Choice Questions (Single Best Answer) and Extending Matching Item questions.

Once you've passed this bit, you can take Section 2.

- **Section 2: Clinical and oral.** A clinical examination with short cases and an oral exam covering clinical scenarios and an academic viva.

More information can be found in Chapter 21 and full specific details are on the Intercollegiate Specialty Board's website (www.intercollegiate.org.uk). Note that there are new regulations for each of the specialties in force from 2012, which mainly restrict the number of attempts at the exam.

Costs

The total amount is payable up front. You set up a personal fee account and pay into that, so if you fail a section, you have to top it up. It also presumably means interest is being earned on your money, but not by you. Failing is therefore very, very expensive.

- Section 1: £520
- Section 2: £1275

References

A Reference Guide for Post Graduate Specialty Training in the UK. The Gold Guide Core Training Supplement (4e) (2010). London: MMC.

Applicant Guide for application and recruitment to medical specialty training in England in 2011 (2010). London: Department of Health.

Core Surgical Training and Experience in Surgical Specialties in England, Paper 31–6 (2010). London: Medical Education England.

http://specialty.walesdeanery.org/

www.cfwi.org.uk

www.intercollegiate.org.uk

www.mmc.nhs.uk

www.mmc.scot.nhs.uk/

www.nimdta.gov.uk/

www.rcseng.ac.uk

Chapter 8
GENERAL SURGERY

Matt Stephenson
General surgical specialty registrar, ST7, South East Thames rotation

Introduction, 140
The subspecialties, 141
The general career path, 142
What's it like being a general surgical core trainee?, 142
Recruitment to specialty training, 143
What's it like being a general surgical specialty registrar?, 143
Courses during general surgical specialty training, 144
Exit exams, 146
What's it like as a consultant?, 146
Reference, 147
Organisations, 147

Introduction

General surgery, as the name suggests is quite a mixed bag. Which other training pathway will make you competent to manage any acute surgical emergency in the middle of the night? Which other specialty enables you to do anything from varicose vein stripping to Whipple's procedures, inguinal hernias to mastectomies? In short, general surgery is the best.

The reality these days, of course, is somewhat divergent from the above. Historically, as a general surgeon your operating list might have started with a thyroidectomy and ended with a below-knee amputation and covered any or every bit of anatomy in between. Not any more unfortunately. An eminent public institution recently debated the motion: 'This house believes that the days of the general surgeon are over'. Subspecialisation within general surgery is expanding all the time and the main subspecialties are:

- colorectal
- upper gastrointestinal (GI)
- breast
- vascular
- transplant
- hepatopancreaticobiliary (HPB)
- endocrine.

Generally through ST3–8 you will rotate through a variety (but not all) of these specialties. Usually in ST5 you will be asked to choose which area to specialise in, and from thereon, mainly only do that specialty, although you will often

The Hands-on Guide to Surgical Training, First Edition. Matthew Stephenson.

still have to cover the general on-call shifts.

Given general surgery is so big and diverse, the different subspecialty options deserve a quick explanation.

The subspecialties

Breast

The increase in popularity and development of better oncoplastic techniques has resulted in a change in the career paths of those wanting to operate on breasts. Whereas in the quite recent past breast surgery would be part of the general surgeon's remit, breast subspecialists with a particular interest in oncoplastic reconstruction are now more the norm at new consultant appointments. Trusts want consultants who can offer the whole range of oncoplastic options, and to acquire these requires subspecialisation and usually a surrendering of your general duties. With the increase in breast cancer screening and political pressure to improve breast cancer services, breast surgery is often under the public microscope. Breast surgery is particularly popular for those wanting a life outside the hospital for such luxuries as raising a family as the out-of-hours work is not too taxing (unless still doing the general on calls). Many cite the reason for not choosing breast surgery as a career as – 'well, once they develop a pill to cure breast cancer all breast surgeons will be out of a job'. There's some truth to that, but alas a cure seems a long way off still, and imagine if they develop a pill to reverse atherosclerosis, a much bigger killer than breast cancer. From stroke physicians to vascular surgeons, we'd all be out of a job.

Colorectal

Colorectal is the largest subspecialty of general surgery and if you want to remain as general as possible, it's likely this is the one for you. The vast majority of colorectal surgeons still do the general emergency take. The colorectal subspecialty has been transformed in recent years by the development of laparoscopic surgery as the standard in most centres for colonic resections. Screening for bowel cancer is also making an impact on services. Even within colorectal surgery there are sub-subspecialties such as pelvic floor surgery, inflammatory bowel disease, intestinal failure, etc.

Upper GI

As with colorectal surgery, laparoscopic upper gastrointestinal resections are replacing open operations in many centres. But there's a significant amount of non-malignant work too, including gallstones and reflux. One of the biggest growth markets in the future is likely to be bariatric surgery (surgery for weight loss, essentially). Upper GI is a relatively small specialty that's also becoming centralised in a smaller number of centres.

Vascular

As with the other specialties, vascular surgery used to be an intrinsic component of general surgery, but many general surgeons have had to surrender their general skills to focus on developments in vascular surgery. The Vascular Society has even formally requested to split vascular surgery off from general surgery altogether in the near future (this will probably take effect around 2013). This is particularly because with the continuing proliferation of endovascular treatments for pathologies previously treated with open surgery, vascular surgeons need to be able to offer their patients the full range of treatments without having to ask for the help of an interventional radiologist. In many units there is a considerable power struggle between radiologists and vascular surgeons as to who will do endovascular aneurysm repairs (EVARs), stenting, etc. In the future (no one knows exactly when yet) it's likely that if you want to be a vascular surgeon you don't become a general surgeon at all and instead follow a new joint specialised vascular surgery and interventional radiology course.

Hepatopancreaticobiliary

This is a competitive, small subspecialty of general surgery performed in a select few centres. You'll be doing some of the biggest operations in existence, such as Whipple's procedures and liver resections. The patients are often very sick and you'll need to be able to manage their medical issues too.

Transplant

Also a very small subspecialty of general surgery, this is a very demanding career to choose. Technically you will have to be able to perform anastomoses on tiny vessels and personally your work–life balance is heavily weighted towards work – when an organ becomes available, wherever that may be, you may be called upon to go get it out of a dying or dead patient. It also demands exemplary complication-free operations when harvesting organs from fit and healthy donors.

Endocrine

Much of the surgery of the thyroid and parathyroid glands has been taken by ENT surgeons; however, some general surgeons still perform these. There is good evidence to say that the more thyroidectomies and parathyroidectomies you do, the better your results, hence some general surgeons have specialised in these along with the other main gland within this subspecialty: the adrenal gland. Laparoscopic adrenalectomies have now become the norm compared with open procedures.

The general career path

After doing foundation years 1 and 2, you'll have to apply for a two-year core surgical training rotation, during which time you'll have to pass the Membership of the Royal College of Surgeons (MRCS) exams. After CT2 you apply for specialty training, therefore entering at the ST3 stage, which runs through to ST8. If you haven't finished MRCS or achieved all of the other entry criteria to ST3 by CT2, it's sometimes possible to do a third CT year and then apply for ST3 from this.

What's it like being a general surgical core trainee?

The nature of the job varies enormously depending on the subspecialty to which you are attached. Breast jobs for instance are pretty quiet, as you have few inpatients, whereas colorectal or vascular jobs can be very busy with lots of unwell inpatients. You will be part of the on-call team, in many hospitals as the first point of referral for GPs or A&E, and usually the first to see and assess acute patients. You'll also be expected to go to clinics where you'll probably find yourself quite supervised, to begin with at least. All importantly, of course, you will also be trying to get to theatre as much as possible to master the essential general surgical operations: appendicectomy, inguinal hernia repair, repair of other kinds of hernia, laparotomies (opening and closing to begin with), draining abscesses, minor operations and the art of assisting well.

You'll also need to be honing your CV on a continual basis, organising audits, publishing a paper or two, attending courses, presenting and studying for your MRCS – all in preparation for the very competitive ST3 applications.

Recruitment to Specialty Training

From 2011, recruitment to ST3 in England and Wales has been through a single national process jointly managed by the London Deanery and the Specialist Advisory Committee in General Surgery. This has the advantage of you not having to fill out separate application forms for all the different deaneries and instead list them in order of your preference.

For the 2011 round of recruitment, information was available from the London Deanery website. You will need to have completed at least 24 months of surgery including at least six months of general surgery (not including foundation years), to have completely passed MRCS, attended Advanced Trauma Life Support (ATLS), Basic Surgical Skills (BSS) courses, etc., as well as the other more generic criteria listed in the person specifications. Of note, you may be advantaged by doing a year of general surgery and no more than four years (more suggests you've not progressed with your career fast enough).

Following the application stage (which comes out annually in February) you may be short-listed if you've ranked high enough and be invited to interview. However, in 2011 there was no short-listing – all candidates were invited to interview as long as they met the long-listing criteria.

There were five different stations with a total examining time (including breaks) of 115 minutes. But these things seem to change every year; find out about how your selection process will work in advance so it's not a surprise on the day.

What's it like being a general surgical specialty registrar?

Mastering the whole range of skills required of you as a general surgeon is daunting. You mainly need to concentrate on the emergency skills in the early years (ST3–5) so you can cope with emergencies in the night, see patients in general clinics and competently manage acute general surgical referrals.

On call, you may be the second busiest person in the hospital after the medical registrar. In all but the quietest hospitals you will be resident on call. You will be expected to operate independently very early on for operations such as appendicectomies (hence the importance of learning these in the core training years) and gradually build up to more advanced procedures. You may find that in the latter years of specialty training your ability to do an extremely wide range of procedures peaks and then falls off to be replaced with the ability to do a certain limited range, really well. A good senior general surgical registrar is often a true general surgeon, until subspecialisation comes along and takes most of it away.

On average you'll attend two clinics a week and be scheduled for at least a full day of operating once a week.

As with the other specialties you will have to be assessed at least annually at an Annual Review of Competence Progression (ARCP) interview (see Chapter 7) to ensure you're ready to progress to the next year.

Courses during general surgical specialty training

There are a huge number of courses for this huge specialty and the more senior you get, the more esoteric the course, but the following should give you an idea of some of the main courses available from the Royal College of Surgeons.

Then there are some more subspecialty-specific courses.

CT1–2	ST3–4	ST5–6	ST7–8 Consultants
Core Skills in Laparoscopic Surgery		13th Bill Owen – Oesophago-Gastric Symposium: 'Meet the Experts'	
	Intermediate Skills in Laparoscopic Surgery (Suturing and Anastomosis)		
		Oesophago-Gastric Cancer Surgery	
Specialist Registrar Skills in Generral Surgery		Thyroid and Parathyroid Surgery	
Common Elective and Acute Problems in the General Surgery of Childhood			
Amputations			
Specialty Skills in Emergency Surgery and Trauma	Endovascular Aneurysm Repair Planning		
		Definitive Surgical Trauma Skills (DSTS)	
		Emergency Surgery for the On-call General Surgeon	
		Bariatric Surgery Techniques (Advanced Laparoscopy)	
Legal Aspects of Surgical Practice			

Source: The Royal College of Surgeons of England

Breast surgery course portfolio

<table>
<tr><th colspan="2">CT1–2</th><th colspan="2">ST3–4</th><th colspan="2">ST5–6</th><th colspan="2">ST7–8
Consultants</th></tr>
<tr><td colspan="4">Specialty Skills in Breast</td><td colspan="4">Advanced Skills in Breast Disease Management</td></tr>
<tr><td></td><td></td><td colspan="3">Specialty Skills in Oncoplastic and Breast Reconstruction Surgery Level I</td><td></td><td></td><td></td></tr>
<tr><td></td><td></td><td colspan="4">Breast Reduction, Mastopexy and Management of Breast Asymmetry</td><td></td><td></td></tr>
<tr><td></td><td></td><td></td><td></td><td colspan="3">Specialty Skills in Oncoplastic and Breast Reconstruction Surgery Level II</td><td></td></tr>
<tr><td></td><td></td><td colspan="4">Aesthetic and Reconstructive Surgical Skills Cadaver Dissection</td><td colspan="2"></td></tr>
<tr><td colspan="8">Legal Aspects of Surgical Practice</td></tr>
<tr><td></td><td></td><td colspan="4">Breast Augmentation</td><td></td><td></td></tr>
</table>

Source: The Royal College of Surgeons of England

Coloproctology surgery course portfolio

<table>
<tr><th colspan="2">CT1–2</th><th colspan="2">ST3–4</th><th colspan="2">ST5–6</th><th colspan="2">ST7–8
Consultants</th></tr>
<tr><td></td><td></td><td colspan="3">Specialty Skills in Coloproctology Stage 1 (ST3–5)</td><td colspan="3">Specialty Skills in Coloproctology Stage 2 (ST6–8)</td></tr>
<tr><td colspan="8">Legal Aspects of Surgical Practice</td></tr>
</table>

Source: The Royal College of Surgeons of England

Vascular surgery course portfolio

<table>
<tr><th colspan="2">CT1–2</th><th colspan="2">ST3–4</th><th colspan="2">ST5–6</th><th colspan="2">ST7–8
Consultants</th></tr>
<tr><td colspan="4">Specialty Skills in Vascular surgery</td><td colspan="4">Advanced Skills in Vascular Surgery</td></tr>
<tr><td colspan="8">Introduction to Endovascular Interventions</td></tr>
<tr><td colspan="8">Amputations</td></tr>
<tr><td></td><td></td><td colspan="6">Endovascular Aneurysm Repair Planning</td></tr>
<tr><td></td><td></td><td colspan="6">Modern Management of Varicose Veins</td></tr>
<tr><td></td><td></td><td colspan="6">Vascular Access for Dialysis</td></tr>
</table>

Source: The Royal College of Surgeons of England

Trauma and emergency course portfolio

CT1–2	ST3–4	ST5–6	ST7–8 Consultants
Specialty Skills in Emergency Surgery and Trauma		Definitive Surgical Trauma Skills for the General Surgeon (DSTS)	
		Emergency Surgery for the On-Call General Surgeon	

All the figures above, and related figures in subsequent chapters, are taken from www.rcseng.ac.uk/education/courses/specialty/gscourses.html.

Exit exams

Most trainees take their exit exams in ST7 or ST8 gaining the letters FRCS (Gen. Surg) after their name.

What's it like as a consultant?

You end your training as an expert in one subspecialty of general surgery but also able to handle all the general surgical emergencies and therefore remain on the emergency general rota as a consultant. However, you are unlikely to be able to find a consultant job that will allow you to continue to practise your specialist art and still do much elective operating in the other general surgical subspecialties. Why? First, each subspecialty has advanced over the years so much that no one surgeon could possibly be expert in all of them. Second, there is some evidence that unless you're doing a minimum of X procedures per year, you won't be as good as someone who is. One of the unfortunate consequences of this is that if all you do all day is breast surgery and ever-diminishing amounts of elective abdominal surgery you deskill at abdominal surgery, yet you will still be called on in the middle of the night to do a difficult Hartmann's procedure. These days consultant jobs will often be advertised as vascular consultant or breast consultant with no general workload at all, even on the emergency front. This has some important implications of job satisfaction for those who hoped to be generalists, variety of work and also the taboo subject of private work. In general, if you're not doing an operation routinely in the NHS, there will be greater obstacles to you doing it in the private sector, which means a substantial reduction in the amount of work that comes your way.

However, there will always be the need for a general surgeon. Even if only because you need someone capable of managing the general surgical take that might include cholecystitis, bowel obstruction, breast abscesses, ischaemic legs, etc. You can't have an HPB, colorectal, breast and vascular consultant all on call separately (although often the patients will then be handed over to a specialist in that area come the morning if more specialist definitive care is needed).

Reference

Paterson-Brown S, Garden JO (2009) *Companion to Specialist Surgical Practice* (8 vols). London: Saunders.

Organisations

The **Association of Surgeons of Great Britain & Northern Ireland (ASGBI)** is the only association covering the whole of general surgery and its subspecialties throughout the UK. There is an annual conference that's worth trying to attend and present in.

If you're interested in breast, the Mammary Fold: www.themammaryfold.com/

If you're interested in colorectal, the Duke's Club: www.thedukesclub.org.uk/

If you're interested in upper GI or HPB, the Association of Upper GI Surgeons (AUGIS): www.augis.org/trainees/trainees.htm

If you're interested in vascular, the Rouleaux Club: www.rouleauxclub.com/

If you're interested in endocrine, the British Association of Endocrine & Thyroid Surgeons (BAETS): www.baets.org.uk/

If you're interested in transplant, the Carrel Club: www.carrelclub.org.uk/

NON-CLINICAL

Chapter 9
UROLOGY

Wasim Mahmalji
Urology trainee, ST3, London Deanery and Kent, Surrey and Sussex Deanery

Introduction, 148
The general career path, 148
What's it like being a urology foundation doctor?, 149
What's it like being a urology core trainee?, 150
Recruitment to specialty training, 151
What's it like being a urology specialty trainee?, 151
Courses during urology specialty training, 154
Exit exams, 154
What's it like as a consultant?, 154
Summary, 155
References, 155
Organisations, 155

Introduction

What exactly is urology? It's a surgical specialty that cares for diseases of the kidneys, ureters, bladder and genitals. Urologists care for both male and female patients of all ages, ranging from newborn babies to the elderly. Most urologists have expert knowledge of 'general' urological problems and procedures; however, it's common for urologists to subspecialise in a particular area; the main areas are highlighted in Figure 9.1.

It's an innovative specialty with surgical methods including open, laparoscopic, endoscopic and robotic techniques. Operating lists vary from all-day inpatient lists, to varied day case surgery.

Because of its varied and dynamic nature it's no surprise that urology is a competitive specialty. As of September 2010, the British Association of Urological Surgeons (BAUS) stated that in England, Wales, Scotland and Northern Ireland there were a total of 329 specialist and specialty registrars and just 800 consultants, suggesting great competition for consultant posts. Each step of the way to a career in urology is competitive and as you progress from FY1 through to registrar it only gets tougher.

The general career path

After doing foundation years 1 and 2 you'll have to apply for a two-year core

The Hands-on Guide to Surgical Training, First Edition. Matthew Stephenson.

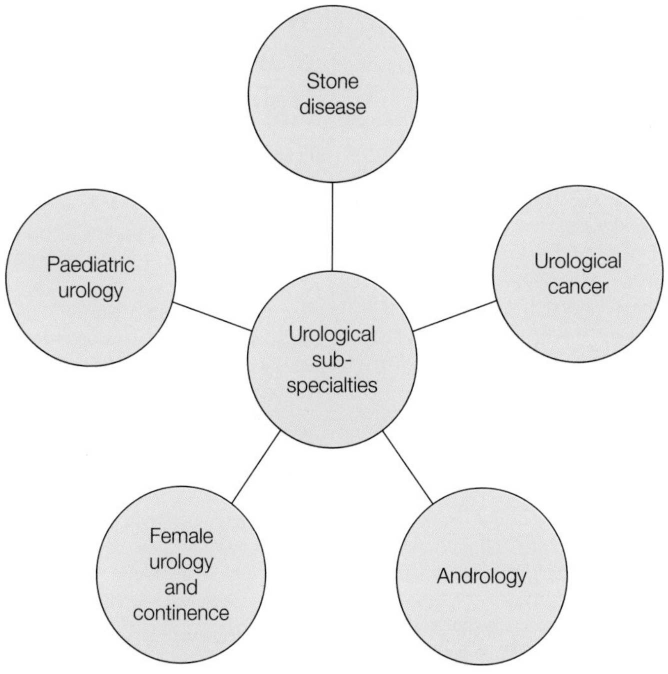

Figure 9.1 The urological subspecialties.

surgical training rotation, during which time you'll have to pass the Membership of the Royal College of Surgeons (MRCS) exams. After CT2 you apply for specialty training, therefore entering at the ST3 stage, which runs through to ST7, one year shorter than most. If you haven't finished MRCS or achieved all of the other entry criteria to ST3 by CT2 it's sometimes possible to do a third CT year and then apply for ST3 from this.

What's it like being a urology foundation doctor?

As with any FY1 job it's busy and you may feel more like an 'admin monkey' than a doctor, but it's what every FY1 has to go through. You can take the positives out of being a urology FY1 by picking up the basics, such as becoming slick at urethral catheter insertion, and learning about the sizes and different properties of different types of catheter, which will help you regardless of career path. Your on calls are usually merged with general surgery and it's unlikely you will be accepting referrals; it will be mainly ward-based problems such as blocked and non-draining catheters.

As an FY2 you're the equivalent of the old 'senior house officer' (SHO) and should 'push on' and develop further clinical and surgical skills. Depending on where you work, the on calls may or may not be merged with surgery. If they are then it's likely you will be much busier. You can expect to see lots of renal colic, retention of urine, haematuria and scrotal pain.

By the end of FY2 you should be confident in hand and instrument knot tying, identifying different sutures and understanding their properties. If possible you should pre-identify cases in theatre that you can be supervised performing, such as flexible cystoscopies, epididymal cysts, hydrocoeles and assisting in larger cases.

If you are serious about a career in urology you should complete at least one urological audit cycle. A common problem is where to get started. A good place to start is by speaking to senior team members or contacting the hospital's clinical audit department for ideas. If you can involve yourself in any publication at this level it will greatly enhance your CV. Being first, second or third author in any published case report, audit or study is very achievable in FY1. It's advisable to try to present research at local or regional level. What can you present? The simple answer is anything urological!

What's it like being a urology core trainee?

Recruitment to CT level is very competitive. Deaneries may offer purely urology-based CT1/2 or combine urology with other specialties. It's essential that you have at least six months of urology experience at CT1/2 level. You must make every effort to make the most of the CT programme if you wish to be competitive for ST recruitment.

- **Courses**: the Royal College of Surgeons Core Skills in Urology modules 1–4 are a must.
- **Audit**: know your audits well, as it's very likely you will be asked about one in any ST interview. Audits should also be urology-specific ideally.
- **Publications**: as with audits you should have a number of publications at this stage, again know them well as you will be asked about them at interview and ideally they should be urological.
- **Presentations**: you should hopefully have presented at local and regional level and should now be aiming at national and international level. Institutions such as BAUS, the European Association of Urology (EAU) and the American Urological Association (AUA) all hold regular meeting that can be presented at.
- **Prizes**: BAUS, the EUA, AUA and the Royal Society of Medicine Urology Section all hold regular meetings and competitions offering prizes that can be entered.

- **Surgical competence**: Ideally you should push for maximum urological exposure in core training. Both elective and emergency surgical skills should be developed. Procedures including flexible/rigid cystoscopy, circumcision, scrotal exploration, supra-pubic catheterisation and any others should be performed in as high a number as possible. You should also be developing skills to manage acute and elective admissions.
- **Examinations**: full MRCS membership is a must – you cannot apply to an ST programme without it. If you are struggling to pass, courses are available to help.
- **Higher degrees**: an MSc at this stage is very possible (see Chapter 7) and will aid any ST application. There are a number of institutes that tailor courses for postgraduates and are flexible offering distance and e-learning, different topics and courses over two to three years.

So if you have completed all the above steps will you be guaranteed an ST3 post in urology? No, nothing is ever guaranteed when it comes to medical job applications. The recruitment process, candidate criteria, job numbers, etc., may all change. But if you have done all of the above as a candidate you will certainly be taken seriously and will be in with a chance.

Recruitment to specialty training

Since 2009, urology ST3 recruitment has been nationally led for England, Wales and Scotland (it is separate for Northern Ireland). In 2011, it was based in the Yorkshire and the Humber Deanery. Applications are usually open from mid-February and close in mid-March. It is fiercely competitive (see Chapter 7). The number of national training numbers (NTNs) varies each year and between deaneries. If invited to interview you will be given specific instructions on the documentation required on the day and the layout of your portfolio. It's worth investing in a professional-looking binder and labelling your portfolio; remember, a small and impressive portfolio is more impressive than a thick set of files with little substance. The interviews in 2010 were divided into six stations (Figure 9.2).

What's it like being a urology specialty trainee?

The training programme is five years in duration and will take you from ST3 to ST7 and possibly ST8; each training year will usually be based at a different hospital. As an ST trainee you are still required to complete a minimum number of DOPS (direct observation of procedural skills), mini-CEXs (clinical evaluation exercises), CBDs (case-based discussions) and a single mini-PAT (peer assessment tool) each year. The exact number will be defined by your programme director and varies from year to year. You are also required to maintain your logbook, recording all the operations you perform; again the number of procedures is outlined by your PD and the more the better, but a rough figure would be 30 transurethral resections

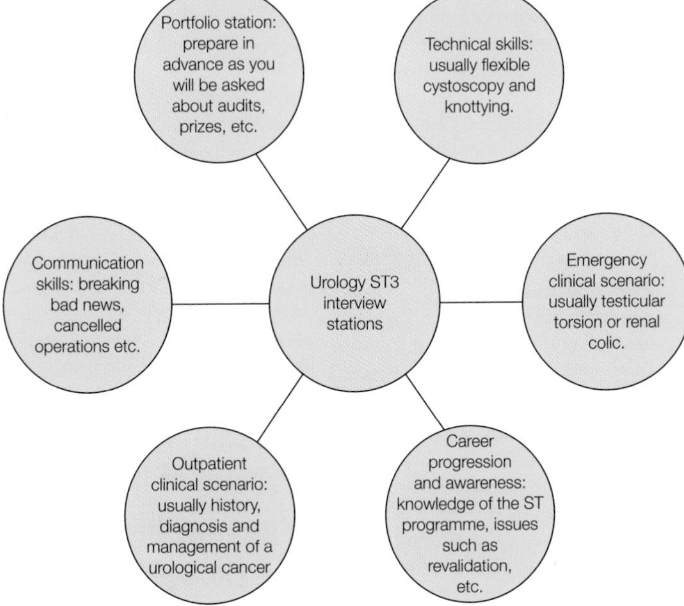

Figure 9.2 ST3 urology interview stations.

of prostate (TURPs) and transurethral resections of bladder tumour (TURBTs).

What's expected at ST3/4

Considered a 'junior specialty registrar' (StR) these are the years where you build your core clinical and urological skills. By the end of ST3/4 you will be expected to be able to do the following.

- **Clinic**: see patients independently and formulate management plans for 'general' or 'common' urological problems.
- **Haematuria clinic**: a 'one-stop shop' where patients have upper tract imaging and flexible cystoscopy. At this stage you should be able to run and manage patients in the haematuria clinic.
- **Day surgery**: perform cystoscopy, bladder biopsy, optical urethrotomy, circumcision, scrotal exploration, hydrocoele repair and epididymal cyst removal unsupervised.
- **Main theatre**: perform simple TURPs, TURBTs, ureteric stent insertion, rigid ureteroscopy simple stone

retrieval and assist in large open or laparoscopic cases.

What's expected at ST5/6

Considered a 'senior StR', these are the years where you develop more advanced clinical and urological skills. By the end of ST5/6 you will be expected to be able to do the following.

- **Clinic**: see more complex patients and offer management plans for prostate, bladder and renal cancer.
- **Day surgery**: perform inguinal orchidectomy, open ligations of varicocoeles and trans-obtruator/vaginal slings unsupervised.
- **Main theatre**: perform difficult TURBTs and flexible ureteroscopy complex stone retrieval; perform simple open nephrectomy, prostatectomy and cystectomy under consultant supervision.
- **The FRCS (Urol)**: it is at this point that most ST trainees think about sitting the exit exam for urology. In order to sit the exam two consultants must act as referees indicating that you are ready.

What's expected at ST7+

By this stage you should be consultant grade; however, it is also an opportunity to define your specialist area in urology and develop more advanced laparoscopic and robotic (generally considered the future of minimally invasive surgery) skills. On completion of the ST programme and if you have been successful in the FRCS, you will be awarded the Certificate of Completion of Training (CCT).

Typical timetable

A typical weekly timetable as an ST3 is shown in Table 9.1. However, as with all the subspecialties it's important to note that with the 48-hour European Working Time Directive (EWTD) timetables are variable and may include/exclude night shifts and on-call patterns.

The on-call shifts as a urology specialty registrar (StR) are variable, depending on the location of the centre and the structure of its urology department. Whether it's the SHO (FY2 or core trainee) or StR who accepts the referrals will differ between centres; however, if it's an 'SHO' referral service it's usually mandatory that they are reviewed by a StR after admission. An area of controversy is the phasing out of StRs working night shifts. This is mainly due to the EWTD limiting StR hours. Effectively what this means is that after 8pm, should the night SHO require support the consultants must provide it.

Table 9.1 A typical weekly timetable as a urology StR

Monday		Tuesday		Wednesday		Thursday		Friday	
AM	**PM**	**AM**	**PM**	**AM**	**PM**	**AM**	**PM**	**AM**	**PM**
Admin	On-call	Theatre	Theatre	Haematuria clinic	Clinic	Theatre	Theatre	MDT	Day theatre

Courses during urology specialty training

The following is a brief description of some of the courses available from the Royal College of Surgeons.

CT1–2	ST3–4	ST5–6	ST7–8 Consultants
Operative Skills in Urology : Modules 1 and 2		Reconstructive Techniques in Urology	
Operative Skills in Urology : Modules 3 and 4		Joint RCS and SFNUU Masterclass in the Management of Detrusor Overactivity	
	Advanced Urodynamics		
	Urological Anatomy for Surgery		Advanced Applied Female Pelvic Anatomy
		Essential Pathology and Radiology for the FRCS Urology	
Legal Aspects of Surgical Practice			
		Penile and Urethral Reconstruction Surgery	

Source: The Royal College of Surgeons of England

Exit exams

As mentioned above, most trainees will consider sitting the FRCS (Urol) between ST5 and ST6. Remember you cannot gain your CCT without it.

What's it like as a consultant?

Once you are a CCT holder you are eligible to apply for a consultant post. Consultants will usually have a urological subspecialty or interest, and work closely with other consultants in their department. As a consultant you are a leader in a team and often have to show leadership qualities and ensure that you are aware of the actions of your StRs and SHOs. Ultimately the consultant is responsible for all patients under their care. Consultants in urology often combine NHS work with a day of private practice. Their week will usually consist of an all-day main theatre operating list, a day surgery list, a number of clinics and a weekly multidisciplinary team meeting. On calls vary for consultants. A consultant may be on call daily or weekly, and as mentioned earlier, after certain hours they may be the only point of contact for the on-call SHO.

For some years now there has been talk of creating 'office' urologists. What this means is that there would be urological surgeons who work in hospitals and have subspecialist interests and there would be polyclinic/GP-based urologists who provide a 'general urology' service (such as TURPS,

TURBTS, etc.). Until now this has not come to full fruition and has met much criticism and obstacles.

Summary

Why did I choose urology? It was more a case of urology chose me. As soon as I was exposed to its varied, dynamic and constantly evolving nature I knew I wanted to pursue a career in a specialty ensuring maximal job satisfaction. It's a noble vocation, often dealing with sensitive patient issues. No two days are the same and operating lists are wide and varied as are its on calls. It's a physically and mentally demanding specialty but one where you can really make a difference to peoples' lives.

References

Mahmalji W, Mukerji G, Abel P, Raza A (2010) A community urology service: fact or fiction? *British Journal of Urology International* **106**(10): 1428–30.

From medical student to specialty trainee, the latest editions of these books will always be useful so are a worthwhile investment:

Reynard J, Brewster S, Biers S. *Oxford Handbook of Urology*. Oxford: Oxford University Press.

Reynard J, Mark S, Turner K, Armenakas N, Feneley M, Sullivan M. *Urological Surgery, Oxford Specialist Handbooks in Surgery*. Oxford: Oxford University Press.

Also the latest British Association of Urological Surgeons (BAUS) and European Association of Urology (EAU) guidelines will help keep you up to date.

Organisations

The **British Association of Urological Surgeons** (BAUS; www.baus.org.uk/), the **European Association of Urology** (EAU; www.uroweb.org/) and the **American Urological Association** (AUA; www.auanet.org/): **t**hree large and reputable institutions. All the websites contain urology specific courses, prizes and meetings.

Senior Urological Registrars Group (www.surg-online.net/): a great resource for SpRs and StRs giving guidance and details on courses meeting etc.

This chapter is dedicated to the Urology Department of York District Hospital, York, England.

Chapter 10
CARDIOTHORACIC SURGERY

Sion Barnard
Thoracic surgery consultant, Freeman Hospital, Newcastle and is the Dean of Cardiothoracic Surgery

Introduction, 156
The general career path, 156
What's it like being a cardiothoracics core trainee?, 156
Recruitment to specialty training, 157
What's it like being a cardiothoracics specialty trainee?, 158
Courses during cardiothoracic training, 158
The exit exam, 159
What's it like as a consultant?, 159
Summary, 159
References, 159
Organisations, 159

Introduction

Cardiothoracic surgery is a broad specialty, encompassing general cardiac surgery, paediatric cardiothoracic surgery and thoracic surgery. In addition, the training and day-to-day practice in several centres also includes heart and lung transplantation, and mechanical heart support. Most operations are coronary artery bypass grafting (CABG), a well-proven procedure for the relief of angina.

The general career path

Entry to higher surgical training in the specialty is at ST3, following at least six months in the specialty in core training; this may change to 10 months in 2012. A number of trainees are appointed at ST3 from outside core, usually those who have been in the specialty for some years, although there is active encouragement for trainees to enter from core. The entry at ST3 is via national selection. There is an expectation that some (4–6 months) general surgery would be done prior to applying to ST3 for cardiothoracic.

What's it like being a cardiothoracics core trainee?

Core training in cardiothoracic surgery varies slightly from centre to centre. Ideally the trainee should have some on-call commitment and should be exposed

The Hands-on Guide to Surgical Training, First Edition. Matthew Stephenson.

to cardiothoracic surgical intensive care, and also have commitments to theatre and outpatient clinics. With national selection established, there are clear operative goals for the core trainee to achieve to be competitive at ST3 and these can be used as part of a learning agreement. There is certainly an expectation that the core trainee will take a number of long saphenous veins, open and close chests via sternotomy or thoracotomy, and do some of the simpler video-assisted thoracic surgery (VATS) procedures such as lung biopsy.

Although there are major textbooks in both major subspecialties, e.g. Kirklin for cardiac surgery and *General Thoracic Surgery* (Shields *et al.*) or *Pearson's Thoracic & Esophageal Surgery* for thoracic surgery, there are more basic books that focus on specific areas for the core trainee. These include Bojar's *Manual of Perioperative Care in Adult Cardiothoracic Surgery* and *Cardiothoracic Surgery* in the Oxford Specialist Handbooks in Surgery series, which is aimed at the more junior or core trainee.

Recruitment to specialty training

Following the Medical Training Application Service (MTAS) fiasco of 2007, cardiothoracic surgery has been heavily involved in national selection, as opposed to the previous system of individual deanery-based applications. The ST3 posts are typically advertised in January following a rigorous process of allocation of posts, the numbers of which are determined centrally by the Department of Health Workforce Planning Group based in Hampshire. Deaneries, through their training programme directors, bid for posts based on the strengths of their rotation and past record of getting trainees through, for example, the FRCS (C-Th) exam, and facilities for training, including delegation rate for operations. These are decided in December, prior to the advert going out in January.

There is a four-week window for ST3 applications, which leads to short-listing (there is about a 60–70% chance of being short-listed). Although the numbers were small in the first year (2008) of the new national selection system, leading to an inevitable small number of trainees who were short-listed, the numbers have increased in the specialty in the past two years with 27 posts in 2011. National selection was hosted in Birmingham for three years until 2010, but with the change of Cardiothoracic Specialist Advisory Committee (SAC) Chair has now moved to Wessex.

One notable change, reflecting the demographics of trainees in the specialty, was in the person specification in 2010. Trainees who might be quite experienced and who have done the Exit FRCS exam while in non-training jobs are now ineligible to apply for training at ST3 level.

The format of the assessments for the short-listed candidate is that on the first morning there is a CV/portfolio review as in a standard interview and in the afternoon there are structured questions regarding the specialty in clinical scenarios, governance issues, etc. The following day there is a series of Objective Structured Assessments of

Technical Skills (OSATS), where operative techniques at a simple level are assessed, and on the final morning, there is a PowerPoint presentation of an audit project and a separate telephone scenario. This gives us several points at which to evaluate the candidate fully. The format has been independently assessed by the University of Birmingham Medical Education Research Group and has been found to be acceptable, particularly in terms of fairness, for the applicant and the assessor.

What's it like being a cardiothoracics specialty trainee?

It is understood that a trainee appointed to ST3 would already have experience in performing some basic parts of the main operations, such as coronary artery bypass grafting and lung resection already. This would allow them to progress to performing most of each operation and the whole of some of the simpler operations, such as coronary artery bypass grafting (one or two) and some of the simpler lobectomies.

As the trainee progresses there will be some pressure to jump ship into either cardiac surgery or thoracic surgery, although many trainees come into the specialty hoping to do both; however, the recent tendency has been to appoint to one or other of these two main specialties. It is expected this trend will continue, but there may still be occasional cardiothoracic appointments made at consultant level in the future.

Currently the specialty has partly implemented peri-Certificate of Completion of Training (CCT) fellowships, so that trainees can get extra training towards the end of their time in the specialty of their choice. The four subjects being looked at particularly are paediatric cardiothoracic surgery, thoracic surgery, transplantation and cardiac surgery. In addition, several hospitals have links with major centres in the US and Canada and senior level training can be arranged in one of these prestigious centres.

Courses during cardiothoracic training

Cardiothoracic surgery course portfolio

<table>
<tr><th colspan="2">CT1–2</th><th colspan="2">ST3–4</th><th colspan="2">ST5–6</th><th colspan="2">ST7–8
Consultants</th></tr>
<tr><td colspan="8">Bypass, Balloons and Circulatory Support</td></tr>
<tr><td colspan="2">Speciality Skills in Cardiothoracic Surgery</td><td colspan="4">Intermediate Cardiac Surgery</td><td></td><td></td></tr>
<tr><td colspan="8">Legal Aspects of Surgical Practice</td></tr>
<tr><td></td><td></td><td></td><td colspan="3">Applied Basic Science for Cardiothoracic Surgical Trainees</td><td></td><td></td></tr>
</table>

Source: The Royal College of Surgeons of England

The exit exam

The exit exam (FRCS C-Th) is typically taken at the end of ST6 (end of the fourth year of registrar training). The pass rate is highest in those who have a national training number (NTN) and lowest in those who are not on a formal training programme. There is increasing pressure, with the new regulations that come into place in 2012, to limit the number of times an applicant can try this exam so that they should enter it only when they are really ready to pass the exam.

What's it like as a consultant?

As a consultant, there is less operating now in most centres than there was in the past. Many consultants now do only three or four operating sessions a week (1.5–2 days). Much of the time is taken up with clinics and multidisciplinary team meetings and a large amount of administration. On calls are quieter than they used to be, partly due to interventional cardiologists, although transplant can still be very busy. However, there is a great career opportunity in transplantation if working through the night appeals to you. It certainly offers more varied – but demanding – practice.

Summary

There is no doubt that cardiothoracics is a rewarding and challenging specialty to be involved in, and this applies not only to cardiothoracic surgery in general, which provides a rich and varied case mix, but also the subspecialties, which are increasingly diverging from each other. Even in transplantation, newer technologies such as ventricular assist devices (VAD) and extracorporeal membrane oxygenation (ECMO) provide increasing opportunities for treatment of end-stage heart and lung failure.

References

Kouchoukos NT, Karp RB, Blackstone EH, Doty DB, Hanley FL (2003) *Kirklin/Barratt-Boyes Cardiac Surgery* (3e). Edinburgh: Churchill Livingstone.

Shields TW, Locicero III J, Reed CE, Feins RH (2009) *General Thoracic Surgery* (7e). Philadelphia: Lippincott Williams & Wilkins.

Patterson GA, Cooper JD, Deslauriers J *et al.* (2008) *Pearson's Thoracic and Esophageal Surgery*. Volume 1 *Thoracic* (3e). Edinburgh: Churchill Livingstone.

Bojar RM (2011) *Manual of Perioperative Care in Adult Cardiac Surgery* (5e). Chichester: Wiley-Blackwell.

Chikwe J, Beddow E, Glenville B (2006) *Cardiothoracic Surgery. Oxford Specialist Handbooks in Surgery*. Oxford: Oxford University Press.

Organisations

Society for Cardiothoracic Surgery in Great Britain & Ireland (www.scts.org).

Chapter 11

ORAL AND MAXILLOFACIAL SURGERY

Richard Burnham
Oral and maxillofacial surgery trainee, ST3, West Midlands Deanery

Introduction, 160
The general career path, 161
What's it like being an OMFS core trainee? 161
Recruitment to specialty training, 163
What's it like being an OMFS specialty trainee in? 163
Courses during OMFS specialty training, 164
Exit exams, 164
What's it like being a consultant? 164
Summary, 165
References, 165
Organisation, 165

Introduction

Oral and maxillofacial surgery (OMFS) is unique among surgical disciplines in that it requires the completion of both a dental and medical undergraduate degree, which as a minimum takes eight years of study and a reasonable portion of your liver to complete. The rewards are massive, both in terms of the kinds of surgery we do and the lifestyle we lead, i.e. on calls don't kill you as a trainee and as a consultant the private practice is good.

What does the discipline of OMFS cover? Well, to the surprise of most medics the list is diverse and includes the following:

- facial trauma
- dentoalveolar surgery
- orofacial cancer
- reconstructive surgery
- orthognathic surgery
- cleft lip and palate surgery
- craniofacial surgery
- skull base surgery
- facial aesthetics
- stereolithography in maxillofacial surgery
- pre-prosthetic and implant surgery
- temporomandibular joint surgery
- facial pain

The Hands-on Guide to Surgical Training, First Edition. Matthew Stephenson.

- oral medicine
- thyroid and parathyroid surgery
- salivary gland disease
- distraction osteogenesis
- maxillofacial prosthetics and technology
- dental treatment of the medically compromised and those with special needs.

This list represents the totality of our workload and it is clear that there is overlap with other disciplines, including plastic surgery, ENT, neurosurgery and dentistry. However, uniquely, our referral base is our friends in general dental practice, and they see some weird and wonderful pathology.

The general career path

As stated above, you have to have a serious love of university to do OMFS, with between 8 and 10 years of university as a requirement. On top of this it's necessary to get your postgraduate exams in surgery and dentistry, both through the Royal College of Surgeons, which is very, very expensive.

The schematic in Figure 11.1 shows the pathway from either starting point, dentistry or medicine, and is as clear as it gets.

Throughout your foundation and core surgical training years it is easy to claw back a bit of time, so that most people in this period tend to be able to drop 1 or even 2 years out of the normal 4 years of foundation and core surgical training. This is achieved by using competencies achieved before returning to medical school, but this is only the case if you wish to jump ahead to an ST3 OMFS. It is really up to the individual how long they go before they have a crack at applying for ST3, but experience is golden and jumping ahead can lead to holes in your broader knowledge base.

What's it like being an OMFS core trainee?

For those of us who did medicine second, being a 30-year-old FY1 is not fun and the core training is ward work with little thanks, so we pile through the Membership of the Royal College of Surgeons (MRCS) exams and apply for specialty training as soon as possible. My friends who did a 'goofy foot' and applied after doing medicine first then dentistry don't need years as a dentist or OMFS SHO, but you need enough skills to be competent to do the on call, as your boss isn't going to be pleased to have to come in and pull a tooth on the emergency list!

It's still possible to apply for core training posts in OMFS, as these historically were run through, but you have to ask what is the added benefit from any standard core surgical training post. Either job will give you the core training one or two years that you need for the CV so that you can apply for ST3.

Core training is a good jump-off point into ST3 applications and gives you a chance to complete MRCS, and as a CT2 OMFS you will do a six-month OMFS job, which can break you back in, but it is an extra two years in an already

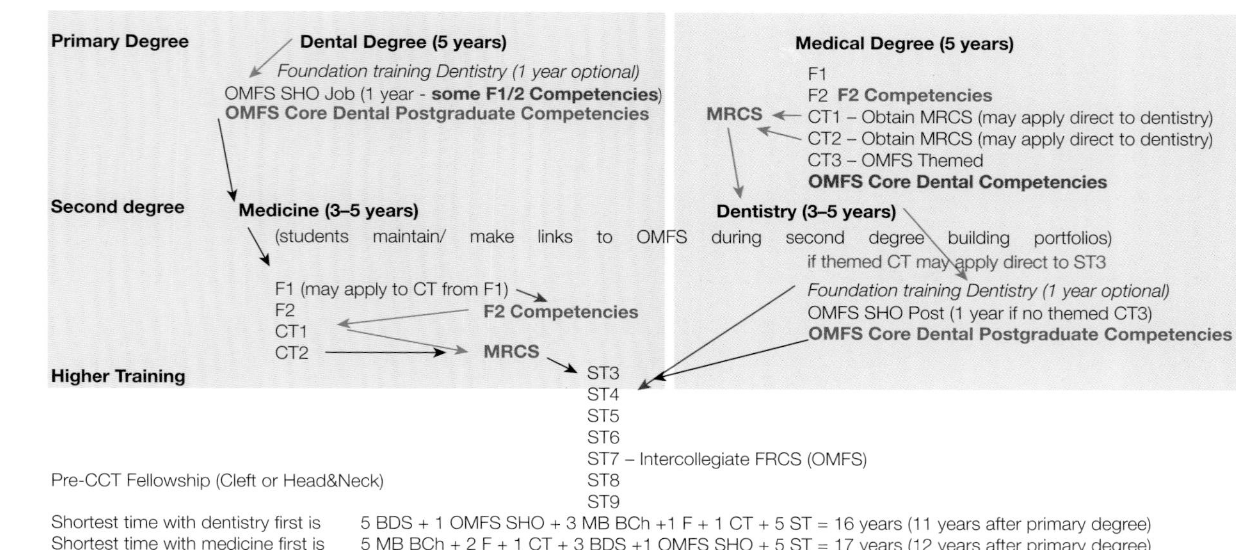

Primary Degree
Dental Degree (5 years)
Foundation training Dentistry (1 year optional)
OMFS SHO Job (1 year - some F1/2 Competencies)
OMFS Core Dental Postgraduate Competencies
Medical Degree (5 years)
F1
F2 F2 Competencies
MRCS
CT1 – Obtain MRCS (may apply direct to dentistry)
CT2 – Obtain MRCS (may apply direct to dentistry)
CT3 – OMFS Themed
OMFS Core Dental Competencies
Second degree
Medicine (3–5 years)
Dentistry (3–5 years)
(students maintain/ make links to OMFS during second degree building portfolios)
if themed CT may apply direct to ST3
F1 (may apply to CT from F1)
F2
CT1
CT2
F2 Competencies
MRCS
Foundation training Dentistry (1 year optional)
OMFS SHO Post (1 year if no themed CT3)
OMFS Core Dental Postgraduate Competencies
Higher Training
ST3
ST4
ST5
ST6
ST7 – Intercollegiate FRCS (OMFS)
Pre-CCT Fellowship (Cleft or Head&Neck)
ST8
ST9
Shortest time with dentistry first is 5 BDS + 1 OMFS SHO + 3 MB BCh +1 F + 1 CT + 5 ST = 16 years (11 years after primary degree)
Shortest time with medicine first is 5 MB BCh + 2 F + 1 CT + 3 BDS +1 OMFS SHO + 5 ST = 17 years (12 years after primary degree)

Figure 11.1 Pathways for training in OMFS. (source: www.baoms.org.uk)

prolonged training pathway. These jobs are very limited with two in Kent, three in London and a few more dotted around the country.

Once you have the basic requirements you can enter the cut and thrust of applications for ST3 OMFS at national recruitment.

Recruitment to specialty training

This became a national recruitment process through the Severn Deanery in 2010, so there is little to go on, but thus far the format has been quite consistent.

It comprises six stations, which are a lot like an Objective Structured Clinical Exam (OSCE), and is extremely fair. There are two of each of the following stations.

- **Portfolio** – ethics, audit, clinical governance, scrutinising your CV.
- **Practical skills** – plate bending, suturing with knowledge testing.
- **Communications** – breaking bad news, phoning the consultant out of hours.

In the 2011 recruitment process for the two stations that dealt with audit and research, they asked for the candidates to bring a handout, which explains an audit and a research project that they have been involved in and the role they played. These were given in with the portfolio. During the two stations they presented on these topics and were then questioned.

I felt that the portfolio station was very important to the panel and is probably heavily weighted, so make sure it's pretty to look at.

The person specifications are not complicated and are listed through the Severn Deanery website. It's necessary to tick every box to get short-listed, but that shouldn't really be too big a headache.

What's it like being an OMFS specialty trainee in?

The five-year training pathway allows for the coverage of all areas, but most hospitals with multiple registrars seem to have a trauma/orthognatic and oncology split.

The average pattern of a working week seems to be:

- four sessions of theatre
- four sessions of clinic
- two sessions of admin.

With operations being performed from day one of your specialty training it's vital to also keep an eye on the books to prevent yourself drowning. It's fair to say that with close supervision specialty trainees are allowed to crack on with much of the surgery and most bosses are happy to teach. Even the head and neck cancer will involve the ST3, if you are prepared.

The only exception to this is the microvascular anastomosis of free flaps, which will require you to have gone on an appropriate course, which can be found through the Royal College of Surgeons website.

The on call for OMFS is non-resident and on average works out at about a one in six, with some nights being quiet and some not so. There is very little need for out-of-hours surgery, but those that do go to theatre are the neck stabbings, failing free flaps and odontogenic infections threatening the airway.

The emergence of the European Working Time Directive (EWTD) has led to cross-cover in many hospitals between OMFS, ENT and plastics, with one 'SHO' grade doctor instead of three. This has led to issues with dentoalveolar trauma, as most doctors really don't have a clue about teeth. But a good local teaching programme will stop 4am calls about avulsed teeth and looks good on the CV.

Courses during OMFS Specialty Training

Oral and maxillofacial surgery course portfolio

Exit exams

The jump-off point is the exit exam of the Fellow of the Royal College of Surgeons in Oral and Maxillofacial Surgery (FRCS (OMFS)), which comprises two exams, one written multiple choice question paper and one clinical, usually taken in ST6. The pain is that it costs £1,700 and it adds stress.

Some trainees add on an extra year to the training pathway to do a fellowship, which can include head and neck oncology, cleft lip and palate or trauma. These last a year and are an excellent chance to learn some more top tips for the field you have chosen to go into.

What's it like being a consultant?

As a consultant you have to declare a specialist interest, which can include the following:

<table>
<tr><th colspan="2">CT1–2</th><th colspan="2">ST3–4</th><th colspan="2">ST5–6</th><th colspan="2">ST7–8
Consultants</th></tr>
<tr><td colspan="4">Emergency Skills Maxillofacial Surgery</td><td colspan="4">Practical Workshop in Temporomandibular Joint (TMJ)</td></tr>
<tr><td colspan="2">Advanced Ward and Peri-operative Management in Oral & maxillofacial Surgery</td><td></td><td></td><td colspan="4">Elective Skills in Facial Trauma</td></tr>
<tr><td></td><td></td><td colspan="3">Basic Surgical Anatomy of the Head and Neck</td><td></td><td></td><td></td></tr>
<tr><td colspan="8">Clinical Digital Photography for Surgeons, Doctors and Dentists</td></tr>
<tr><td colspan="8">Legal Aspects of Surgical Practice</td></tr>
<tr><td></td><td></td><td colspan="6">Cleft Surgery Workshop</td></tr>
<tr><td></td><td></td><td colspan="4">Non-Invasive Techniques and Injectable Substances</td><td></td><td></td></tr>
<tr><td colspan="3">Operative Skills in Ear, Nose and Throat Surgery</td><td></td><td colspan="4">Transoral Laser Surgery - Liverpool</td></tr>
</table>

Figure 11.2 Oral and maxillofacial surgery Royal College of Surgeons course portfolio. Source: The Royal College of Surgeons of England

- head and neck oncology
- trauma
- temporomandibular joint
- orthognathics
- salivary gland
- cleft lip and palate

It is up to the individual consultant which of the above list they take as an interest and that may not be limited to just one area. The choice is partially dictated by service needs. It is often the case that the work splits into 'hard' tissue work and 'soft' tissue work. It is the decision of each consultant and each trust to design the job plan, but this is the same with all surgery. On top of this, basic OMFS cases are added, which are the teeth and cysts.

The on call is relatively easy in terms of the amount of time you're called upon and the private practice is excellent, so consultants tend to have a good life. As a bonus, often our patients are well (except those with cancer), so you aren't faced with bed-blocking social issues or dying patients.

Summary

My reasons for choosing OMFS are simple: I didn't want to be stuck as a dentist, which is the equivalent of being a GP to any surgeon. Having completed dental school and medical school the world was still my oyster and I could have done anything, not just OMFS, and to be honest about half of us do, with anaesthetics being very popular. However, I kept thinking:

1. well patient
2. clear-cut diagnoses
3. very varied surgery
4. good on call
5. there are still consultant jobs
6. **not** a ridiculous completion ratio
7. private practice as a consultant.

My only warnings to those of you who think you can do it are that it takes a long time, there is an increase in dentally qualified oral surgery consultants (stealing our jobs) and workforce planning does not show a huge expansion needed.

If you think this is for you, register your interest with the British Association of Oral and Maxillofacial surgeons and good luck.

References

Coulthard P, Koron R, Kazakou I *et al*. (2000) Patterns and appropriateness of referral from general dental practice to specialist oral and maxillofacial surgical services. *British Journal of Oral and Maxillofacial Surgery* **38**(4): 320–5.

www.baoms.org.uk/document.asp?id=373&detail=2

www.baoms.org.uk/page.asp?id=384

www.baoms.org.uk/page.asp?id=47

www.rcseng.ac.uk/education/courses/liverpool-practical-microvascular-surgery-course

www.severndeanery.nhs.uk/recruitment/vacancies/specialty-recruitment/oral-maxillofacial-surgery/person-specification/

Organisation

Membership of the British Association of Oral and Maxillofacial Surgeons (BAOMS; www.baoms.org.uk) is a must.

NON-CLINICAL

Chapter 12

EAR, NOSE AND THROAT SURGERY (OTORHINOLARYNGOLOGY – HEAD AND NECK SURGERY)

James E Mitchell
ENT specialty registrar, ST6, St George's Hospital, London

Introduction, 166
The general career path, 167
What's it like being an ENT core trainee? 167
Recruitment to specialty training, 168
What's it like being an ENT specialty trainee? 168
Courses during ENT specialist training, 169
Exit exams, 169
What's it like being a consultant? 170
Summary, 170
References, 170
Organisations, 170

Introduction

Ear, nose and throat (ENT) is a popular choice of surgical career. It's a broad and diverse specialty with patients ranging from infants to the elderly. The surgery is particularly diverse, from delicate and precise surgery to the ear, facial plastic surgery, endoscopic sinus and skull base surgery, to major head and neck resection and reconstruction for cancer. ENT surgery frequently involves the use of gadgets such as microscopes, endoscopes and lasers. A significant proportion of the ENT surgeon's work is outpatient based, and this also utilises a plethora of instruments. ENT surgeons provide complete medical and surgical care for their patients. ENT has a number of subspecialties:

- otology, neurotology and skull base
- rhinology
- facial plastics
- laryngology
- head and neck
- paediatric otolaryngology.

Depending on the subspecialty, ENT surgeons work closely with speech and language therapists, audiologists, oncologists, plastic surgeons, maxillofacial

The Hands-on Guide to Surgical Training, First Edition. Matthew Stephenson.

surgeons and other specialists, often in multidisciplinary teams. Most ENT surgeons are involved in clinical and academic research alongside their clinical work.

The general career path

During the first two foundation years, trainees will undertake six four-month posts in surgical and medical specialties. Some rotations will contain a four-month placement in ENT. If you are interested in ENT it would be useful to undertake a foundation programme that includes ENT, but this is not essential for career progression.

The next stage comprises of two years of core surgical training (CT1 and CT2). This period will contain four- or six-month posts in different surgical specialties where you will gain a broad surgical experience. You will need to pick a programme that contains at least a six-month placement in ENT. Better still, select a programme that is tailored to a career in ENT. These programmes include specialties that are more relevant to ENT, such as plastic surgery, neurosurgery and maxillofacial surgery.

To be eligible to apply for specialty registrar training you will need to have passed the Membership of the Royal College of Surgeons (MRCS) exam and also the Diploma in Otolaryngology during the foundation or core surgical training years. However, there are two options unique to ENT trainees:

- sit the MRCS exam and the Diploma in Otolaryngology – Head and Neck Surgery (DOHNS) exam separately. Obtaining the generic MRCS qualification will leave your career options open to other surgical specialties *or*
- if you are certain that your only career path is ENT, then sit MRCS-ENT exam. This consists of Part A (multiple-choice questions) of the MRCS and Part B (Objective Structured Clinical Exam) of the DOHNS.

What's it like being an ENT core trainee?

Most core trainees find their first ENT job a very steep learning curve. ENT is very equipment dependent and it takes time and training to get used to the tools of the trade. It would be advisable to read an introductory ENT book before your first post, such as one of those listed in the References section. Better still, attend an introduction to ENT course. If you're lucky, your local department will organise its own course or even pay for you to attend one – it's worth asking.

Core training ENT posts involve an element of ward work, on-calls, emergency clinics, and the opportunity to get involved in theatre and outpatient clinics. Most ward work is administrative and of general medical care, typical of any surgical post. Common conditions presenting to the on-call ENT CT are epistaxis, tonsillitis, quinsy, ear infections and foreign bodies in their ear, nose or throat. These conditions account for the majority of your on-call workload. The acute airway is one emergency that causes anxiety for CTs. These patients usually require prompt involvement of the on-call ENT registrar and anaesthetist.

Many ENT 'emergencies' can safely be seen the next day in an emergency clinic. Much of the work in these clinics is treating ear infections, recurrent nose bleeds and nasal injuries. Make the most of opportunities to participate in operations and see outpatients in clinics. An experienced CT will learn how to perform a tonsillectomy, adenoidectomy and insert grommets. Becoming familiar with the wide range of ENT conditions seen in outpatients will be invaluable when starting out as a specialty registrar.

Recruitment to specialty training

Recruitment to ENT specialty training is very competitive. Competition ratios are typically around 14:1 (applications: places). In addition to achieving the exams mentioned above, candidates will need to have undertaken at least 24 months of surgical training at CT level, of which at least six months must be in ENT. Beware that there is a planned policy of penalising candidates who have undertaken prolonged periods of training in ENT without securing a national training number (NTN). Generally a maximum of 18 months is allowed. More than this may result in points being deducted from your application ranking score. Therefore, if you have achieved 18 months training in ENT posts and have not yet got a specialty training place, you would be better off gaining experience in related specialties.

An alternative would be to undertake research or a higher degree to enhance your competitiveness. Selection centres look for evidence of research and audit involvement. Because ENT is so competitive, most successful candidates will have undertaken at least one audit per year and published several papers. Although these do not have to be in ENT-related topics, if they are, this further demonstrates commitment to the specialty. Attendance at relevant ENT courses will also enhance your chances of success.

Currently, recruitment in England is via an annual national selection process. Scotland and Wales run separate selection processes. Thirty-two places were available in England for 2011. If your initial application is successful, you will be invited to the selection day which usually comprises of six stations. These stations include a portfolio/CV station, research skills, communication skills, ENT emergency management scenario, ENT outpatient management scenario and a practical skills station.

What's it like being an ENT specialty trainee?

Specialty training lasts six years (ST3–8). Most training programmes will involve moving around different hospitals every one to two years in order to gain full experience in the range of ENT surgery.

Most ENT services are delivered via a 'hub-and-spoke' model. This is where one base 'hub' hospital deals with all major surgery and emergency admissions and other surrounding 'spoke' hospitals have only outpatient or day surgery work. Therefore, travelling between hospitals during the week, or within any day, is common.

During the early years you will learn how to assess and manage common ENT symptoms in clinics, such as nasal blockage, dizziness, throat symptoms, neck lumps, etc. You will learn how to perform procedures such as sinus and septal surgery, myringoplasty and submandibular gland excision. During ST4–6 trainees will perform more advanced procedures such as thyroidectomy and cholesteatoma surgery. In the later stages of ST6–8 more complex surgery is undertaken, such as laryngectomy, parotidectomy and rhinoplasty.

A typical week will involve four theatre sessions and three to four clinics. Usually, one of these clinics will be specialized, e.g. head and neck cancer or paediatric airway. Registrars will typically have two to three sessions a week without clinical commitments, allowing time to undertake research/audits and higher degrees.

All posts will have an on-call commitment that is usually worked over a 24-hour period (or 48 hours at weekends). In general, ENT on-calls are not busy compared with other surgical specialties. Most calls can be dealt with over the phone and many registrars will be able to be on-call from home provided they live close to the hospital. Many ENT conditions can safely wait until the next day. However, severe epistaxis, post-tonsillectomy bleeding, airway emergencies and some aerodigestive foreign bodies often need to be dealt with promptly, and this will require an operation, usually performed by the on-call registrar.

Courses during ENT specialist training

Most specialty registrar (StR) training programmes will have regular regional training sessions. Many StRs will undertake higher degree courses alongside training. Most trainees (and some CT1/2s looking to improve their CV for StR applications) take the following courses. Many different institutions run these types of course both within the UK and abroad.

- Endoscopic sinus surgery course
- Temporal bone dissection course
- Facial plastic surgery course
- ENT radiology
- Head and neck dissection course
- Paediatric ENT course
- Audiology/Otology/Balance courses
- Laser courses
- Research skills/statistics courses
- Teaching skills courses/management courses

Exit exams

During the final two years of training, ST7–8, the FRCS (ORL) exit exam is taken. This consists of two written papers (multiple choice and extended matching items questions) and a subsequent viva/practical exam. A high level of skill and knowledge is required and the overall pass rate for specialty trainees is around 60%.

Once the FRCS (ORL) is achieved, most trainees will undertake a 'fellowship' year in their subspecialty of interest.

During training, specialty registrars will continue to undertake audits, research and higher degrees. At the end of six years of successful specialty training, you will be awarded the CCT (Certificate of Completion of Training), enabling you to apply for consultant posts.

What's it like being a consultant?

Currently, competition for ENT consultant posts is fierce. There has been an expansion of ENT registrar posts over the past five years, but the expected expansion in consultant posts has not been so forthcoming. There are currently 565 consultant ENT surgeons and 337 ENT specialty registrars in the UK, and there is a bottleneck of approximately 60 fully trained ENT surgeons who have yet to find a consultant post. Given this situation, many are trying very hard to improve their competitiveness with higher degrees, multiple publications/international presentations, etc. Although the out-of-hours component of work is less demanding, the additional endeavour to being appointed to a consultant post is particularly onerous.

The working week will be similar to that of a registrar at the end of training. The type of work undertaken will depend on whether the work is more generalist or as a subspecialist. It is much more common for ENT consultants to be subspecialists now. As with all consultant posts, there is a significant additional administrative and management role. The out-of-hours emergency work is generally less onerous than in other specialties. The specialty lends itself fairly well to working part time and is thus popular with female surgeons planning families.

Summary

Surgeons in training usually choose this specialty because of its variety and ever evolving use of technology. ENT surgeons are usually considered too friendly and approachable to be surgeons! Although competition is tough and achieving a successful career takes an enormous amount of hard work, most will accomplish a good work–life balance.

References

Corbridge RJ (1998). *Essential ENT Practice A Clinical Text*. London: Hodder Arnold.

Dhillon RA, East CA (2006) *Ear Nose and Throat and Head and Neck Surgery An Illustrated Colour Text*. Edinburgh: Churchill Livingstone.

Lyons M, Singh A (2005) Your First ENT Job: A Survivor's Guide. Oxford: Radcliffe Publishing.

Web links to ENT courses

www.entuk.org/medical_students/foundation/11.03.13%20app

www.rcseng.ac.uk/education/courses/ent_surgery.html

www.wxmec.org.uk/courses/IntroENT.html

Organisations

Association of Otolaryngologists in Training; www.aotent.com/

British Association of Otolaryngology – Head and Neck Surgery; www.entuk.org/

Chapter 13
PAEDIATRIC SURGERY

Max Pachl
Paediatric surgery specialty registrar, ST6, Birmingham Children's Hospital and is one of two national trainee representatives for paediatric surgery

Introduction, 171
The general career path, 172
What's it like being a paediatric surgery core trainee? 172
Recruitment to specialty training, 172
What's it like being a paediatric surgery specialty trainee? 174
Courses during paediatric surgery specialty training, 175
Exit exams, 176
What's it like as a consultant? 177
Summary, 177
References, 178
Organisations, 178

Introduction

Paediatric surgery includes neonatal surgery, paediatric general surgery, paediatric urology, paediatric oncology surgery and paediatric trauma. It continues to be the only surgical discipline in which one can practise general surgery without being, for example, a purely upper gastrointestinal (GI) surgeon, or purely lower GI, as happens in adult 'general surgery' practice.

One day's operating can involve things as varied as excision of a lung abnormality, repair of a diaphragmatic hernia, a laparotomy on a premature baby, formation of a colostomy and repair of an inguinal hernia. Paediatric surgeons operate on patients from the extremes of prematurity such as babies born at 24 weeks gestation weighing 500 g or less, to young adults who are 17 years of age.

And for those of you with a child's mentality, there is nothing like having a mock light sabre fight with a four-year-old on the ward or performing a minor procedure under local anaesthesia while the patient watches *Harry Potter* or *Toy Story*. It helps if you know the names of characters in popular children's programmes, and even if you're not a big football fan, talking about last night's game with a 10-year-old is a good way to win trust from your young patient.

Paediatric surgery is a small speciality with fewer than 140 consultants in the UK and approximately 110 trainees at varying stages of training. Fewer than 10 ST3 posts come up each year at present and this is certain to decrease in the next few years as there is currently an abundance of trainees. Twenty-five training numbers will be removed from the system in the years up to 2018 in England and Wales.

The Hands-on Guide to Surgical Training, First Edition. Matthew Stephenson.

Operating on children is a fascinating and challenging experience, their anatomy and physiology is akin to what you learn at medical school. They have not yet been affected by the rigours of age-related diseases.

The general career path

In the current climate a core training rotation in paediatric surgery is essential, and it's almost impossible to find a six-month stand-alone post in paediatric surgery. In 2010, there were 15 core training rotations in paediatric surgery nationally. The pathway to your Certificate of Completion of Training (CCT) is similar to other specialties and takes the form of FY1–2, CT1–2, ST3–8.

What's it like being a paediatric surgery core trainee?

Paediatric surgery core training is encompassed within a rotation that will usually include paediatric or neonatal intensive care along with paediatric surgery and occasionally adult general surgery. Clearly the number of placements depends on whether the rotation is based on four- or six-month attachments.

You will have exposure to the length and breadth of paediatric surgery and be expected to complete a number of workplace-based assessments (WBAs).

Generally speaking there are no FY1s in paediatric surgery, only FY2/CT1–2 and above. The FY2/CT1–2 will undertake the majority of the tasks in paediatric surgery that in adult surgery would be expected to fall within the remit of an FY1.

Prior to beginning your attachment in paediatric surgery there are a number of useful books that are appropriate (see References). This list is by no means exhaustive and will depend on your previous exposure to the specialty.

Essential courses to have attended at the stage of application for an ST3 post are Advanced Paediatric Life Support (APLS) or Paediatric Advanced Life Support (PALS). Desirable ones include Advanced Trauma Life Support (ATLS), Basic Surgical Skills or equivalent and Care of the Critically Ill Surgical Patient. (CCrISP).

You will need to have completed the Membership of the Royal College of Surgeons (MRCS) exams prior to applying for an ST3 post. It can be difficult when you're doing paediatric surgery attachments, especially when attempting Part 2. It's therefore vital to get to as many adult surgical clinics as possible to consolidate your learning and examination techniques.

Recruitment to Specialty Training

Recruitment is at a national level (England, Wales, Scotland and Northern Ireland) on a yearly basis and at present normally takes place in April or May. It is currently led by the Yorkshire and the Humber Deanery. It takes the form of an Objective Structured Clinical Exam (OSCE)-like assessment with a number of different tables/rooms and at present it assesses the following categories:

- CV and portfolio
- career progression
- academic abilities and experience
- clinical/teamwork
- clinical judgement
- communication
- skills

These may change in forthcoming selection rounds. Competition is fierce and the ratio of applicants to jobs is high (see Chapter 7).

Essential criteria for selection at ST3 include at least 24 months experience in surgery (not including foundation modules but including paediatric or neonatal critical care), of which at least six months has been in paediatric surgery. Desirable criteria include up to six months neonatology or critical care experience; at least six months' experience in paediatric surgery in United Kingdom; up to one year in paediatric surgery/urology, or general surgery at ST3 level.

Note that both the essential and desirable criteria include six months of paediatric surgery. Six months' experience in the UK is desirable, but not essential.

Although these criteria say that either paediatric or neonatal critical care (PICU/NICU) are acceptable, NICU is probably more useful long term and will help in your day-to-day activities, especially in units where neonatal medical support is off-site, such as Birmingham and Sheffield for example.

Going to national training sessions, conferences and the like also helps to 'get your face known' in our small specialty. Although getting a national training number (NTN) is based on an objective assessment, it can only help to meet consultants in the specialty who can advise on what chances you stand of getting one.

Training centres in paediatric surgery are organised into regional consortia which provide a broad exposure to paediatric surgery. Each consortia contains one or more children's hospitals.

- **Northwest**: Liverpool, Manchester.
- **Northern Ireland**: Belfast.
- **Yorkshire/East Midlands/Northern**: Newcastle, Leeds, Hull, Sheffield, Nottingham, Leicester.
- **Midlands & West**: Birmingham, Bristol, Cardiff.
- **South East**: Chelsea and Westminster, Royal London, Lewisham, St George's, King's College, Great Ormond Street, Evelina, Southampton, Brighton, Oxford, Cambridge, Norfolk and Norwich.
- **Republic of Ireland**: Dublin.

A NTN is issued by a deanery within the consortium and this equates to your base hospital. This is because all the deaneries except London have only one children's hospital within their catchment area. NTNs are allocated at national recruitment and are based on ranking scores from the interviews and on preferences declared at application. The higher your ranking, the better the chance of achieving your preferred consortium. At present NTNs from England, Northern Ireland and the devolved nations are allocated at national recruitment.

What's it like being a paediatric surgery specialty trainee?

The training programme covers the required six years of higher surgical training (ST3–8) within a single consortium. You are expected to spend at least two years of the six training outside your base hospital. One or both of these will be at another of the centres within your consortium and one may be an Out Of Programme (OOP) year. OOPs can be as training (OOPT), which can be either inside or outside the UK; experience (OOPE), which is generally a programme that is outwith clinical training (such as management); or research (OOPR).

There is an Annual Review of Competency Progression (ARCP) that must be satisfactory to progress to the next stage of training. Currently there is a requirement for a specific number of WBAs to be completed for each year of training.

- **ST3–ST4** should complete four case-based discussions (CBD), four mini-clinical evaluation exercises (mini-CEX), two surgical direct observation of procedural skills (SDOP) and 12 procedure-based assessments (PBA).
- **ST5–ST8** should complete six CBDs, four mini-CEXs and 12 PBAs.

One multi-source feedback (MSF) should be completed at ST3, ST5 and ST7. If these are not completed then the trainee will receive an automatic outcome 2 at ARCP.

Procedures

By the end of ST3/ST4 you should be able to carry out surgical procedures in the following groups (depending on placements) under supervision or independently.

- **Laparoscopy**: appendicectomy, for impalpable testis, ligation of varicocele.
- **General surgery of childhood**: inguinal herniotomy, hydrocele, circumcision, umbilical/epigastric hernia repair, pyloromyotomy, appendicectomy.
- **GI**: rectal biopsy, manual evacuation, upper GI endoscopy, percutaneous endoscopic gastrostomy (PEG) placement/removal, open gastrostomy, fundoplication.
- **Neonatal**: intestinal resection/anastomosis, diaphragmatic hernia repair, correction of malrotation, stoma formation, closure of gastroschisis.
- **Thoracic**: insertion open/percutaneous chest drain, thoracotomy.
- **Oncology**: central venous line placement, cervical lymph node biopsy, salpingo-oopherectomy.
- **Urology**: insertion of suprapubic catheter, cystoscopy

By the end of ST5/ST6 you should be able to carry out surgical procedures in the following groups (depending on placements) under supervision or independently

- **Laparoscopy**:fundoplication,cholecystectomy, pyloromyotomy, insertion of gastrostomy.
- **GI**: fundoplication, right hemicolectomy, subtotal hemicolectomy, small bowel resection for Crohn's disease,

laparotomy for reduction of intussusception.

- **Neonatal**: closure of gastroschisis/exomphalos, diaphragmatic hernia repair, correction of malrotation, laparotomy for necrotising enterocolitis (NEC), laparotomy for simple meconium ileus, duodeno-duodenostomy, neonatal inguinal herniotomy.
- **Thoracic**: resection of congenital cystic adenomatous malformation (CCAM), decortication of empyema, resection of mediastinal mass.
- **Oncology**: tumour nephrectomy.
- **Urology**: cystoscopy, nephrectomy, heminephrectomy, pyeloplasty, vesicostomy formation/closure, repair distal hypospadias.

By the end of ST7/ST8 you should be able to carry out surgical procedures in the following groups (depending on placements) under supervision or independently.

- **Laparoscopy**: nephrectomy.
- **General surgery of childhood**: laparotomy for trauma or adhesions.
- **GI**: pull-through for Hirschsprung's disease.
- **Neonatal**: laparotomy for simple/complex meconium ileus, repair of tracheo-oesophageal fistula (TOF).
- **Oncology**: resection of neuroblastoma.
- **Urology**: repair proximal hypospadias, bladder augmentation.

Indicative numbers

There used to be a specific number of procedures in generic groups that had to be carried out during training in order to be considered for the award of CCT. These will be overhauled in the next few years and a number of index cases in modified groups will be selected that will reflect trainees' overall experience in specific areas and will be blueprinted to both the curriculum and the e-logbook.

Timetable

A typical weekly timetable as an ST3 or above may include:

- a daily morning ward round, with or without consultant supervision
- two or three theatre sessions
- at least one general clinic
- one admin session
- one study/teaching session
- other sessions dependent on training requirements.

There is a significant out-of-hours commitment when on-call. Partly this is due to the fact that the majority of children would be assessed by ST3 or above prior to admission or discharge. There is also the fact that children can present at any time of day or night and some conditions, such as intussusception for example, are only encountered in an emergency setting. On calls are therefore imperative to gain experience in emergency paediatric surgery.

Courses during paediatric surgery specialty training

There are a plethora of courses for trainees, many of which are stage appropriate or specific and there are three sets of national training days per year. As there are a small number of trainees in each deanery we don't have deanery training days, but instead have sets of national training days in varying locations throughout the UK which last for two days. The national training days occur in spring and autumn, with one other session at the British Association of Paediatric Surgeons (BAPS) congress, which is normally held in July.

As paediatric surgery is a close-knit specialty you meet the same people at courses and training days. Most trainees will know many others, if not by name then at least by face. There is the opportunity to become friends or acquaintances with many trainees and this continues into consultant practice.

Relevant courses include, but are by no means limited to, those listed in Table 13.1. Trainees can go on these courses at any time of their training, but the level at which they are best taken are shown in the last column.

Exit exams

Most trainees would undertake the exit exam (FRCS (Paed)) in year five of their

Table 13.1 Courses relevant to paediatric surgery training

Course	Location	Aimed at
GOS Laparoscopy course	Great Ormond Street	ST3 and above
Practical management of paediatric trauma	Oxford	ST3 and above
BAPES Endosurgery course	Leeds	ST3 and above
Dundee Laparoscopy course	Cuschieri Centre, Dundee	ST3 and above
BAPS Oncology course	London	ST3 and above
Basic sciences in paediatric surgery	RCS England	ST5 and above
BAPU Urology course	Cambridge	ST5 and above
Oxford Neonatal course	Oxford	ST5 and above
Anorectal workshop	Amsterdam/Cincinnati	ST6 and above
EITS (IRCAD) videosurgery course	Strasbourg, France	ST6 and above

training scheme, i.e. ST7. Application requires at least two UK consultant referees who confirm that you are eligible and ready to take the exam.

What's it like as a consultant?

Once you've achieved your CCT you can practise as a consultant paediatric surgeon or consultant paediatric urologist. Some urologists are involved in the general surgery rota and so will continue to undertake emergency paediatric general surgery. Some will not be involved in the general surgery rota and will only undertake paediatric urology. There is some crossover between the roles in that both will undertake so called elective 'general surgery of childhood' procedures such as inguinal herniotomies and patent process vaginalis (PPV) ligations.

There are a few post-CCT fellowships available in paediatric urology and, while not essential to attain a post as a paediatric urologist, they are highly desirable and recommended.

As a consultant you would be expected to have a subspecialty interest. These can be developed over time and include:

- oncology (normally includes venous access procedures)
- colorectal
- thoracic
- minimal access (although this is rapidly being removed as most if not all current trainees achieving CCT will be competent in a large number of minimal access procedures)
- upper GI
- hepatopancreaticobiliary (HPB) (specific 'liver' centres at Birmingham, Leeds and King's College only, although some procedures are undertaken in other paediatric centres)
- bladder exstrophy and epispadias (Manchester and Great Ormond Street only).

While on call, consultant paediatric surgeons are in hospital out of hours more often than their colleagues in adult surgery. This involves both assessment and performing procedures on neonates and children out of hours. After the NCEPOD report of 2003 out-of-hours operating has been reduced and as a consequence those children who require an out-of-hours procedure tend to be the most critically ill. This is combined with the fact that many congenital anomalies are rare and some are only seen once or twice a year or less. The on-call registrar may therefore have no experience with some of them.

Having said all that, a consultant's job is very rewarding and constantly challenging. Even as a senior consultant, there are clinical conditions and variations of anomalies that have never been seen before. In this surgical specialty more than any other, lifelong learning is a clinical reality.

Summary

Paediatric surgery is a constantly challenging speciality even with the common conditions that we deal with. It's always stimulating and never mundane. Many would say that the neonatal side of the job is the most interesting, given that we deal with babies with multiple congenital problems ranging from being born with an oesophageal atresia or congenital diaphragmatic hernia, to being born with an ano-rectal malformation (although most of these anomalies occur in less than 1 in 5,000 live births and so are fairly rare).

The length and breadth of the specialty is quite amazing and once you start investigating fetal development it's astounding that congenital anomalies happen as rarely as they do. Operating on a premature baby who weighs 500 g is also part of the job along with operating on the 16-year-old who weighs 95 kg. No two days are ever the same.

It is not a job for the faint hearted and dealing with children with cancer is never fun, but it can be very rewarding to remove a tumour and know that you have achieved a cure for that patient who can then have another 70 years or so to live. Clearly it's impossible to save everyone, and dealing with the death of a child can be very difficult, but it's part and parcel of what we do.

It does, I think, take people of a particular personality type to become a paediatric surgeon. Sensitivity is massively important and how you come across to the child can sometimes mean the difference between an easy day and a hard one. Their interaction with you and your team can occasionally define their relationship with the medical community for the next few years or in some cases decades, so it's vital to get it right first time.

It's a job that I would highly recommend to anyone who is considering surgery as a career.

References

Davenport M, Pierro A (2009) *Paediatric Surgery* (Oxford Specialist Handbooks in Surgery). Oxford: Oxford University Press.

Glick PL, Pearl RH, Irish MS, Caty MG (2000) *Pediatric Surgical Secrets*. Philadelphia: Hanley and Belfus.

Hutson JM, Woodward AA, Beasley SW (eds) (1999) *Jones' Clinical Paediatric Surgery: Diagnosis and Management*. Oxford: Blackwell.

Sinha K, Davenport M (eds) (2010) *Handbook of Pediatric Surgery*. London: Springer.

Organisations

British Association of Paediatric Endoscopic Surgeons, BAPES, www.bapes.org.uk

British Association of Paediatric Surgeons, BAPS, www.baps.org.uk

British Association of Paediatric Urologists, BAPU, www.bapu.org.uk

Childrens Cancer and Leukaemia Group, CCLG, www.ukccsg.org/

European Association of Paediatric Surgeons, EUPSA, www.eupsa.org/

European Society for Paediatric Urologists, ESPU, www.espu.org/

International Paediatric Endosurgery Group, IPEG, www.ipeg.org

Trips, www.traineesinpaediatricsurgery.org/; Trips is the website for UK paediatric surgical trainees. The idea is to bring all resources that are relevant to the trainee under one roof. It is hosted by BAPS and contains information on courses and training days. It also has links to relevant organisations along with news, exam information, resources and access to the yahoo forum for trainees.

World Federation of Associations of Paediatric Surgeons, WOFAPS, www.wofaps.co.za/

Chapter 14
NEUROSURGERY

Sophie J Camp
Neurosurgery specialty registrar, ST5, Charing Cross Hospital, London

Introduction, 179
The general career path, 180
Recruitment to specialty training, 180
What's it like being a neurosurgery specialty trainee? 181
Courses during neurosurgery specialty training, 181
Exit exams, 184
What's it like as a consultant? 184
Summary, 185
References, 185
Organisations, 185

Introduction

'Neurosurgery is an arrogant occupation', the words of Frank Vertosick an American neurosurgeon whose book *When the Air Hits Your Brain* I strongly recommend to those planning a career in this specialty. It details some of the more challenging cases he encountered during his years as a neurosurgeon, which in themselves are fascinating. It also reveals the mentality of the neurosurgeon, how they learn to cope with operating when there is no margin for error. As he puts it, 'Neurosurgeons do things that cannot be undone'.

Neurosurgery, broadly speaking, entails the diagnosis, assessment and surgical management of disorders of the nervous system. Typically, this is taken to comprise operations in and around the brain and spinal cord. The peripheral nervous system is not exclusively the domain of the neurosurgeon. Many specialties, including neurosurgeons, plastic surgeons, orthopaedic surgeons and, specific to the upper limb, specialist hand surgeons, undertake surgery on peripheral nerves.

Neurosurgery covers the subspecialties of

- neuro-oncology
- vascular neurosurgery
- skull base surgery
- complex spinal surgery
- functional neurosurgery
- trauma
- paediatric neurosurgery.

The Hands-on Guide to Surgical Training, First Edition. Matthew Stephenson.

General career path

Neurosurgical training currently comprises eight years of specialty training (ST1–8), divided into three stages: initial, intermediate, and final.

The initial stage (ST1–3) follows the two foundation years, with junior doctors able to apply at any stage within the three years, i.e. you do not necessarily have to apply straight from FY2, but can undertake stand-alone jobs first, making you eligible to apply at different stages from ST1 to ST3. To date, neurosurgery remains a run-through specialty. It is not uncoupled, like general surgery or trauma and orthopaedics, therefore once a national training number (NTN) has been allocated, and assuming competencies are met, progression is inevitable (and this can be from as early as ST1).

At the initial stage (ST1–3), fixed term specialty training appointments (FTSTA) are also available as stand-alone one-year appointments. The person specifications are similar for the stand-alone and run-through posts. The distinction between ST1, ST2 and ST3 manifests in the duration of experience in neurosurgical-related training, competencies achieved, and obtaining Membership of the Royal College of Surgeons (Table 14.1).

Recruitment to specialty training

Recruitment is currently undertaken at a national level, currently coordinated by the Yorkshire and the Humber Deanery, via Objective Structured Clinical Evaluation (OSCE)-style stations and entry can be at any of the stages from ST1 to ST3. Table 14.1 indicates the ST level that is appropriate to apply for, depending on experience.

Useful surgical skills can be acquired from placements in general surgery, plastic surgery, trauma and orthopaedics, ear nose and throat surgery, and cardiothoracics. Together with neurology, neuro-intensive care, neuroradiology,

Table 14.1 The different requirements for the initial stages of neurosurgery training

	ST1	**ST2**	**ST3**
Neurosurgery experience	<18 months*	≥12 months*	≥24 months*
Competencies	FY	CT/ST1	CT/ST2
MRCS	N/A	N/A	required

*MRCS – Membership of the Royal College of Surgeons; FY – foundation years; CT/ST – core training/specialty training; *not including foundation modules.*

and accident and emergency medicine, these fields provide a knowledge base of pre- and postoperative management of the neurosurgical patient. This means that, if at the FY2 stage you do not get a FTSTA or ST1 post, stand-alone jobs may be undertaken which may aid subsequent application(s) for run-through training.

What's it like being a neurosurgery specialty trainee?

Due to the European Working Time Directive (EWTD), many hospitals now operate a full shift system. As a ST1–3 time is occupied with the management of both pre- and postoperative ward patients. There is individual unit variation with regard to outpatient clinic duties, although these do provide a good forum for learning. Many ST1–3 trainees gain much of their operating experience out of hours. However, at this time there is typically cross cover with neurology patients.

The intermediate stage covers ST4 and ST5, which entails general neurosurgical training. Although there may be regional variation, unlike most other specialities, ST4 is generally the first 'registrar' year. Dependent on the unit and catchment area, from ST4 to ST8 out-of-hours surgery is the norm rather than the exception. In the ST4–8 years time is split between operating, outpatient clinics and on-call/emergency cover.

ST6–8 comprises advanced neurosurgical training, incorporating a year of special interest training, when time can be spent in a subspecialty of interest. This may be in the form of a fellowship overseas if desired.

Table 14.2 details the procedures expected to be performed and the level of expertise required during each stage of training. Progression to the next ST level is determined by the Annual Review of Competence Progression (ARCP), at which logbooks are scrutinised, competencies are reviewed via workplace-based assessments and additional facets of training, such as teaching, research and audit, are evaluated.

Courses during neurosurgery specialty training

There are a number of courses that are useful at various stages of neurosurgery training, as detailed below.

1 The programme of neurosurgery courses held at the Royal College of Surgeons of England (www.rcseng.ac.uk).

2 Neurosurgical Approaches to the Cranial Compartments held at The Royal College of Surgeons of Edinburgh (www.rcsed.ac.uk) ST3–8.

3 Leeds Neurosurgical Department Neuroanatomy Courses (www.leedsneuroanatomycourses.co.uk) ST3–8.

4 Cambridge Lectures in Neurosurgical Anatomy (www.clna.org.uk) ST1–8.

5 British Neurosurgical Trainee Courses (www.neurosurgerycourse.co.uk) ST4–8.

6 European Association of Neurosurgical Societies Training Course (www.eans.org/pages/home) ST4–8.

Table 14.2 Schedule of essential operative competencies taken from the neurosurgery syllabus (www.iscp.ac.uk)

Surgical approach	Initial	Intermediate	Final
Burr hole	3	4	4
Craniotomy – convexity	2	3	4
Craniotomy – pterional	1	3	4
Craniotomy – midline supratentorial	1	3	4
Craniotomy – midline posterior fossa	2	3	4
Transsphenoidal approach	1	2	4
Lateral posterior fossa	1	2	4
Lumbar fenestration	2	4	4
Laminectomy	2	3	4
Insertion of lumbar drain	3	4	4
Tapping/draining of CSF reservoir	3	4	4
Application of skull traction	2	4	4
Image guidance/Stereotaxy set-up	2	4	4
Insertion of intracranial (ICP) monitor	3	4	4
Burr hole evacuation of CSDH	3	4	4
Elevation of depressed skull fracture	2	4	4
Craniotomy for traumatic haematoma (ICH)	2	3	4
Craniotomy for spontaneous intracerebral haematoma (ICH supratentorial)	1	3	4

Table 14.2 (*Continued*)

Surgical approach	Initial	Intermediate	Final
Craniotomy for spontaneous intracerebellar haematoma (ICH infratentorial)	1	3	4
Insertion of ventricular drain/access device	3	4	4
Insertion of VP shunt	2	3	4
Revision of VP shunt	1	2	4
Supratentorial tumour biopsy	2	3	4
Craniotomy for supratentorial intrinsic tumour/metastasis	1	3	4
Craniotomy for posterior fossa intrinsic tumour/metastasis	1	2	4
Craniotomy for convexity meningioma	1	3	4
Excision of intradural extramedullary tumour	1	2	4
Lumbar microdiscectomy	1	3	4
Anterior cervical discectomy	1	3	4
Insertion of paediatric EVD	1	2	4
Evacuation of paediatric intracranial haematoma (ICH)	1	2	4

Level of competency: 1 – has observed; 2 – can do with assistance; 3 – can do whole but may need assistance; 4 – competent to do whole without assistance and manage complications. CSF – cerebrospinal fluid; ICP – intracranial pressure; CSDH – chronic subdural haematoma; ICH – intracerebral haematoma; EVD – external ventricular drain; VP – ventriculoperitoneal.

<table>
<tr><th colspan="2">CT1–2</th><th colspan="2">ST3–4</th><th colspan="2">ST5–6</th><th colspan="2">ST7–8
Consultants</th></tr>
<tr><td colspan="3">Operative Skills in Neurosurgery</td><td></td><td colspan="4">Minimally Invasive Intracranial Neurosurgery</td></tr>
<tr><td></td><td colspan="3">Clinical Skills in Spinal Assessment and Management</td><td colspan="3">Spinal Revision FRCS</td><td></td></tr>
<tr><td></td><td></td><td></td><td colspan="3">Surgical Approaches to Pituitary Lesions</td><td></td><td></td></tr>
<tr><td colspan="8">Neurosurgery Week</td></tr>
<tr><td></td><td></td><td></td><td></td><td colspan="4">Technical Advances to Skull Base Surgery</td></tr>
<tr><td></td><td></td><td></td><td colspan="5">Neuro-Oncology</td></tr>
<tr><td colspan="6">Elective Skills in Facial Trauma</td><td></td><td></td></tr>
<tr><td></td><td></td><td></td><td></td><td colspan="4">Technical Tips and Error Avoidance in Spinal Surgery (TTEASS)</td></tr>
<tr><td colspan="8">Legal Aspects of Surgical Practice</td></tr>
<tr><td colspan="8">Decision Making and Judgement in Spinal Surgery</td></tr>
<tr><td colspan="8">Neurological Anatomy</td></tr>
<tr><td colspan="8">Neuroradiology</td></tr>
<tr><td colspan="8">Approaches for Intracranial Surgery</td></tr>
</table>

Source: The Royal College of Surgeons of England

Exit exams

During the final stage the exit exam, i.e. the Intercollegiate Examination in Neurological Surgery, FRCS (SN) is undertaken. This is usually taken at the ST7 or 8 level. It comprises a written part of two papers (110 multiple-choice questions in two hours; 135 extended matching items [EMI] questions in 2.5 hours) and clinical component (long case of 30 minutes; short cases over 30 minutes; and three 30-minute orals covering operative surgery and surgical anatomy, investigations of the neurosurgical patient and the non-operative clinical practice of neurosurgery). The exam takes place twice a year hosted by different neurosurgical units within the UK.

What's it like as a consultant?

The rewards of a consultant post are more autonomy regarding case mix, operating schedules and time management. However, intra/inter-hospital politics and bureaucracy pose an increasing burden. Most consultant neurosurgeons subspecialise, i.e. their elective work is predominantly in one of the aforementioned categories. Emergency work covers all areas, and as a consultant, attendance in the operating theatre may be required dependent on trainee surgical ability. Neurosurgery is very much a consultant-led service, and life and death decisions are generally made by the boss whatever hour of the day or night.

Summary

Neurosurgery is a fascinating and immensely rewarding specialty. Managing critically ill patients and operating where the stakes are so high is a tremendous responsibility. The big positive is that there are few specialties where a patient can walk into an outpatient clinic intact and you know that you and your team are responsible not just for the patient's ability to function, but for their very being!

References

Firlik KS (2006) *Brain Matters: Adventures of a Brain Surgeon*. London: Weidenfeld & Nicolson.

Fuller G (2008) *Neurological Examination Made Easy* (4e). London: Churchill Livingstone Elsevier.

Greenberg MS (2010) *Handbook of Neurosurgery* (7e). New York: Thieme.

Kaye AH (2005) *Essential Neurosurgery* (3e). Oxford: Blackwell Publishing.

Liebenberg WA, Johnson RD (2010) *Neurosurgery for Basic Surgical Trainees* (2e). Hippocrates Books.

Rhoton AL (2002) The posterior fossa: microsurgical anatomy and approaches. *Neurosurgery* (September Supplement).

Rhoton AL (2002) The supratentorial cranial space:microsurgical anatomy and surgical approaches. *Neurosurgery* (October Supplement)

Samandouras G (2010) *The Neurosurgeon's Handbook*. Oxford: Oxford University Press.

Vertosick F (2008) *When the Air Hits Your Brain*. New York: Norton & Co.

Organisations

It is always useful to belong to specialty-specific organisations, not just for the CV, but to keep informed of developments in the field and changes to training/practice. A few of these such organisations are detailed below.

American Association of Neurological Surgeons (www.aans.org)

British Neurosurgical Trainees Association (www.e1v1m1.co.uk)

Congress of Neurological Surgeons (www.cns.org)

European Association of Neurosurgical Societies (www.eans.org/pages/home)

Society of British Neurological Surgeons (www.sbns.org.uk)

Chapter 15
ORTHOPAEDICS

Iain Findlay
Orthopaedic specialty registrar, ST7, King's College Hospital, London

Introduction, 186
Subspecialties, 187
The general career path, 187
What's it like being an orthopaedic core trainee? 188
Recruitment to specialty training, 188
What's it like being an orthopaedic specialty trainee? 189
Courses during orthopaedic specialist training, 190
Exit exams, 190
What's it like as a consultant?, 190
Reference, 192
Organisations, 192

Introduction

Orthopaedics is the Marmite of medicine: you either love it or hate it. The butt of many a medical joke, orthopods do have to be thick skinned. However, they do tend to be among the most contented doctors in the hospital. Civilised rotas, no long ward rounds, varied clinics with generally happy patients and plenty of operating all make this the sensible career choice.

It is a truly unique specialty with a very different training scheme and weekly schedule to all other medical careers. Put simply, orthopaedics is about operating and fundamentally that is why you want to be a surgical trainee. The volume of surgery and variety of operations is vast. Trauma lists are getting busier; the population is ageing and the demand for elective procedures exponentially increasing. Registrars are expected to have a minimum of 400 cases in their logbooks every year.

Training progresses rapidly. ST3-level registrars concentrate on becoming comfortable with basic trauma, guided by their consultants and more senior registrars. Over the years this progresses to becoming comfortable with most aspects of trauma, while developing experience with elective surgery. This continues throughout ST4 to ST8, and during a fellowship with an emphasis on subspecialty training, the aim being to produce consultants with well-rounded experience and a specialist interest in areas that complement an orthopaedic department.

The Hands-on Guide to Surgical Training, First Edition. Matthew Stephenson.

Subspecialties

Hip and knee

Total hip and knee replacements are two of the most successful operations ever developed. Thousands are carried out each year, with constant research to improve function and longevity. Revision surgery of joint replacements that are worn out is also a major undertaking. The other end of this subspecialty involves soft tissue arthroscopic surgery and ligament reconstruction, allowing work with younger, very high-function patients.

Foot and ankle

This is a hugely evolving area with a complex range of treatment principles and operations. Hard as it may be to believe, even bunion surgery is full of dilemmas and debate. Foot and ankle surgery also extends to major reconstructive surgery, especially in rheumatoid patients.

Upper limb

Something for everyone: arthroscopic surgery, joint replacement, trauma, nerve decompressions and tendon repairs. This is the subspecialty to put paid to any jokes about brutes with hammers. Demanding an expert knowledge of anatomy, upper limb surgery is full of subspecialties of subspecialties.

Spine

There is a huge overlap with neurosurgery. Many major centres employ both varieties of surgeon with the aim of providing a multidisciplinary approach to this very complex area. As a general rule of thumb, orthopods tend to be more involved in stabilisation of the spine with metalwork, but will still perform discectomies and decompressions. Just the sort of operating to test even the steadiest of hands.

Paediatrics

Tends now to be based in tertiary referral centres. This is a sign of the complexity of problems that have to be dealt with. It is perhaps different to other areas of orthopaedics in that the outpatient management is as demanding as the operative management.

Trauma

If this is what you fancy, find a hospital near a motorway, dry ski slope, sports ground and a nursing home! A post in a major trauma centre will deal with all the trauma you can dream of.

The general career path

After doing your foundation years, you require experience in orthopaedics as a core trainee before you progress. Fortunately, almost every hospital will have an orthopaedic department. After successfully passing your Membership of the Royal College of Surgeons (MRCS) exams you can apply for specialty training. This is essentially where your orthopaedic specific training begins. Running from ST3 to ST8 you will rotate around a variety of district and central teaching hospitals. Each post is split into two six-month subspecialty placements. After a taster of all of these, you tailor your training in your final few years towards your area of interest and then after a year or two of fellowships to refine your skills you are ready to be a consultant.

What's it like being an orthopaedic core trainee?

The true answer is, it depends. You need to be lucky, and on the negative side, trainees may find themselves mainly fulfilling on-call and ward duties. There is a high turnover of patients, who are often elderly with complex problems. Many units now work with a Care of the Elderly service to help juniors. Once the wards are under control, try and gain experience in all aspects of orthopaedics.

Enthusiasm goes a long way. No one has ever turned down an extra pair of hands in fracture clinic. The same goes for theatre time, get stuck in and involved. Build up your confidence in theatre, beginning with assisting and wound closure. With this, and with help from your seniors, you should begin to be able to cope with simple cases. Ankle fractures and hip fractures are the cases you should concentrate on to begin with. Have an idea of the principles of their treatment and try and learn the steps of their operative fixation. This makes it much easier for your consultant or registrar to take you through the procedure.

The easiest place to shine, or look like an idiot, is in the trauma meeting. Your main role as a core trainee is seeing and organising the management of A&E referrals. Every morning every case is presented by the on-call team in the trauma meeting. A clear concise history and examination and a management plan (with help from your registrar) will mark you out to all the consultants present.

Recruitment to specialty training

Speciality training is currently recruited nationwide in England, coordinated by the Yorkshire and the Humber Deanery. Wales and Northern Ireland run a similar process independently, but in Scotland recruitment is still run through from ST1. The application process is via application forms followed by short-listing and interviews for the selected candidates. Successful candidates will then be matched to preferred deaneries. However, be aware that this process has changed almost every year since the start of Modernising Medical Careers (MMC) implementation. Keep your wits about you and investigate the specifications of your local deanery and the colleges. The British Orthopaedic Trainees Association (BOTA) is also very helpful.

Essentially, experience in orthopaedics and related specialties is mandatory, and it is a very competitive field. You need to tee up your portfolio to make it stand out. Publications are the traditional way to do this. They show commitment and interest in the field, but can also feel like an elusive holy grail. The chances of you coming up with an appropriate prospective randomised control trial, passing it through ethical approval, collecting the data, writing it up and then having it published are rather slim in the short period of time available. Therefore, speak to your consultants early about their projects and offer to help out. Most will have research half finished or data ready to be analysed. Look for case reports as they have a much quicker turnover. Team up with other core or specialty trainees to share the workload. Presentations at educational meetings are also invaluable. The turn-around time for these is also much quicker than for publications.

Attend suitable courses, not just Advanced Trauma Life Support (ATLS) and Basic Surgical Skills (BSS). The AO Principles of Fracture Management Course (currently £995) is strongly recommended. It may be a bit expensive, but the combination of dry bones workshops, tutorials and lectures will soon have you feeling confident.

The actual recruitment procedure changes every year. It is now becoming clear that short-listed candidates will attend a structured clinical interview. The interview panel will organise various stations to assess your suitability and commitment.

- A portfolio review station to assess your academic achievements.
- A structured interview assessing your commitment to and knowledge of orthopaedic training.
- Various clinical scenarios and viva questions.

The last thing you want is to be asked these questions for the first time at interview, so get your registrars and consultants to prepare you as much as possible.

What's it like being an orthopaedic specialty trainee?

It's easy to be overwhelmed. Trauma meetings rattle through the previous day's admissions, with management decisions made immediately; clinics are busy and varied; and theatre lists packed full of cases. Take things one step at a time. First of all make sure you are comfortable with the management of your consultant's patients and aware of their subspecialty. Ask them early about their preferences for postoperative regimes and specific patient concerns.

The next stage is to make yourself as comfortable as possible with trauma, especially out-of-hours emergencies. For most rotas other than major trauma centres you are non-resident. This is brilliant for training: you don't miss out on your consultant's theatre list or teaching sessions by being resident on night shifts for a week for instance and it avoids the hospital canteen and dingy on-calls rooms. However, to put your mind at rest and avoid disasters in the middle of the night, always find the on-call FY2 or CT before you leave the hospital or go to your on-call room.

- Make sure they have your **contact details**.
- Make sure they know who is the **consultant on call**.
- Advise them about any **orthopaedic emergencies** that they should contact you about **immediately** (especially compartment syndrome, open fractures, irreducible dislocations, cauda equina syndrome, septic arthritis, displaced supracondylar fractures in

children, fractures with neurovascular compromise).

It follows that you should have a plan of attack for all of the above emergencies, but never take anything to theatre out of hours without letting the on-call consultant know.

As a general aim of training you should be comfortable with the vast majority of trauma operations by ST8. This time span indicates the huge range of operations and techniques that are required. It should also give the more junior trainees a certain perspective on their learning curve. Try and build up your logbook right from the very start. Scrub in with all your colleagues, more senior trainees and consultants to gain as much experience as possible. One word of warning: be careful even of 'straightforward cases'. Every case is different and every consultant and registrar has a story about a hip hemiarthroplasty, dynamic hip screw or ankle fracture that made them sweat.

Each trainee is expected to do six months of every subspecialty. This will give you a taster of orthopaedics in preparation for the exit exam and before fellowships are decided upon. It also means that new skills have to be learnt in every post, both in theatre and outpatients. The key is to keep your training well balanced. Even if you are 100% sure that knee surgery is for you, pace your six-month knee postings out over the six or so years of your training. Make sure that you get to experience a broad spectrum of cases. There always tends to be a degree of cross cover in clinics and theatre, and the sooner you can get familiar with most facets of the job, the more comfortable life will be.

As you progress in your training, hopefully there will be areas of interest that you wish to pursue. Tailoring your later posts to work with consultants with similar interest will allow you to continue your development.

Courses during orthopaedic specialist training

The following orthopaedics courses are run by the Royal College of Surgeons Figure 15.1.

Exit exams

The Fellowship of the Royal College of Surgeons (FRCS) (Tr and Orth) is the bane of all trainees' lives. It is sat at around the ST7 and ST8 stage and comprises to two parts.

- Two written papers of mutiple-choice questions (MCQs) and extended matching items (EMI) questions.
- A viva exam of clinical cases and oral exams in trauma, paediatrics and hands, adult elective orthopaedics and the dreaded basic sciences.

Most training circuits arrange teaching guided to preparation for this exam. It is undoubtedly a slog, but with early preparation and working in small groups it can be made slightly less painful.

What's it like as a consultant?

Every consultant post varies. New consultants work to provide an efficient and

<table>
<tr><th colspan="2">CT1–2</th><th colspan="2">ST3–4</th><th colspan="2">ST5–6</th><th colspan="2">ST7–8 Consultants</th></tr>
<tr><td colspan="2">So you want to be an Orthopaedic Surgeon (F1–2)</td><td colspan="2">Surgical Approaches to Upper and Lower Limb</td><td colspan="3">Spinal Revision FRCS</td><td></td></tr>
<tr><td></td><td colspan="2">Core Skills in Operative Orthopaedic Surgery</td><td></td><td></td><td></td><td></td><td></td></tr>
<tr><td colspan="4">Basic Techniques in Arthroscopic Surgery</td><td></td><td colspan="3">Revision Hip Surgery</td></tr>
<tr><td colspan="4">Primary Hip Replacement</td><td colspan="4">Advanced Arthroscopy Wrist Workshop</td></tr>
<tr><td colspan="4">Primary Knee Replacement Surgery</td><td></td><td></td><td></td><td></td></tr>
<tr><td colspan="4">Current Concepts in External Fixation in Trauma</td><td></td><td></td><td></td><td></td></tr>
<tr><td colspan="3">Hip, Ankle and Distal Radial fractures</td><td></td><td></td><td></td><td colspan="2">Masterclass in Foot and Ankle Surgery</td></tr>
<tr><td></td><td colspan="3">Clinical Skills in Spinal Assessment and Management</td><td colspan="4">Technical Tips and Error Avoidance in Spinal Surgery (TTEASS)</td></tr>
<tr><td colspan="2">Clinical Skills of Examining Orghopaedic Patients</td><td colspan="6">Tibia Masterclass - Nail, Plate, Ilizarov: The Unsolved Problem</td></tr>
<tr><td></td><td colspan="2">Hand Surgery</td><td></td><td></td><td></td><td></td><td></td></tr>
<tr><td></td><td></td><td colspan="4">Aesthetic and Reconstructive Surgical Skills Cadaver Dissection</td><td></td><td></td></tr>
<tr><td colspan="8">Legal Aspects of Surgical Practice</td></tr>
<tr><td></td><td colspan="5">Basic Ilizarov Method course</td><td></td><td></td></tr>
<tr><td colspan="8">Decision Making and Judgement in Spinal Surgery</td></tr>
<tr><td></td><td></td><td colspan="4">Spinal Microsurgery</td><td></td><td></td></tr>
<tr><td colspan="8">Amputations</td></tr>
<tr><td></td><td></td><td></td><td colspan="3">Advanced Skills in Hand and Wrist Surgery</td><td></td><td></td></tr>
<tr><td></td><td colspan="5">FRCS (Tr & Orth) Viva Course for Orthopaedic Surgeons</td><td></td><td></td></tr>
</table>

Figure 15.1 Orthopaedics Royal College of Surgeons course portfolio.
Source: The Royal College of Surgeons of England

useful service for their trust. The week is split into half-day sessions with usually three operative (two elective and one trauma) and three outpatient (two elective and one fracture). Consultants tend to use their other sessions for extra theatre lists, teaching, specialist clinics and admin work. Many consultants begin with a more general interest in their subspecialty and then refine their practice over time. This allows for continued development in operative techniques, patient management and research.

The key behind being an orthopaedic consultant is working as a team with your other consultants to maintain an efficient and successful department. The specialty is subspecialised so the aim is not to be able to manage every single patient, but rather to offer an area of expertise and provide a high-level service. This can be refined during your career, hopefully allowing you a rewarding and satisfying career.

Reference

Young AF, Caesar BC, David LA. A career in trauma and orthopaedics. www.bmjcareers.com

Organisations

American Academy of Orthopaedic Surgeons (www.orthoinfo.aaos.org)

British Orthopaedic Association (www.boa.ac.uk)

British Orthopaedic Trainees Association (www.bota.org.uk)

Chapter 16
PLASTIC SURGERY

Sofiane Rimouche
Plastic surgery specialty registrar, ST6, North Western rotation and President of the UK Plastic Surgery Trainees Association (PLASTA)

Introduction, 193
The general career path, 194
What's it like being a plastic surgery core trainee? 194
Recruitment to specialty training, 195
What's it like being a plastic surgery specialty trainee? 196
Courses during plastic surgery specialty training, 197
Exit exams, 198
What's it like as a consultant? 198
References, 199
Organisations, 199

Introduction

Plastic surgery is a craft specialty concerned with reconstructing both form and function with aesthetic considerations. It deals with a wide breadth of both elective and emergency conditions, including:

- acute hand trauma
- congenital hand deformities
- cleft lip and palate
- craniofacial anomalies
- hypospadias surgery
- elective hand and upper limb surgery
- lower limb reconstruction
- burns management
- cancer resection and reconstruction in all areas of the body, including head and neck, breast, trunk and pelvis.

In addition, there's body contouring reconstruction following bariatric surgery.

Plastic surgery is a technical specialty. The use of microsurgical techniques and understanding of the blood supply of the skin and soft tissues is essential. The specialty prides itself on research and innovation, which is fundamental for specialty development, progress and providing patients with best care possible. Certainly 'nip and tuck', or aesthetic/cosmetic surgery, is also a significant branch within plastic surgery, which is the only subspecialty where there is formal training and assessment throughout.

Plastic surgery is more than a science, it is an art. The surgeon's skills, innovations and artistic touch are essential in dealing with individual patient problems. There is a significant interaction with other surgical and medical

The Hands-on Guide to Surgical Training, First Edition. Matthew Stephenson.

colleagues. The plastic surgeon is an essential member of various multidisciplinary teams. Plastic surgery is unique in terms of the breadth of practice and patients' age span from infants to the elderly. There is no doubt that it's a very competitive specialty, and commitment and hard work are essential. It's also not for the faint hearted. However, the rewards are enormous. Most of your patients are grateful. The surgery you perform is interesting, exciting, challenging and varied. There is scope for academic positions and research interests. The on call can be busy, but certainly manageable, and as a trainee or a consultant your lifestyle is reasonable. Private practice is also good for those who wish to pursue it. And calling yourself a plastic surgeon is definitely cooler than calling yourself brain surgeon!

The general career path

In the past, it used to take an average of 14 years after medical qualification to become a consultant plastic surgeon. However, with recent changes in medical and surgical training following Modernising Medical Careers (MMC) implementation, training has been shortened. After doing foundation years 1 and 2, you'll have to apply for a two-year core surgical training rotation, during which time you'll have to pass the Membership of the Royal College of Surgeons (MRCS) exams. After CT2 you apply for specialty training therefore entering at the ST3 stage, which runs through to ST8. Although some candidates may progress directly from core training to specialty training, most will require you to spend further time consolidating the CV, either in stand-alone clinical fellow positions, registrar positions (locum appointment for service [LAS] or locum appointment for training [LAT]) or research positions prior to obtaining a national training number (NTN).

What's it like being a plastic surgery core trainee?

Core training posts in plastic surgery involve an element of ward work, on calls, trauma clinics (if available), and opportunities to get involved in theatre and outpatients. In many hospitals you are the first point of referral for GPs or A&E, and usually the first to see and assess acute patients, including hand trauma, facial trauma, soft tissue defects, and infections and burns. Most plastic surgery patients are usually well. However, if you work in a burns unit your patients have the potential to be very unwell.

In the beginning it's likely to be daunting due to the breadth of the specialty. However, as with any other surgical specialty, it's a steep learning curve. It's important to apply common sense, be safe and ask for help if unsure. Most plastic surgery units will have local guidelines and run induction programmes. It's essential that you familiarise yourself early on with the basic assessment and management of hand and facial trauma, burns and patient monitoring following microsurgical procedures such as flaps and replanted parts.

We are surgeons and love operating, so you must maximise your surgical exposure by trying to get to theatre as much as possible to master the essential surgical skills such as wound debridement and exploration, suturing and plastic surgical techniques such as skin grafting and microsurgery. There's a lot to learn and I highly recommend having the basic skills courses (see the Courses section) under your belt early and also purchase a pair of surgical loops (initially get a cheap pair, you can buy them for about £100 via the internet). During core training you may want to focus on becoming comfortable with basic operations such as basic hand trauma, skin grafting, local flaps and running local anaesthetic lists.

You'll also need to be honing your portfolio on a continual basis, organising audits, publishing a paper or two per year, going on courses, presenting and studying for your MRCS – all in preparation for the very competitive ST3 applications.

Recruitment to specialty training

From 2008, recruitment to ST3 has been through a single national process jointly managed by the London Deanery and the Specialist Advisory Committee in Plastic Surgery. You will need to have completed at least 24 months of surgery including at least six months of plastic surgery (not including foundation years), to have passed MRCS, attended Advanced Trauma Life Support (ATLS) and Basic Surgical Skills (BSS) courses, etc., as well as the other more generic criteria listed in the person specifications. Over the past three years there were between 15 and 30 NTNs on offer each year.

The online application form is standard. The main subsections include:

- clinical experience
- commitment to the specialty
- audit
- research
- clinical governance
- presentations
- papers
- management
- leadership
- teaching and communication skills.

A detailed guide on how to fill the application form, person specification and the scoring criteria/sheet used for the short list are available from the London Deanery website. It's important to study these forms well in advance and gear your portfolio towards filling each box.

Following the application stage you may be short listed if you've ranked high enough and be invited to interview. This has recently taken the form of a structured interview comprising three separate sections. The first section is divided into two-part clinical scenarios (two or three) and the second one is on audit, research and teaching. The second section of the interview candidates are given a topic and asked to prepare a short presentation to the panel. You may also get further clinical scenarios which could test skills such as communication. The last part of the interview is on the evaluation/critique of a research article.

So how do you add value to your portfolio? It's helpful to show commitment to the specialty from early on. At medical student stage you need to make sure you undertake a plastic surgery placement if you can, or organise a taster week. You could also intercalate and undertake a year of research on a plastic surgery-related topic. Make contact with your local plastic surgery unit and offer your services to help out with audit and research activities. This also applies to foundation doctors and core trainees. Some units offer a foundation post in plastic surgery; try and obtain one of these positions or consider spending your taster week (available to all foundation doctors in FY2) in a plastic surgery department. An alternative is to apply for an academic foundation post where you may be given a choice of undertaking a four-month research project of your choice, which of course it has to be in a plastic surgery-related topic.

Although it's no longer essential to undertake formal research after obtaining the MRCS (e.g. MD or PhD), as there is a separate academic pathway, you may want to consider it anyway as it will make you competitive not only for gaining an NTN, but also for consultant posts, and it enables you to learn very valuable skills. An alternative is to consider a part-time higher degree such as an MSc in surgical sciences at Imperial or an MSc in wound healing and tissue repair at Cardiff. In addition, consider educational and management degrees which will be a very attractive alternative. Please don't forget the 3As, which I believe to be essential, be Affable, Available and Able.

What's it like being a plastic surgery specialty trainee?

The wide breadth of the specialty and the knowledge and skills you need to learn can be daunting in the beginning. On call is varied, depending on the size of the unit. It can be very busy in the larger units. Usually, you will be non-resident on call and operating in the middle of the night is infrequent. Most of the emergency operating will involve dealing with hand, lower limb and facial trauma, soft tissue coverage and infections in all age groups. In addition, major burns could keep you busy. You will be expected to operate independently very early on for operations such as hand and facial trauma (hence the importance of learning these in the core training years) and gradually building up to more advanced procedures. Similar principles apply to elective work. It's important to master the basic procedures early on and build up your expertise. Usually most trainees rotate through all major subspecialties.

On average you'll attend two to three clinics a week and be scheduled for at least a full day of operating once a week, a trauma list and a local anaesthetic list.

You will be expected to continue to be involved with audit, research, presentations, publishing and educational activities.

The British Association of Plastic Reconstructive and Aesthetic Surgery (BAPRAS) in conjunction with the Department of Health is in the process of developing an e-learning plastic surgery resource (eLPRAS). This is an exciting development and will cover all of the plastic surgery curriculum, including multiple-choice practice questions. This will be an extremely valuable educational and revision resource.

As with the other specialties you will have to be assessed at least annually at an Annual Review of Competence Progression (ARCP) interview (see Chapter 7) to ensure that you're ready to progress to the next year. Certain units will arrange a yearly mock exam.

Most plastic surgery trainees will undertake a pre-Certificate of Completion of Training (CCT) fellowship, either a national or an international one (see Chapter 21).

A number of plastic surgery-related MScs and diplomas have been developed. These are suitable for specialty trainees. They include:

- hand diploma
- Masters in oncoplastic breast surgery
- postgraduate diploma in burns surgery
- postgraduate diploma in Aesthetic surgery.

Life as a plastic surgery specialty registrar is fun and rewarding. However, one potential drawback, depending on your rotation, is a long commute or you may even need to relocate between cities during your training as plastic surgery services are provided at a regional level (one unit usually serves several cities). In addition, it's estimated that most trainees spend on average around £30,000 on fees, loops, courses, books and meetings during the course of their training.

Courses during plastic surgery specialty training

There are a huge number of both national and international courses for this diverse specialty. The following should give you an idea of the main courses you should consider attending if you have the opportunity.

Medical students

- BAPRAS Undergraduate Day (career forum course, free)

Foundation/Core training

- Basic Skills courses: Core Skills in Plastic Surgery (RCS) or Essentials in Plastic Surgery by MY Plastic Surgery Course (Wakefield)
- Emergency Management of Severe Burns (British Burns Association)
- Hand surgery course: Basic Skills in Hand Surgery (RCS) or Foundation in Trauma Hand Surgery by MY Plastic Surgery Course (Wakefield)
- Hand fracture fixation course: main three courses are Leicester, Derby or AO Leeds courses
- Microsurgery course: main three courses are Canniesburn, Northwick Park or Ganga India courses

Specialty training

- Advanced BAPRAS plastic surgery courses: each series has six two-day courses which run over three years. This course series cover most of the plastic surgery curriculum
- British Society for Surgery of the Hand (BSSH) hand instructional courses: each series has six two-day courses which run over three years. This course series cover the entire hand surgery syllabus.
- RCS aesthetic reconstruction courses: each series has nine one-day courses which run over three years. This course series cover most of the aesthetic surgery curriculum.
- Flap dissection courses: the main courses are Canniesburn, North East and RCS Bristol course.
- Royal Society of Medicine (RSM) plastic surgery section courses: a number of one- or half-day courses that may also be useful.
- Exam courses: main courses are Canniesburn, Norwich and WAPS Birmingham courses.
- Specialised courses: there are a significant number of other specialised courses; the BAPRAS, Plastic Surgery Trainees Association (PLASTA) and RCS websites are a good source for obtaining information.

Exit exams

Most trainees take their exit exams in ST7 gaining the letters FRCS (Plast) after their names. The exam involves both a written and a clinical part. Details are available on the Intercollegiate Examination Board website, www.intercollegiate.org.uk. It's important to note that from 2012 new restrictions apply where you have to pass the written part within two years of your first sitting and you are only allowed three attempts at the clinical Part. A useful online revision resource is frcsplast.

What's it like as a consultant?

After obtaining your CCT, you are eligible to have your name on the GMC Plastic Surgery Specialist Register and therefore entitled to practise as a consultant plastic surgeon in the UK. Consultant practices vary depending on the size of the unit and subspecialty interest. As with other surgical specialties, developing an area of interest or even subspecialising is becoming the norm rather than the exception. These are the main subspecialty interests in plastic surgery:

- breast
- burns
- clefts
- cosmetic/aesthetics
- craniofacial
- ear reconstruction
- facial re-animation
- general paediatrics
- head and neck
- hand and upper limb
- lasers

- lower limb
- post-bariatric reconstruction
- soft tissue sarcoma
- skin oncology
- urogenital.

Consultants usually have one or two areas of interest or subspecialisation. However, due to the breadth of the specialty and need for on-call cover, most consultants provide a general plastic surgery service covering microsurgical reconstruction, hand trauma, lower limb trauma, general paediatric, wounds management and burns. In the larger units there is a move towards separating burns and other general plastic surgery on call, including hand trauma. As mentioned earlier, operating during the night is infrequent, especially with most trusts providing protected consultant-led trauma lists during the daytime. The on call can occasionally be busy but certainly manageable. Opportunities for private practice, usually in the form of aesthetic/cosmetic surgery, are also available for those who choose to pursue it. As mentioned earlier you get to work on a regular basis with other colleagues from different specialties. Most consultants work in teaching hospitals and also offer services, usually in the form of clinics, to peripheral district general hospitals.

Most plastic surgeons enjoy their job and the type of surgery they perform. The surgery is varied, interesting, challenging, stimulating and fun. I consider myself lucky to practise the art of plastic surgery and highly recommend pursuing this career. If you are interested in surgery, you will not regret it.

References

Barts and The London postgraduate diplomas in: Burn Care, www.icms.qmul.ac.uk/courses/burn%20care/index.html; and Aesthetic Plastic Surgery, www.icms.qmul.ac.uk/courses/aesthetic%20surgery/index.html

Courses organised by the Royal College of Surgeons, www.rcseng.ac.uk/education/courses/specialty/plastic.html

Courses run at Canniesburn Hospital, www.canniesburn.org/courses.html

E-Learning for Plastic, Reconstructive and Aesthetic Surgery, www.e-lfh.org.uk/projects/e-lpras/index.html (E- LPRS)

MY Plastic Surgery course, www.myplasticsurgerycourse.org/

North East International Flap course, www.northeastflapcourse.co.uk/

Northwick Park Microsurgery course, npimr.org/workshops

Ganga Medical Centre course, www.gangahospital.com/microsurgery/new/institute.html

Online resource for FRCS preparation, www.frcsplast.com/

Royal Society of Medicine Plastic Surgery Section meetings, www.rsm.ac.uk/academ/smtps.php

West Midlands Advanced Plastic Surgery Course UK, www.wapscourse.co.uk/index.html

Organisations

BAAPS (British Association of Aesthetic Surgeons; www.baaps.org.uk/): specialty trainees with NTNs can join as trainee members for only £50 per annum, which you can get back on the fee of the yearly scientific meeting if you attend. Trainee membership may become a pre-requisite for future full membership.

BAPRAS (British Association of Plastic Reconstructive and Aesthetic Surgeons; www.bapras.org.uk/): I highly recommend joining as a junior (foundation or core trainees) or specialty trainee (NTN). It costs £190 per annum. You can also join as a medical student. As a member you receive 63% discount on the scientific meeting fees and a substantial reduction to the Advanced Courses fees. You also receive a copy of the *Journal of Plastic Reconstructive and Aesthetic Surgery* (JPRAS). Fantastic value for the £190. Even if not a member the website is an excellent educational resource.

BBA (British Burns Association; www.britishburnassociation.org/): you can become a trainee member.

BSSH (British Society for Surgery of The Hand; www.bssh.ac.uk/): trainee membership cost £105 per annum. You get the European Journal of Hand Surgery as part of the membership.

Craniofacial Society of Britain and Ireland (www.craniofacialsociety.org.uk/)

PLASTA (Plastic Surgery Trainees Association; plasta.org.uk/): an excellent resource for general chat with other trainees, obtaining up-to-date information on politics, training, fellowships and courses. Membership is free.

Chapter 17
APPLYING FOR JOBS

Matt Stephenson

Introduction, 201
Key principles in applying for jobs, 201
Portfolio, 202
Curriculum vitae, 208
Application forms, 209
Interviews, 210
Common questions, 213
Getting career advice, 217
Coping with failure, 217
References, 218

Introduction

Applying for a job in surgery doesn't start the day the job applications are advertised. It started on your first day at medical school. If your career has been, ahem, hitherto inauspicious – today's the day to get your house in order. Preparation is key to succeeding in getting the job you want. If you've published a paper this year, completed an audit cycle and gone on a couple of courses, congratulations, you're about average. What you need is to set yourself apart from the crowd.

If the next round of job interviews seems a long way off: it's ages until you need to apply for core training, ST3 seems a lifetime away, or you're ST4 now and consultant interviews aren't for years – good – now's the time to start putting your application together. If you're juggling a full-time job and life in general, the notice given before interviews sometimes isn't enough time to polish your shoes, let alone complete a new audit and publish a paper.

But how, practically, can you start applying for a job when the application form isn't going to come out for several years? Well obviously you can't exactly – that's where the professional portfolio comes in (see later).

However, there are several themes common to surgical job applications regardless of the level applied for and these will be discussed in this chapter; the specifics of each level are dealt with in Chapters 5–7.

Key principles in applying for jobs

There are a few general principles to consider when it comes to applying for jobs/rotations, the theme common to all of them is to prepare and organise yourself early.

The Hands-on Guide to Surgical Training, First Edition. Matthew Stephenson.

1 Keep a **calendar/diary** to remind you of all the forthcoming dates when jobs are out (see the relevant sections of Chapters 5–7 for approximate dates for each level) and deadlines for applications to be in.

2 Choose **one single email address** and stick to it (i.e. not a trust email address which you can't check at weekends and will change if you move posts); all applications will require an email address so it had better be one that you check regularly and that you're not going to change.

3 **Bookmark on your web browser** the relevant body you'll be applying to next, e.g. the relevant deanery for ST3 applications to general surgery, and keep an eye on developments.

4 Ensure your **CV and portfolio** are kept as **up to date** as possible to help you fill in sections of the application forms more easily when the time comes.

5 **Download and view** the application forms at the **earliest opportunity** once they're released (this usually requires pre-registering); some of the questions require a good deal of thinking and the more time you have to think the better.

6 **Read all of the guidance** provided with the application forms and adhere closely to it.

7 Read through the **person specifications** to ensure you're going in at the right level.

8 **Prepare** thoroughly for the **interview**.

9 Keep **checking your emails** regularly for offers; time to reply is likely to be limited.

10 Throughout the process, don't leave anything until the **last minute**.

Portfolio

Portfolios these days have usurped the curriculum vitae (CV) as the primary documentary evidence of your achievements, the CV is merely relegated to a section of the portfolio. If your portfolio is bursting with relevant pages, applying for and getting the right job for you is considerably easier.

But portfolios aren't just for applying for jobs, they are also crucial evidence of your continued progression through training. They are therefore required for Annual Review of Competence Progression (ARCP) meetings for core and specialty trainees, so don't assume once you've got on to a rotation that you can dispense with it, it's something you will continually add to as you go along. It is a living document.

First, invest in a decent case to put your portfolio in. It's amazing at interviews how many people turn up with a battered old lever-arch file. It doesn't make it look like you've made much of an effort. Second, organise the sections properly in a sensible order with marker tabs between sections and an index at the front to help you find something quickly. Your interviewer will almost certainly take your portfolio from you to read it. Third, don't annoy them by making it difficult to locate something, or by putting vital documents all in a plastic sleeve that they then have to empty to look at.

Your portfolio needs to speak volumes. It should not only contain the usual vital documents but also convey your:

- enthusiasm as a doctor
- willingness to learn and train

- ability to reflect
- career looks well planned
- pride in your achievements
- organisational skills.

In addition to these you should demonstrate how you follow the principles of Good Medical Practice as outlined in the document of the same name published by the General Medical Council (GMC). Rather than organise your portfolio into sections equating to the principles, the easiest way to do it is to include a **mapping document** which points the reader to a section of your portfolio that demonstrates how you're following the principles of Good Medical Practice. This is particularly important later on in your career for appraisals, and including it at this stage shows your understanding of the overarching principles expected of doctors, and that you get the idea that these days no one trusts doctors on their word alone, they have to prove it. Once again, thanks for that Dr Shipman, *et al*.

Table 17.1 Ways in which you can show you are meeting Good Medical Practice standards

Domain of GMP	Examples of how you might prove it
Good Medical Care	Logbook Mini-peer assessment tools (PATs) Personal development plans Certificates of completion of stages of training, e.g. Foundation Achievement of Competency Document (FACD) Reflections on practice/complaints/critical incidents, etc.
Maintaining Good Medical Practice	Attendance at teaching sessions Attendance at courses Exam certificates Record of clinical governance/research activities Record of good use of study leave
Relationships with patients	Thank you letters Mini-PATs Patient questionnaires Complaints and how they were handled
Relationships with colleagues	Mini-PATs Other reviews from your consultant/trainer/assigned educational supervisor Other 360 degree assessments

Table 17.1 *(Continued)*

Domain of GMP	Examples of how you might prove it
Teaching and training	Record of teaching sessions you've been involved with Certificates of teaching on a course Feedback forms about your teaching Teaching courses you've been on
Probity	Via a statement as below
Health	Via a statement as below

There are some standardised ways of presenting part of your portfolio, such as through the Intercollegiate Surgical Curriculum Programme (ISCP) website. If you have kept up to date with all the form filling requested on the ISCP website, you can generate a PDF file which can form part of your portfolio. It would be divided into the following categories:

- global objectives
- learning agreements
- personal development plans
- case-based discussion (CBD) list
- CBD summary
- clinical evaluation exercise (CEX) list
- CEX summary
- procedure-based assessment (PBA) list
- PBA summary
- direct observation of procedural skills in surgery (SDOPS) list
- SDOPS summary
- evidence
- topics and progress
- logbook operations summary (ISCP)
- mini-PATs and multi-source feedbacks (MSFs).

This in fact provides only part of the portfolio. It covers just the in-house assessments, learning agreements and a logbook summary. It's then up to personal preference exactly how you structure the rest of your portfolio, and it depends on the stage you're at. Also you cannot for instance include a section on prizes unless you've won some. It's really up to you how you organise it, but make sure you include roughly the following.

- **Cover:** an attractive front sheet displaying your name and stating that it's your portfolio
- **Index/Contents page**
- **Section 1: Personal details** and basic things such as GMC number, on a single page.

■ **Section 2: Mapping document** for Good Medical Practice Principles. See above.

■ **Section 3: Statement of Health and Probity**. A page simply stating your signed declaration that you are healthy and fit to practise and not the subject of criminal investigations. Various versions are available to download such as from the ISCP website.

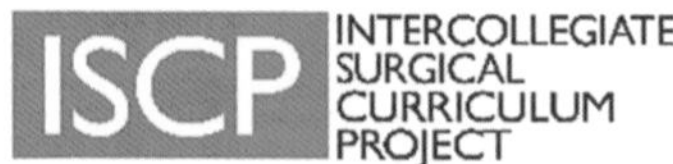

Statement of health and probity

Surgeons are dedicated to providing the best and most up to date care of their patients. They are morally accountable for their actions. Their conduct is guided by professional values and standards against which they are judged. All doctors, including those in training, must have integrity and honesty, and must take care of their own health and well-being so as not to put patients at risk. This is clearly laid out in *Good Medical Practice* (GMP).

As a trainee member of the profession of surgery these values and standards apply to you. It is essential that you understand your responsibility and accountability to your profession, to the surgical team and your employer. You must read the relevant sections of GMP before completing the self declaration forms. At the beginning of each placement, please confirm with your signature and the date that you comply with the Probity declaration (1.1 and 1.2 and the Health declaration 2.1 and 2.2).

1. Probity declaration

1.1 Professional obligations

I (the trainee) accept the professional obligations placed upon me in paragraphs 48 to 58 of *Good Medical Practice.*

1.2 Convictions, findings against you and disciplinary action

I (the trainee) confirm that since my last assessment / appraisal I have not, in the UK or outside:

- Been convicted of a criminal offence or have proceedings pending against me.
- Had any cases considered by the GMC, other professional regulatory body, or other licensing body or have any such cases pending against me.
- Had any disciplinary actions taken against me by an employer or contractor or have had any contract terminated or suspended on grounds relating to my fitness to practise.

Probity declaration 1.1 and 1.2

Signature of Trainee .... Date ....

Name of Trainee ....

Source: *www.iscp.ac.uk*

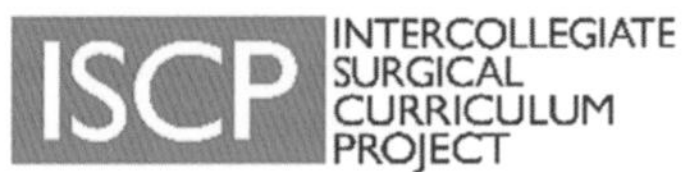

2. Health declaration:

2.1 Professional obligations

The GMC's guidance in *Good Medical Practice* regarding serious communicable diseases says that if a doctor has a serious condition which they could pass on to patients or colleagues they must have any necessary tests and act on the advice given to them by a suitably qualified colleague about necessary treatment and/or modifications to their clinical practice. Moreover, if their judgement or performance could be significantly affected by a condition or illness, physical disease or by taking medication, they must take and follow advice from a consultant in occupational health or another suitably qualified colleague on whether, and in what ways, they should modify their practice.

I accept the professional obligations placed on me in paragraphs 59 to 60 of *Good Medical Practice* and regarding serious communicable diseases.

2.2. Regulatory and voluntary proceedings

Since my last assessment / appraisal **I have not,** in the UK or outside:

- Been the subject of any health proceedings by the GMC or other professional regulatory or licensing body.
- Been the subject of medical supervision or restrictions (whether voluntary otherwise) imposed by an employer or contractor resulting from any illness or physical condition.

Health declaration 2.1 and 2.2		
Signature of Trainee	....	Date ....
Name of Trainee	....	

IMPORTANT NOTE:
If you are unable to sign the above declarations then you must discuss the matter with your Assigned Trainer or Programme Director immediately.

Figure 17.1 Example of a statement of health and probity, taken from the ISCP website. Source: www.iscp.ac.uk

■ **Section 4: Your curriculum vitae (see later)**. Most of the rest of the portfolio is really just an expanded version of your CV, so this forms a nice summary of the rest of the contents. It's sensible in fact to make the order of the contents of the CV roughly the same as the order of the contents of the portfolio.

■ **Section 5: Important certificates (originals)**. Simply as proof you've done them. Sadly no one trusts anyone on their word any more, even in medicine.

- Primary medical qualification
- Other degree qualifications such as an intercalated BSc
- Current GMC certificate (make sure it's in date)
- MRCS certificate if you have one already

- Completion of Foundation Competencies

■ **Section 6: Certificates for the courses you've been on,** particularly:

- Basic Surgical Skills (BSS)
- Advanced Trauma Life Support (ATLS)
- Advanced Life Support (ALS)
- Care of the Critically Ill Surgical Patient (CCrISP)

■ **Section 7: Results of post-graduate examinations**. Include letters telling you that you've passed (with the score you got if it's any good).

■ **Section 8: Courses or professional meetings attended**. Have you been to any conferences? Any regional meetings? Any drug rep lectures? Have a page to list all these and then insert the certificates of attendance for each meeting (almost all meetings of all descriptions now provide such certificates of attendance as they recognise the shift towards having to provide this evidence). Make sure you pick your certificate up at these events and put it straight into your portfolio before you lose it.

■ **Section 9: Publications and presentations**. Publications are still valued highly by interview panels. If you have several, have a sheet listing them all in the usual format and then print out the original papers themselves. Indicate if they have been presented at any national or international meetings (see Chapter 19 for more details).

■ **Section 10: Audit**. Include summaries of all the audits you've been involved in and what your role in them was. Were they presented in any directorate meetings at morbidity and mortality meetings for instance? Did you complete the audit loop? Have they changed practice? Some people even keep the agendas of directorate meetings at which they were presented if their name is on it. Certainly keep a copy of the summary of the audit itself in the portfolio.

■ **Section 11: Prizes and awards**. If you've managed to get a prize, make a big song and dance about it by giving it its own section. If you have several, all the better.

■ **Section 12: In-house assessment forms and learning agreements**. The ISCP website can be used for this section. This will be quite a large section and you may want to subdivide it if it's not already subdivided (i.e. if you haven't used the ISCP website). Include all the workplace-based assessments you've completed along with any current learning agreements and evidence of competencies. Currently, interview panels (and ARCP panels too) are putting a huge amount of weight on workplace-based assessments (whatever you may think of them). Make sure that you keep up with filling them out as you go along with your job.

■ **Section 13: Logbook**. This is a uniquely important part of job applications for surgical trainees. Make sure you keep it up to date as you go along, it's most unpleasant having to trawl through theatre logbooks for months retrospectively, especially if nobody bothered to put your name in if you were just assisting. Use an internet-based logbook such as that on www.elogbook.org. Be meticulously accurate about it and never ever lie, people have been caught out before and there would be grave consequences. Don't just include a print-out of all the procedures; you must include a consolidation sheet that summarises how many of each operation you've: (a) assisted with; (b) supervised trainer scrubbed; (c) supervised trainer unscrubbed; (d) performed; (e) trained a junior trainee to do.

- **Section 14: Teaching**. Include certificates for teaching on courses or feedback forms from students.
- **Section 15: Letters from patients**. If you've received any letters of thanks from patients, students or even staff, keep them.
- **Section 16:** Evidence of **reflective practice**. You can include a short section on reflective practice by talking about certain unusual clinical or non-clinical situations that have arisen and how you handled them. It doesn't have to be an essay, but anything showing you have insight into your practice and have the ability to reflect and improve is good.
- **Section 17: Extracurricular** activities. Include any Olympic gold medals or Oscars you may have won.

Curriculum vitae

The CV used to be the only way to tell a potential employer about yourself. Back in the days when you would apply directly to a hospital department for a job, you would usually be asked just to send in a covering letter, perhaps a basic application form and several copies of your CV. Application forms and portfolios have now usurped the CV in medicine; however, you still need a CV for your portfolio. It provides a good overview of the contents of your portfolio and is still favoured by many senior surgeons. It remains the standard way of applying for consultant posts and, for many trust posts that are not part of the main training schemes.

Some basics

- **Paper type** – choose a good-quality heavy paper printed at a high quality setting on your printer.
- **Font** – choose an easy-to-read font. The Serif style of font like Times New Roman tends to be less easy to read than the Sans Serif style of font like Arial, but this is less traditional. It's down to personal preference.
- It must be **well structured** with clear headings, which should be in a larger font.
- **Staple or bind together** – don't display each page in separate plastic sheets which are then inserted into your ring binder portfolio. This makes it difficult to take them out, especially if more than one person on the panel wants to have a look.
- **Print** more than one copy (for the reason above).
- **Up to date** – make sure you've deleted any old, out-of-date entries. If you used to be an avid opera goer but haven't seen a show for five years it will be awkward if they ask you what you've been to see recently.
- Run a **spellchecker** before printing.

Suggested sections

It's down to personal preference how you organise your CV and this may be affected by your own circumstances, strengths and weaknesses, but it should be arranged logically. It's sensible if it roughly mirrors your portfolio in terms of order, but here, in no particular order, are some suggested sections.

- **Personal details**
  - Name
  - Address
  - Home and mobile telephone number
  - GMC number
  - Professional memberships
- **Career aims**
  - A basic statement summarising where you're at in your training and where you want to be
- **Employment history**
  - Chronological beginning with most recent. State whether jobs were approved training posts
- **Pre-university examinations**
  - The more senior you become the less relevant this is and may be relegated to a single line
- **Undergraduate examinations**
  - Include the marks you got if you think it will help
- **Postgraduate examinations**
  - State the stage you're at with MRCS and whether you've passed the first part or both parts
- **Prizes** and **awards**
- List of **courses** attended
  - Don't forget about non-surgical ones like resuscitation training
- **Professional meetings** attended
  - For example the Association of Surgeons of Great Britain and Ireland (ASGBI) conference
- **Research** and **publications**
  - Include all that have been submitted. The interviewers are used to everyone saying they've submitted something or some work is in progress, especially if nothing's published already. Make sure you can back it up with evidence such as an email acknowledging receipt of the submission
- **Audit**
  - Include your role and whether the audit loop was closed
- **Teaching**
  - List your teaching activities, have you taught on any courses (if so, hopefully you got a certificate for it)?
- **Miscellaneous**
  - Journal Club
  - Extracurricular activities
- **Referees**
  - Include at least two, one of whom should be your current consultant

Application forms

Providing specific advice about filling in application forms is challenging, given that they vary depending on the specific grade and from year to year. In essence, you need your application form to stand out from the crowd, so consider very carefully how your answers sound, rewriting them as many times as necessary. The most crucial thing about your answers is to look at the **person specifications**, particularly the 'Personal skills' section and make sure that you're demonstrating as many of those characteristics in your answers as possible.

At least some of the questions come up in most application forms, for example 'Give details of outstanding achievements outside the field of medicine' and 'What experience do you have of teaching?', so save your answers to these to re-use on other forms if you're applying through more than one application process. This is likely to be less relevant now if national selection remains the norm as opposed to separate deanery applications.

In many specialties the application form has become much less of a priority for selection and indeed in 2011, for example, there was no short-listing for core surgical training, just long-listing. As long as you fulfilled the basic criteria for long-listing (i.e. primary medical degree, etc.) you would be invited for interview. There is currently a trend away from application forms as it's felt by many that they are inferior to physical selection centre processes (interviews, Objective Structured Clinical Examinations [OSCE], etc.) and that it's better to just invite everyone for interview.

Nevertheless, great care still needs to be taken to fill them in properly. Failing to put that you have passed your MRCS examination in the correct section of the form for ST3 applications, for example, has in the past resulted in immediate failure to meet long-listing criteria and hence no interview, which seems pretty harsh.

Interviews

The interviewers are looking to assess a number of things at interview and this varies to some degree according to the level for which you're applying. However, there is one fundamental feature at all levels from foundation to consultant – would they trust you to look after their patients? Aside from how many publications you've had or prizes you've won, do you seem like a safe, competent, honest doctor? This comes across in so many more ways than can be measured in the objective points scoring system now present at interviews. Much of it will come across in your demeanour, your dress, body language, rate of speech, confidence and many more unwritten or unspoken ways.

Of course there are no boxes on the interviewer's piece of paper to score you for all of these, they are highly subjective and officially they can't directly add up to points (or the withholding of points). However, if an applicant turns up to interview dressed as a pirate, bellowing their answers while performing cartwheels, even if they give perfect 10 out of 10 answers to all questions, it's very unlikely they'll be given the job. In other words, even though interviews now are more structured and there are marking systems in place, your interviewers are still human beings, and the marks they give will be influenced by the general impression you give, not just the detail of what you say.

In some specialties it is now the norm to have to give a pre-prepared presentation to the interview panel. Some specialties now have interviews in an OSCE style in which you rotate around different stations, some of which will include assessments of technical ability. Objective Structured Assessments of Technical Skills (OSATS) are also used in some selection processes, such as in ST3 applications to cardiothoracic surgery. Make sure you know exactly what to expect before you turn up on the day and if possible get advice from candidates who have gone through the process before.

Dress

First impressions are crucial. Few things give a poorer first impression than being dressed unconventionally or not appearing meticulously well groomed. You should wear a smart, conventional dark grey or black suit with polished shoes. If it has to be pin-striped, the stripes should be very subtle. Men should wear a non-eye catching tie, be clean-shaven with their hair cut short. You should look the part.

Body language

This may be obvious, but in an interview where the nerves are getting the better of you, your subconscious will take over and change your body language without you noticing. You must appear relaxed, but not so relaxed you slouch, and you must appear keen, but not so keen you're perched on the edge of your chair. Adopt a comfortable position without crossing your legs or your arms, this comes across as defensive. Unbuttoning your jacket helps make you appear open. Either hold your hands together in front of you or rest them on the table if there's one in front of you.

Equally, you shouldn't obsess over your body language, but if you can control it up to a point it will help. Be sure to shake every one of the panel members' hands on arriving and be sure to make eye contact with them at the same time and smile. Remember their names as you're introduced and try to call them by it later on in the interview – it makes anyone feel special being called by their name. If you didn't catch it first time, don't ask again.

Practice

In the past, trainees would tend to get a lot more interview practice as it was commoner for everyone to take six-month stand-alone SHO jobs or other middle-grade jobs. Now it's possible that having completed your foundation years you only have two interviews stages left before applying for consultancy: entry into core training and then specialty training. So you probably won't be quite so accustomed to interviews, but then neither will any of the other applicants. So take every opportunity for interview practice, ideally with a senior consultant who has experience of interviewing. Nobody likes role play, but try to make the most of experiences like this. It is possible to prepare roughly what you would say for many common interview questions, at least as a starter sentence, and trying these out on people really helps you decide if your answer makes any sense.

Prepare psychologically

Make sure you get a good night's sleep beforehand and attempt a decent breakfast if you can. Don't go to work on the morning of an interview, your trust should give you time off to prepare. If you have a long way to travel it's usually worth staying somewhere local the night beforehand, as public or private transport are both unpredictable and you don't need the stress of fearing being late too.

Take some deep breaths before being called in to the interview room. Remind yourself of all the positive aspects of your application and why you're so great. Ignore the size of other people's portfolios (they are often filled with entirely irrelevant rubbish). Plan something for afterwards that you can look forward to, to keep you feeling and appearing optimistic.

Know the facts

Make sure you know how you would answer all the common questions often asked at interview; this takes some preparation. Your answer doesn't have to be perfect in content, in fact at least some of the panel probably won't really be listening. They want to see that you've thought it through and you're delivering a structured answer.

Regarding clinical questions, of course, knowing the facts can be more important, and assuming you're applying for the appropriate level it's unlikely you'll be asked something that will completely knock you for six, as it will almost certainly be something commonly encountered at your stage of training. In general the interviewer wants to see that you can think logically around a problem and, above all, that you sound safe.

Questions

It's generally advised that you should ask questions of the interviewers, because it suggests that you're interested enough to have thought of a question. These days, however, because you don't apply to a specific hospital, rather to a deanery or indeed nationally, you can't ask 'will I have the opportunity to participate in Prof X's new extraordinarily exciting research project on lipoproteins and macrophages?' Any questions you could possibly think of will almost certainly be covered in the guidance notes, or the interviewers wouldn't know. Best avoided unless you can really think of something sensible.

Portfolio

Ensure your portfolio is immaculately presented and organised (see Portfolio section).

Know the system

Make sure you understand exactly how the system will work; this varies according to the level applied for and is subject to change year on year. Some interviews for instance are comprised of an OSCE system and others will simply involve rotation through three different areas of questioning. It helps to have as few surprises as possible on the day.

Know the panel

It is sometimes possible to contact those organising your interviews to find out who will be on the panel. This is sometimes helpful in that you can find out a little about their specialist interests and make sure you don't put your foot in it. For instance, saying that you've avoided doing a vascular surgery job because you don't like the smell of gangrenous extremities will win you no favours if your interviewer is a professor of vascular surgery (but it just might in the right jovial circumstances with colorectal surgeons). Even if you don't know specifically who will be on the panel it sometimes helps to know how many people there will be and in what capacity, for instance are there any lay people there. Will you be facing three people on the panel or 12? Again, it helps to have as few surprises as possible on the day.

Know the venue

If at all possible, do a dummy run to the venue the day before if you've never been there. Make sure you know how to get there and how long it will take.

Consider going on an interview course

There are many interview preparation courses available from medical student level through to consultant. These can provide an excellent opportunity to practise answering questions in front of a panel – role play that can be excruciating at the time but will pay off, especially if you receive useful feedback about your technique.

Common questions

The same old questions pop up over and over again, and the following list is by no means exhaustive. You should aim to prepare the first line or two of your answer to as many of the questions as you can (note that there's a lot of overlap between many of these questions, so you won't have to come up with that many answers); the interviewer is likely to drift off shortly anyway. There's also a lot of overlap between the different sections of questions; they could have all been listed together, but some attempt has been made to divide them up. In answering them, remember again what the person specifications are for that post, and try to fit them into your answer to score maximum points.

Remember that often there is no right or wrong answer, and particularly if they throw you a curved ball; they're looking to see if you can logically and coherently come up with an answer and don't get completely flummoxed. There will of course be variations on these questions depending on the level you're applying for, but not as much as you would think. For instance, a question such as 'What have you done that you're most proud of?' fits all levels and comes up with remarkable frequency. More commonly nowadays questions tend to be scenario based, i.e. you are presented with an awkward clinical or non-clinical situation to see how you would handle it. Again, they'll be marking you in accordance with the person specifications, so try to make your answer demonstrate, for instance, your calm judgement under pressure and your 'capacity to think beyond the obvious'.

Portfolio

- What is exceptional about your CV/Application/Portfolio?
- What part of your CV/application/portfolio are you most proud of?
- Name three areas of your portfolio you would like to improve over the next year.

- How many [insert operation] have you done this year? [referring to the logbook]
- There doesn't seem to be much in the research section.
- Tell us about [something in your portfolio].

Career plans

- What made you go into surgery?
- What is your long term-career plan?
- Where do you see yourself in 10 years time?
- Why do you want to do [insert specialty]?
- What have you done to prepare yourself for a career in [insert specialty]?
- What do you have to offer to [insert specialty]?
- What do you like about [insert specialty] and what do you dislike?
- What are the challenges facing [insert specialty] over the next 10 years?

Personal/General

- List three adjectives that best describe you.
- What would your friends/colleagues/patients say about you?
- What are your main strengths?
- What is your main weakness?
- What's your biggest achievement?/What have you done that makes you proud?
- What skills have you gained that will make you a good surgeon?
- What are the qualities of a good surgeon?
- Which placement have you particularly liked/disliked?
    - How do you measure success as a surgeon?
    - Would you be happy being an average trainee?
    - What have you done that is different to anyone else applying?
    - What makes you the best candidate for the job?
    - What do you think will be your biggest challenge in your training?
    - Tell us about the best consultant you've worked with.
    - Tell us about the worst consultant you've worked with.
    - What do you do to relax?
    - What experiences outside work have you found useful in your career?
- What makes you angry?
- How do you handle stress?
- How do you cope with pressure?
- How do you recognise when you are stressed?

Communication

- Give an example of a situation where your communication skills made a difference to clinical care.
- Have you had any communication skills training?
- How can you improve your communication skills?

■ Give an example of a situation where you failed to communicate well. What happened?

Working with colleagues and patients

■ You're about to finish five long days in a row on call and it's Friday 8pm, the doctor coming on to relieve you telephones to say he's got diarrhoea and vomiting so can't come in and asks you to do his shifts. What do you do?

■ Do you work better as part of a team or on your own?

■ What experience have you had working with a multidisciplinary team?

■ What makes a good leader?

■ What makes a team work well?

■ Have you experienced good leadership in the past from a colleague? What was good about it?

■ What is the difference between a manager and a leader?

■ Tell us about your experience of managing a team.

■ Tell us about a situation where you showed leadership.

■ How would you motivate your team?

■ Describe a situation where you had to give negative feedback to a colleague.

■ Give an example of a situation where your work was criticised. How did you handle it?

■ How would you cope if a complaint is made against you?

■ How would you approach the issue of a non-performing colleague?

■ How would you handle a situation where you had a disagreement with a nurse over the management of a patient?

■ What would you do if a patient disagreed with your treatment approach?

■ How do you react if a patient makes a suggestion about their treatment having researched it on the internet?

■ What difficult decisions have you made in a clinical setting, give a recent example?

Research and clinical governance

■ Is research important?

■ What is research?

■ Do you think all trainee surgeons should do research?

■ What obstacles do trainees face in trying to do research?

■ Tell me about your research experience.

■ Tell me about some interesting research you read about recently?

■ How did you organise your research project?

■ How do you go about setting up a randomized clinical trial?

■ What is evidence-based medicine?

■ How does evidence-based medicine affect [insert specialty]?

■ What are the pros and cons of evidence-based practice in surgery?

■ What are the different levels of evidence available?

■ What does impact factor mean?

- How many publications have you had this year?
- What is your understanding of the term 'clinical governance'.
- What is audit?
- Tell me about your audit experience.
- What is the difference between audit and research?
- What is the audit cycle?
- How does clinical governance affect patient safety?
- Do you think clinical governance is useful or is it just more bureaucracy?
- Who, in your hospital, is responsible for clinical governance?
- What is clinical risk management?
- What is a near miss? Can you give an example of one you experienced recently?
- What happens to critical incidents forms once they have been submitted?

NHS/Political issues

- What is NICE? What do they do?
- Tell us about a NICE guideline that you use in your practice.
- What is the National Patient Safety Agency?
- What do you know about the European Working Time Directive?
- What can you tell me about appraisals?
- What's the WHO surgical checklist? Is it important?
- What do you know about revalidation?
- What is the difference between assessment and appraisal?
- Is the expanding role of nurses a benefit or a danger to the medical profession?
- What is the difference between a protocol and a guideline?
- What do you think about management issues? Do you think it's something surgeons should be involved with?
- What is informed consent?

Teaching and training

- Tell us about your teaching experience.
- Have you had any formal training in teaching?
- What is problem-based learning?
- Now that trainees have less time for training how do you intend to get fully trained?
- What measures have you taken to improve your training?
- How do you identify your training needs?
- You're not getting enough opportunities in theatre with a particular consultant, how do you approach it?
- What e-learning resources do you use?
- What courses have you been on recently? What courses are you planning on attending in the next year?
- How did you keep your skills up to date during you research/career break?

Ethical issues

- How would you handle a problem doctor?

- You suspect a colleague/your consultant has come to work drunk, what do you do?
- One of you colleagues is always late for work. What do you do?
- How would you handle a patient who refuses to be treated by one of your colleagues because of his ethnicity?
- You see a patient verbally abuse a nurse. How do you handle it?
- Your consultant mentions something to a patient that you believe to be wrong. How do you react?
- You have suspicions that one of your colleagues has been stealing hospital property. What would you do?

Clinical

- You're on call on a weekend and in theatre with a patient anaesthetised on the table. Your consultant has said that he's happy for you to do [insert operation] when he arrives, but he's late. Simultaneously you're called by A&E to say a patient has come in with [insert condition] and by the wards about another patient with [insert problem]. What do you do?
- What is the biggest mistake that you have made in a clinical setting?
- Tell me about an interesting case you have managed recently? What went well?

Getting career advice

Useful career advice is often hard to find. Ask your seniors first but bear in mind they are likely to be biased towards (or even against) their own specialty, they may also be out of touch with current career issues. There are a number of internet options. Some generic information is available on www.medicalcareers.nhs.uk and www.support4doctors.org and more surgery specific advice on http://surgicalcareers.rcseng.ac.uk.

Coping with failure

Succeeding in job applications is open to a huge amount of luck and the system can be exceedingly harsh, especially if you've set your heart on a career in surgery. The system these days of, effectively, one chance per year is a particularly tough 'all or nothing' affair. Don't give up too easily, some of the very best surgeons have had to cope with rejection at some stage and had to keep applying, albeit when opportunities came around more frequently.

Ask yourself honestly why you didn't get the job, and even though it can be painful, ask around of the people you know that did get a job to see what they're offering that you're not. Forensically analyse your portfolio in the same way as the interviewers have and try to be as objective as possible. Have you simply not done enough research? Enough cutting? Enough workplace-based assessments? If so, fix it. Was your interview style too nervous? Your answers on clinical governance too vague? If so practise your interview style. Consider going on an interview course. Use the failure as an opportunity to revolutionise your portfolio and set yourself the aims that in the next year, before the next application round, you will have done X number of publications and audits, etc., or that you're going to spend every spare minute hanging around theatres building up the logbook.

Of course despite all of this, not everyone can get on in surgery, there simply aren't enough training posts in the UK for those that want to do it. First, you may wonder why you would want to stay in a small island of such inclement weather anyway and venture off to where there are more training opportunities in surgery, such as Australia or New Zealand. However, if emigrating isn't an option and surgery is the only thing you can envisage doing and you can't get a training post then you'll have to consider non-training jobs in the form of locum appointments or trust grades. Even though these are not formally training posts, they can be just as effective in getting you trained. At the end of the day the job is essentially the same as a training one – same patients, same colleagues, same duties – there just isn't the same onus of responsibility on the trust to train you and there is no deanery-related support. It is still possible to have a career as a surgeon without following the formal training pathway and there is also the option of getting onto the specialist register via Article 14 (see Chapter 21) if you have your heart set on becoming a consultant.

Finally, if the reality of your career prospects doesn't match up to your dreams, this can be a heartbreaking truth to accept. You need support around you: family, friends and you may want to think about the following:

- your GP
- Doctors Support Line 0844 395 3010 organised by the Doctors Support Network
- Surgeon-to-Surgeon helpline 020 7869 6212 organised by the Royal College of Surgeons
- support4doctors.org
- BMA Doctors for Doctors service 08459 200 169
- Royal Medical Benevolent Fund can provide financial support, on www.rmbf.org or by contacting a case worker directly on 020 8540 9194
- Samaritans 08457 90 90 90.

References

surgicalcareers.rcseng.ac.uk
www.iscp.ac.uk
www.medicalcareers.nhs.uk
www.mmc.nhs.uk

Chapter 18
FLEXIBLE TRAINING AND WOMEN IN SURGERY

Flexible training, 219
Maternity leave, 220
Women in surgery, 221
References, 224

Flexible training

Tamzin Cuming

Introduction

Officially known as less than full-time training (LTFT) to emphasise the pro-rata basis of it, training part time in surgery is an option for anyone (yes, even men!) who has 'a well-founded reason'. It's occasionally been used by surgical trainees with other major interests, e.g. sports or ballet. In reality, LTFT training is mainly to enable you to have children during training and split your time better between kids and work, and is principally taken up by women. It needn't be for ever, but it can be for as long as your kids are dependent (age 11, apparently). You can also use it if you have other dependants such as sick parents or your own health issues. It's helpful to be on a training scheme but not essential – locum appointments for training (LATs) can be part time, and trust doctors can make local arrangements. Most doctors who work less than full time are ST3+, although foundation year doctors can go part time and 33% of LTFT trainees are ST1–2.

So, what are the options for how you do it? As a trainee, you are encouraged to job share ('slot share'), where two people each working 50 or 60% of training share one ordinary full-time post; or alternatively you can go solo and do reduced sessions where you work say 80% of a full-time post. As these are part of 'normal' training jobs, you don't have to get special educational approval. If you want to create a new job as an 'extra pair of hands' (supernumerary) you now have to get this educationally

The Hands-on Guide to Surgical Training, First Edition. Matthew Stephenson.

approved beforehand. Also this latter option has to be fully funded by the deanery, and many areas can't afford them. Sort it out a long time in advance, or take one that has been set up (and approved!) already. This kind of thing is coordinated by the programme director, although knowledge about flexi training can be patchy among surgeons. Luckily there are websites that cover this subject area so at least you can be up on it, and some deaneries have knowledgeable LTFT staff or deans who can really help.

You no longer have to train at least 50%, although in fact most people do. This means half the hours and half the on call of the full-timers. Whether you have to do on call depends on the specialty and the training committee. If you are heavily pregnant, or breast-feeding then in some circumstances you'll be let off the on call, but it isn't a given. Obviously, if you train at 50% you have to do it for twice as long, in other words specialty training that would normally take six years will take 12 years. More likely, if you worked, say, three years at 70% you would extend a six-year programme by 11 months.

Difficulties with part-time working include communication with full-timers and job-share partners, and having good enough childcare. This can be a particular problem if you want to alternate days on a weekly basis to divvy up the operating equally in a job share (it wouldn't be fair for example if you always worked the Thursday and Friday and your job-share partner always did the Monday and Tuesday, and those are the operating days). In surgery, your first task is to find a job-share partner; look out for anyone at meetings who is pregnant or considering it. It's how I found my job-share partner. Despite a good job share, you can face difficulties in surgery with a system that inherently values extra effort as a sign of commitment. The bosses find it hard to take you seriously when you seem to be 'never there'. The best way over this is to find a genuinely supportive consultant in the region to work for – often, but not always, female. Approach them first informally. Word of mouth helps identify good 'flexi' trainers.

If you are planning a family, it's wise to obtain a national training number (NTN) first, as time to write papers, attend conferences and do research is limited in the early years of bringing up kids – despite what you (and your training committee) may believe, it's not possible for most people to write up a PhD during their maternity leave.

Maternity leave

Read up on it before you get pregnant! You can do with having worked for the NHS for six months before you get pregnant, as this will affect your rights. If you move jobs on a rotation it doesn't affect your rights, but if you are between rotations it can do. The NHS has to extend your contract if it expires just before you deliver. You have certain rights, which are common to all NHS workers. These include maternity leave of up to a year. Regarding maternity pay – be warned, it's for 39 weeks only, and the last 13 are at a pretty low level. Not many people know that three months of your maternity leave can be counted as training.

A personal angle

I've had three children during training – having got pregnant just as I got my training number (ST3 equivalent). I've tried it all: taken time out, worked one day a week, three days a week, gone back to training full time and finally worked in a slot share. Although some people do work full time with kids, I chose to work part time, and was supported in this by consultants, male and female, and by my partner. Financially, it works out similarly to full time – the extra money goes on childcare. Don't expect it to be an easy option – but then any mother will tell you that having kids is hard work, and having a job to come back to is a relief sometimes. Still, I get to see my kids and be a normal 'mum', as well as progressing in surgery.

Women in surgery

Ginny Bowbrick

Female surgeons have come a long way since the days of Dr James Barry (born 1797), who was forced to pretend to be a man in order to follow a surgical career. Extraordinarily, her deception was only discovered after her death. The first woman to obtain the Fellowship of the Royal College of Surgeons in England by examination was Eleanor Davies-Colley in 1911, and although women have sat on Council and held the position of Vice President of the Royal College of Surgeons of England, we still await the first female president of a surgical college.

WinS (Women in Surgery) was formed in 2007 and took over from WIST (Women in Surgical Training) which had been in existence for some 15 years. It states that its mission is 'to encourage, enable and inspire women to fulfil their surgical ambitions'. It aims to do this by raising the profile of women in surgery, understanding the issues faced by female surgeons, encouraging a positive attitude and changing negative ones, and providing advice, guidance and pastoral support for women at all stages of their career.

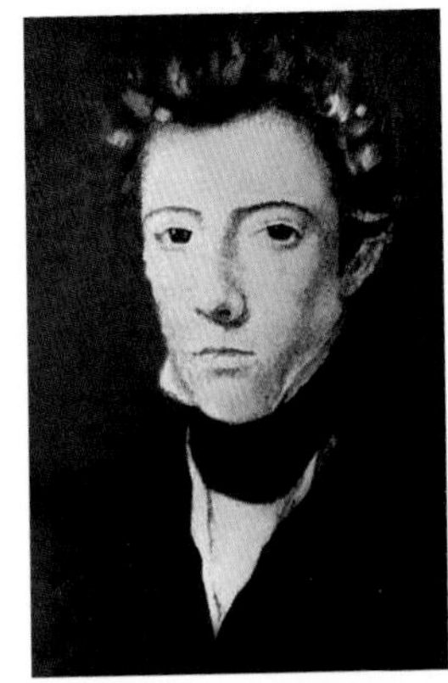

Figure 18.1 James Barry in the early 19th century. Source: Science Photo Library

However, with females now comprising more than half of all medical school graduates, why is the percentage of women choosing a surgical career and achieving consultancy so low in proportion? It can only be because surgery is not perceived by the majority of women to be a career they can follow. This is supported by Glynn and Kerin, who surveyed medical students and junior doctors on issues that would influence career choice and found that for women, lifestyle factors are the chief deterrents for choosing surgery as a career.

This is against the background of improvements in flexible training and not-whole-time working (otherwise known as part time). For a woman to pursue a career in surgery must be viewed as no different to a woman in any other profession, for instance a woman wishing to become a barrister or chair of a board in business. In fact, the report from the Royal College of Physicians in 2009 suggested a less favourable situation in professions such as law, dentistry and veterinary medicine than in medicine and that 'the main challenge ahead is no longer barriers to entry or delays to the career progression of women' – this is substantiated by the fact that young women have consistently been more likely to have a preference for general practice from an early stage.

The Royal College of Physicians undertook a two-year review to examine the changing gender balance in medicine and examine the implications for the profession in light of the changing dynamics of its workforce. Of note it found that the proportion of women among consultants varied across the specialties from more than 40% in paediatrics and public health to less than 10% in surgery. As there are fewer women at consultant level it therefore follows that there are fewer women in leadership roles, with an even smaller number on NHS trust boards as medical directors. This again doesn't reflect the true diversity of the profession.

At registrar level this study showed that the number of women in medicine rose from 11% to 18% between 1996 and 2006 and it is anticipated that within a decade women may make up the majority of newly certified trained specialists and therefore consultants in all specialty groups except radiology, ophthalmology and surgery. The report showed that while there were more male consultants in the surgery group than in any other group (at almost 25% of all male consultants) just under 6% of all female consultants were in this group. Within surgery there was a particularly poor female representation at consultant level in general surgery, cardiothoracic surgery, neurosurgery, urology, and trauma and orthopaedic surgery.

There are challenges to be broached for all women in surgery, apart from the constant juggling of home life and children for those who are mothers. Bloor *et al*. wrote a rather controversial paper in 2008 suggesting that female hospital consultants are '20% less productive than their male colleagues'. In a time of healthcare commissioning this would be viewed unfavourably by managers even if it meant a better service is being offered if, for example, women are spending more time with their patients. But the cause for the difference was unclear and was seen across all specialties; however, research such as this does little to promote women's place in the profession.

So what is the reality? From a personal perspective it never occurred to me 25 years ago when I decided to follow a surgical career as a medical student that it would not be possible as a woman to do so. I knew that I wanted to be a surgeon after assisting at my first operation, which was an appendicectomy. A minor setback was when in competition with a male colleague for a surgical house job the consultant at my teaching hospital stated he wanted the one who played rugby! So I reapplied six months later and was successful that time. Fortunately this couldn't happen now, in part thanks to changes in equality and diversity laws.

If you do not have a 'burning desire' to be a surgeon then you should rethink. I always suggest the 3am test to my trainees who are unsure about following a career in surgery – in other words if you are up at 3am how will you feel about it, especially thinking ahead to when you're in your forties, fifties or even sixties. If you don't have overwhelming enthusiasm in the daytime then you won't be happy to be in theatre in the middle of the night operating, although the out-of-hours demands of some specialties such as breast surgery aren't so onerous. This applies whether male or female.

Not all female surgeons will choose to have children and if they do choose not to their career pathway will be no different to a man's. Having children does complicate a surgical career in practice, but it doesn't make it impossible. I've chosen to work part time at 32 hours a week (which is equivalent to eight programmed activities, whereas a whole-time consultant will typically work 10 to 12). I enjoy my days in mother mode at the school gates talking to the other mums, although this is complicated by the fact that I'm a single mother and in addition, two of my children have special needs. Life is a case of constantly juggling and balancing my children and surgical career while finding a few moments for myself.

I also chose to have my children at the end of my surgical training as I was concerned about working part time as a trainee. This of course raises all the problems of leaving motherhood to later in life, with age-related lower fertility rates and the associated pregnancy-related problems for the mother, such as gestational diabetes, and also birth defects, especially those involving chromosomal abnormalities such as Down syndrome for the baby. In your early twenties it's easy to put off thinking about having children, but the biological clock does exist in the thoughts of most women at some stage of their life. Of women trying to get pregnant without using fertility drugs or in vitro fertilisation at age 30, 75% will get pregnant within one year, and 91% within four years; at age 35, 66% will get pregnant within one year and 84% within four years; and at age 40, 44% will get pregnant within one year, and 64% within four years. These figures are for pregnancies ending in a live birth and take into account the increasing rates of miscarriage in older women.

So where to start if you are thinking of following a surgical career? I would recommend a look at the WinS section of the Royal College of Surgeons of England website. They are able to advise you from before applying to medical school. They run workshops, as well as giving advice to those at medical school or already on a surgical career pathway. Most women find it easier to have a role model, which is true for whichever pathway in medicine you choose, and again if you have no one in mind the WinS office will point you in the right direction. It doesn't have to be a woman either.

There is no reason for a woman not to have a fulfilling career in a specialty as rewarding and stimulating as surgery – your gender does not preclude you but your preconceptions of surgery may.

References

Bloor K, Freemantle N, Maynard A (2008) Gender and variation in activity rates of hospital consultants. *Journal of the Royal Society of Medicine* **101**: 27–33.

Cuming T, Evans R, Bowbrick V (2010) Job sharing. BMJ Careers 29 June (http://careers.bmj.com/careers/advice/view-article.html?id=20001162).

Glynn RW, Kerin MJ (2010) Factors influencing medical students and junior doctors in choosing a career in surgery. *The Surgeon. Journal of the Royal Colleges of Surgeons of Edinburgh and Ireland* **8**(4): 187–91.

NHS employers have a maternity fact sheet with a flow chart (www.nhsemployers.org/Aboutus/Publications/Pages/MaternityIssuesForDoctorsInTraining.aspx)

Royal College of Physicians (2009) *Women and Medicine: the future*. London: RCP. (www.rcplondon.ac.uk/Pubs/contents/bd2d994a-7d38-465f-904a-21a70cdc7d9c.pdf).

Royal College of Surgeons of England information (http://surgicalcareers.rcseng.ac.uk/flexible-working/training).

WebMD Fertility Treatment Less Successful After 35 (www.webmd.com/content/article/89/100183.htm).

West Midlands LTFT training website (www.westmidlandsdeanery.nhs.uk/Home/LessThanFullTimeTrainingFlexibleTraining.aspx).

Women in Surgery, Royal College of Surgeons of England (http://surgicalcareers.rcseng.ac.uk/wins/mission-goals#).

Chapter 19
ACADEMIC SURGERY

Amyn Haji

Overview, 225
Academic surgery for interviews and vivas, 225
How do I get a publication? 230
Research in practice, 230
References, 232

Medicine, the only profession that labours incessantly to destroy the reason for its existence
James Bryce (British academic)

Overview

This chapter is intended to give you an overview of the important academic surgical issues that you may face throughout your core and specialist training. It should offer you an insight to the pathway of academic surgery should you wish to pursue this path. Alternatively, for many of you who do not wish to dedicate your career to academia, you will still face academic hurdles at all stages of your surgical career with interviews, audit and publications being only some of the challenges.

Surgery historically has been heavy on research. The ability to churn out papers or to have spent precious years of your life at a lab bench pipetting growth factors or staining cell markers, has been deemed helpful to a surgical career. Being an avid researcher may not make you a technically better surgeon, but it's worth paying attention to as it will provide you with the opportunity to supervise your own research students in the future and also most of your seniors will have been through a system that values research.

Academic surgery for interviews and vivas

Reviewing a paper

Several interviews now expect **critical appraisal** of a peer-reviewed publication as part of the interview process. In fact, paper review also forms part of viva voce surgical examinations, in the Fellowship of the Royal College of Surgeons exit exams for instance.

The Hands-on Guide to Surgical Training, First Edition. Matthew Stephenson.

The candidate should note that on reviewing a paper, examiners do not expect only a summary of the content of the paper. It's imperative that you consider the **clinical relevance** of the study. Below is a simple checklist that will provide you with a structure for evaluating any manuscript.

1 **General issues**

- **Which journal** is the publication in? Is it reputable? The latter does not necessarily indicate that the study is well conducted and of high quality.
- **Who** wrote the paper? Do they or their institution have a good academic record?
- Is the paper **interesting and relevant**?
- What **level of evidence** is this? (see later in chapter)
- What is the **impact factor** of the journal? The impact factor (IF) is a measure reflecting the average number of citations to articles published in the journal. It's determined on an annual basis and gives a proxy for how important that journal is within that specialty. You would hope to get your own publication into a journal with a high impact factor. It can be calculated using the following formula:

$$\text{IF for 2008} = \frac{\text{number of times articles published in 2006/7 cited by journals in 2008}}{\text{Total number of citable articles published in 2006/7}}$$

(Please note that the citation index is the index of citations between publications, allowing the reader to establish which later documents cite which earlier documents.)

2 Does the **abstract** reflect the content of the paper? Is it clear and concise?

3 **Introduction**

- Does the background or introduction address the relevant points and pose the relevant questions?
- What is the **hypothesis** and was this clearly stated?
- What are the aims and the **primary and secondary outcomes**?

4 **Methodology**

- Was there an **appropriate group** of patients/subjects studied?
- Is there any **selection bias**?
- Were these patients a **representative** group encountered in general surgical practice?
- How were patients **recruited**?
- What were the **inclusion** and **exclusion criteria**?
- Is the **sample size justified**?
- Was a **power calculation** done with an appropriate study design?

For **randomised controlled trials**:

- **How** was randomisation performed?
- Were the groups treated **equally** other than for the experimental intervention?
- What were the **outcome measures**?

- Was a **power calculation** performed and an appropriate sample size sought?
- Were the patients and healthcare professionals **blinded** to the treatment?
- Are all patients who entered the trial accounted for? Are there any **missing data**?
- Are **side effects** and **adverse outcomes** clearly stated?
- What was the **duration of follow-up**?

Statistics:

- Are the **methods described clearly**?
- Are **appropriate tests** used for the data presented?
- Was the analysis performed as per **protocol** or on an **intention to treat** basis? These terms and the distinction are important to understand. For example, if a study was comparing outcomes between laparoscopic and open colorectal surgery and some patients were converted from laparoscopic to open surgery. With an analysis per protocol design, patients who were converted would be treated as the same as the open group, whereas they would remain in the laparoscopic arm for analysis in an intention to treat design. In other words, if you intended to treat them with a laparoscopic operation to begin with, you should still count them in that group even if they end up with an open operation.

5 Results

- Are the results set out **clearly**? Are they presented in a biased manner?
- How large is the **treatment effect**?
- Is there sufficiently long **follow-up?**
- Are significant complications excluded from the analysis?
- Is there a **Type I** or **Type II** error?

Type I error: the study shows a difference between the samples when, in fact, there isn't one.

Type II error: a difference is in fact present between the samples but the study methods failed to show one.

6 Discussion

- Were the **aims** of the study fulfilled?
- What are the **novel observations**?
- Are **errors** in the paper **discussed**?
- Is there appropriate comparison made with a sound **literature review**?
- Are the **conclusions justified**?
- Can the results be **generalised to other populations**?
- What do you think of the paper? **Would you publish it**?

Key academic topics or definitions you may be asked during an interview or viva

1 What are the different levels of evidence based on type of study design?

There are several classification systems in use for the hierarchy of evidence. These include the following.

(a) Scottish Intercollegiate Guidelines Network (www.sign.ac.uk/guidelines/fulltext/50/annexb.html)

(b) Oxford Centre for Evidence-based Medicine (www.cebm.net)

(c) American College of Chest Physicians (www.biomedcentral.com)

(d) Australian National Health and Medical Research Council (www.nhmrc.gov.au)

(e) US Task Force on Community Preventative Services (www.thecommunityguide.org)

Although there are various classifications, they all have the same basis.

- Level 1 – randomised controlled trials (RCTs)
  - 1a meta-analysis of RCTs
  - 1b RCT
- Level 2 – non-randomised studies
  - 2a control study but no randomisation
  - 2b quasi-experimental study
- Level 3 – non-analytical studies, e.g. case reports, case series
- Level 4 – expert opinion

2 Define sensitivity

Sensitivity is the proportion of those with the disease who test positive in the study group (a/a+c).

3 Define specificity

Specificity is the proportion of those without the disease who test negative in the study group (d/b+d).

	Disease present	**Disease absent**
Positive result	True positive (a)	False positive (b)
Negative result	False negative (c)	True negative (d)

4 What is the difference between the mean and the median?

The **mean** is the sum of all the values divided by the number of observations and it is sensitive to outliers.

The **median** is the middle value when all observations are ranked from lowest to highest and it is less sensitive to outliers.

5 What is the standard deviation?

Standard deviation is the measure of scatter or variability of the data distribution and measures the degree to which an individual value deviates from the population mean. It is not dependent on sample size.

6 What is relative risk (RR), absolute risk reduction (ARR) and number needed to treat (NTT)?

RR = likelihood of experiencing the outcomes in the group with the risk factor divided by the likelihood of experiencing the outcomes in the group without the risk factor.

ARR = this represents the percentage of patients who did not have the adverse outcomes because of absence of risk factor.

NNT = this is the inverse of ARR. It represents the number of patients that must be treated to prevent the occurrence of one case.

7 What is the difference between odds ratio and relative risk?

Odds ratio is defined as the probability of experiencing an outcome divided by the probability of not experiencing the outcome. It is favoured for case-controlled studies and retrospective studies.

Relative risk is the intuitive measure of differential likelihood of disease. It is often used in randomised clinical trials or cohort studies.

8 What is confidence interval (CI)?

Confidence intervals provide a useful tool to determine a range of values in which parameters of the target population are likely to lie. For example, a 95% CI represents a range of values that will include the true population parameter in 95% of all cases.

9 What does the null hypothesis mean and what is the P value?

Null hypothesis = no difference exists between study groups.

Alternative hypothesis = there is a significant difference between study arms.

The P value is statistically significant if it is smaller than the threshold of statistical significance, usually set at 0.05. P values depend on standard deviation and the sample size. The larger the difference between the groups, the smaller the standard deviation, or the larger the sample size, the more significant the P value.

10 Describe some types of study

Randomised controlled trials (RCTs)

RCTs are the gold standard for evaluating the effectiveness of an intervention and minimise the risk of confounding factors. There is a 22-item checklist developed to encourage better reporting of RCTs namely the Consolidated Standards of Reporting Trials statement (CONSORT).

Quality of RCTs are assessed using the Jadad scale which is a validated scale that assesses the methods used to obtain double blinding, random assignment and a description of dropouts by the intervention group. Jadad is scored from 1 to 5, with scores less than 2 indicating lower quality studies.

Observational studies

These studies include case-control and cohort studies. There are guidelines published to improve the quality of reporting of observational studies similar to the CONSORT statement. This is termed Strengthening the Reporting of Observational Studies in Epidemiology (STROBE).

The quality of such studies is evaluated using three criteria which include study group selection, group comparability and outcome measures using a scale developed in collaboration between the Universities of Newcastle

(Australia) and Ottawa (Canada) – the Newcastle-Ottawa Scale.

11 What is a meta-analysis?

A **meta-analysis** is a systematic review that uses statistical methods to integrate the findings of several studies into a collection of data. This statistical procedure can quantitatively define the degree and direction of an association. There are various steps taken to conduct a meta-analysis.

1 Subject selection.

2 Retrieval of primary studies.

3 Evaluation of study quality and selection of studies to be used.

4 Selection of either the Fixed Effects statistical model, which assumes that there is no heterogeneity between individual trials, or the Random Effects model. The latter is probably more appropriate in surgical research as this takes random errors and other sources of variation into consideration.

5 Evaluation of heterogeneity.

6 Results of meta-analysis evaluated for reproducibility or sensitivity testing to ensure that the result is not influenced by bias.

How do I get a publication?

It is not often easy to be successful in publishing your manuscript in a reputable journal, and it is not unusual to try several journals before gaining acceptance. There are a number of resources to help you in structuring a manuscript in order to maximise your chances of a positive peer review, for example the *British Journal of Surgery* 'How to write a paper' series of online articles and conference workshops. However, the main difficulties often lie in identification of a suitable research project and dedicating sufficient time to this task amidst a busy clinical schedule. Nowadays, numbers of publications seem to feature in the selection process of most clinical posts and, therefore, it is important to maximise on this and utilise every opportunity during your training.

First, be proactive and enquire whether there are any research projects available by asking the consultants and senior trainees individually. There may be some projects that have been started by previous trainees that you could finish. Alternatively, be on the lookout for unusual case reports at audit meetings, surgical handovers, radiology meetings and clinics, and offer to write up these reports at the earliest opportunity. Working in collaboration with other colleagues increases your chances in being successful with publications and should be encouraged, as long as each of you has a defined role, which should be stated while preparing your manuscript. Motivation for producing papers is often difficult. Producing a list of deadlines for abstract submission to surgical meetings may continuously remind you to be persistent in your approach.

Research in practice

Competition for core and specialty training posts and indeed consultant surgical appointments is fierce and it is therefore no surprise that trainees need to maximise their clinical and academic experience throughout medical school and post qualification. It is often difficult to outline advice about academia as this will differ from individual to individual. Irrespective of the advice given, all doctors in training need to maximise their involvement in clinical audit and peer-reviewed publications. These should be undertaken during clinical training, even if you are not contemplating a career in academic surgery. Prior to embarking on a period of formal research and all the time and money this involves, or entering an academic route of training, it's prudent to determine where you would like to practise as a consultant surgeon and whether you wish to be actively involved in undergraduate and postgraduate education. This may reflect on whether you wish to pursue a higher degree, as the requirements for securing a consultant job in a university teaching hospital as a lecturer may be different to those needed for another establishment without the same credentials.

There are various academic programmes available for trainees, both full and part time, and also within and separate from formal academic fellowships. Some of these opportunities are outlined in this chapter.

Academic training pathways

There are training opportunities during specialist training which are competitive for doctors who wish to pursue an academic pathway in surgery. There are integrated academic training programmes which include the following.

- **Academic Clinical Fellowships (ACFs):** these are competitive-entry training posts that offer clinical duties for 75% of the programme and research for the remaining 25% over a three-year period for surgical trainees. These posts are designed for trainees early on in their career pathway and will be awarded a national training number (NTN) and recognised as an academic trainee.
- **Clinical lectureships:** these posts are for trainees more advanced in their specialty training and require the candidate to have already undertaken a research degree such as a MD/MS or PhD. The post has 50% clinical commitment and 50% research study. The programme runs for four years and it is expected that the post holder would have completed their specialty training during this time.

Research degrees

There are several part-time and full-time posts available that are suitable for surgical training. These can be undertaken prior to starting your specialty training or during time out of programme later on in specialist training for a period of two to three years. The route that you choose to take will depend on your personal circumstances and also whether you are initially successful in obtaining a NTN. A formal research degree at an earlier stage in your career will make you more competitive at both core and specialist training interviews. On the other hand, research later on in your surgical training could help you focus your research on your clinical interests, which may help you in securing a consultant post in that same specialty. Whichever path you choose to take, some research interest – educational, basic science or clinical – will benefit you at some stage in your surgical career.

Masters in surgical education

Teaching and educational interest is something that everyone states on their CV and application forms. Formalising this interest by undertaking a degree in education distinguishes you from your colleagues. Masters in Surgical Education are available both part time, usually over two years, or full time for a one-year period. Examples of such programmes include those from Imperial College (www3.imperial.ac.uk/edudev/programmes/medsurged) and from the University of Dundee. The latter programme is in collaboration with the Association of Surgeons of Great Britain and Ireland (www.asgbi.org.uk/en/postgraduate_qualifications/medical_education__university_of_dundee.cfm).

Masters in Surgical Science or Practice (MSc Surgical Science)

The majority of universities offering medical undergraduate education offer an MSc either part time over two or three years or full time over one academic year. Some of the part-time courses are integrated during the first three years of specialist surgical training such as that offered by Kent, Sussex and Surrey Deanery at the University of Kent. This requires regular attendance to complete a modular programme in two years with a research dissertation in the final year. If time is a constraint for you, then a part-time distance learning MSc may be more appropriate, such as that offered by the University of Edinburgh. (www.essq.rcsed.ac.uk/site/2741/essq_overview.aspx#onl).

Doctorate of Medicine Research (MD(Res)) and Doctorate of Philosophy (PhD)

Although all universities offer full-time research degrees, it's often difficult to arrange a suitable research post with adequate funding and supervision. An MD is often more suited to those wishing to undertake clinical research, whereas basic science is more often than not a requirement for a PhD thesis. However, there are exceptions and any project with substantial weight could pass as a PhD.

Advertisements for such posts are usually advertised in NHS jobs or in the British Medical Journal Careers, but do look out for jobs advertised as 'Research Fellow' as well, as these may have the potential to offer you the opportunity to take things further formally. It is often recommended to write to and visit the professorial units looking for opportunities to undertake either an MD or a PhD. Formal funding for MD posts are hard to come by and you may need to carry out some clinical duties or participate on the emergency rota.

References

www.biomedcentral.com

www.cebm.net

www.nhmrc.gov.au

www.sign.ac.uk/guidelines/fulltext/50/annexb.html

www.thecommunityguide.org

Chapter 20
OTHER ISSUES IN SURGICAL TRAINING

Matt Stephenson

Who's who and what's what? 233
Recent historic changes to surgical training, 239
New Deal and the European Working Time Directive, 241
Money, 243
References, 249

When I review my own professional life and its many satisfactions, the greatest are not the surgical operations I have performed, nor the thousands of patients that I have cured, but the successful young surgeons whose instruction and training I have directed

George Heuer (American surgeon, 1882–1950)

Who's who and what's what?

There are many professional bodies, groups and individual roles involved in surgical training that may appear a mystery – what do they do exactly? How can they impact on your training? It always pays to know who your enemies are… Not enemies, of course, no. One means to say those groups that don't on the surface appear to do much, but which behind the scenes have important parts to play in improving surgical training. The subject may even pop up now and again in interviews.

So who is actually responsible for the quality of training? Well the situation is in a certain amount of flux and there are many possibilities for how things will go in the future, but currently it falls under the following four bodies.

- The General Medical Council (GMC) (formerly PMETB): responsible for overall **quality assurance (QA)**.
- Postgraduate deanery: responsible for **quality management (QM)**.
- Royal College: input into **quality management (QM)**.
- Local trusts: local education providers are responsible for **quality control (QC)**.

PMETB (now absorbed into the GMC)

On 30 September 2005 a new independent non-governmental organisation

The Hands-on Guide to Surgical Training, First Edition. Matthew Stephenson.

was born. Its name was the Postgraduate Medical Education and Training Board. It replaced the Specialist Training Authority (STA), the previous regulatory body which will be familiar to senior trainees. It set about trying to assess, improve and standardise the curricula of all the different specialties, medical and surgical. On 1 April 2010 it was absorbed into the GMC on the recommendation of the Tooke enquiry. The GMC now has the role of PMETB – PMETB no longer exists but is still frequently referred to in non-up-to-date documentation. The GMC also has the role of enrolling you on the specialist register once you have your Certificate of Completion of Training (CCT).

The GMC's role has now been extended to 'secure and maintain standards in postgraduate medical education and training in the UK'. The GMC is now the body responsible for approving posts and programmes as training jobs as opposed to non-training jobs, i.e. counting towards the eventual Certificate of Completion of Training

Postgraduate deanery

The deanery is responsible for implementing the curricula approved by PMETB. It must work with the local healthcare providers, usually the trusts, and also with the royal colleges (the Royal College of Surgeons in our case), to quality manage postgraduate training. This is usually assisted by educational contracts between the deanery and the trust. The following is a list of deaneries:

- East Midlands (North and South)
- East of England Deanery
- London Deanery
- Northern Deanery
- North Western Deanery
- Mersey Deanery
- Wessex Deanery
- Oxford Deanery
- Kent, Surrey and Sussex Deanery
- South West Peninsula Deanery
- Severn Deanery
- West Midlands Deanery
- Yorkshire and the Humber
- Wales Deanery
- West of Scotland Deanery (covering the West of Scotland programme)
- South East Scotland Deanery (covering the East of Scotland programme)
- Northern Ireland Deanery

Royal College of Surgeons

The Royal College of Surgeons is our professional body, the membership of which we gain by passing the MRCS exam, the fellowship of which we later gain by passing the FRCS exam. There are three royal colleges in the UK (with one more in the Republic of Ireland):

- the Royal College of Surgeons of England (also covers Wales and Northern Ireland)
- the Royal College of Surgeons of Edinburgh
- the Royal College of Physicians and Surgeons of Glasgow.

The roles of the Royal College of Surgeons are laid out on its website (here from the England website):

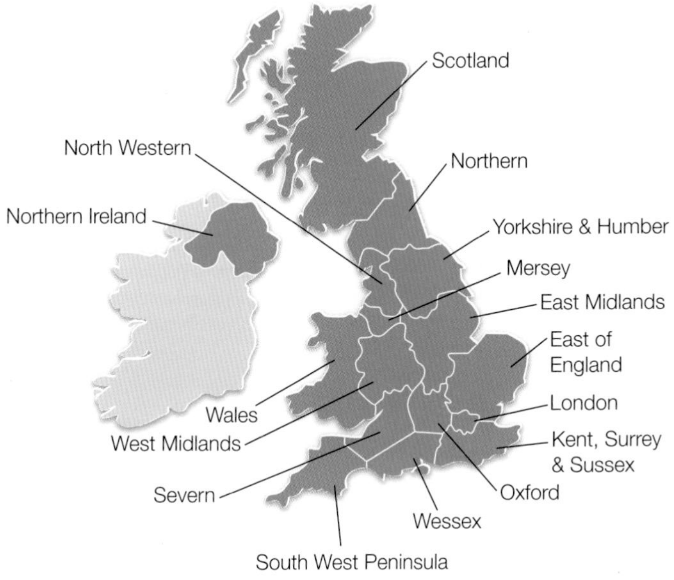

Figure 20.1 The UK postgraduate deaneries.

What the Royal College of Surgeons do

- Supervise training of surgeons in approved posts.
- Provide educational and practical workshops for surgeons and other medical professionals at all stages of their careers.
- Examine trainees to ensure the highest professional standards.
- Promote and support surgical research in the UK.
- Support audit and evaluation of clinical effectiveness.
- Provide support and advice for surgeons in all stages of their careers.
- Provide a mechanism whereby trusts can seek independent advice.
- House a current and historical information resource centre for surgeons in the library and museums.
- Act as an advisory body to the Department of Health, health authorities, trusts, hospitals and other professional bodies.
- Collaborate with other medical and academic organisations in the UK and worldwide.
- Seek to convey the importance of, and provide support for, good, effective communication and interpersonal relationships between patients and surgeons.

What The Royal College of Surgeons don't do

- Register or license surgeons to practise nor have responsibility for disciplinary actions; this is the responsibility of the General Medical Council (GMC).
- Process complaints from patients; this is another responsibility of the GMC or a function of individual hospitals.
- Recommend individual surgeons to patients or offer patients medical advice; the College recommends that patients always seek referral through general practitioners.

Local trusts

The hospital for whom you work and who are charged with providing you with training, among the other responsibilities of any other employer. You are paid by both the deanery and also the trust; your job therefore has both training and service elements.

Who's who?

Training programme directors (TPDs)

TPDs organise, manage and direct specialty training programmes, including core training and specialty training. They will have the support of a local faculty including assigned educational supervisors (AESs). They will oversee the stages of a surgical trainee's progression through training.

Surgical tutor

This is a consultant employed by the trust to ensure, on the ground, that training is being implemented and acts as a link between the trust, the deanery, the school of surgery and the royal college.

Head of school

The head of a school of surgery is jointly appointed by the Royal College and the deanery.

Assigned educational supervisor

This is a consultant who will normally have between one and four trainees under their supervision at any one time. They are there to help you set and achieve your educational objectives using learning agreements and help with other aspects of your training.

Clinical supervisor

A consultant answerable to the AES and the most direct link to training. This is usually the consultant for whom you work.

Other organisations

There are a number of other organisations that are also involved in surgical training, often with mysterious acronymic titles.

JCST

The Joint Committee on Surgical Training is an advisory body to the Royal Colleges of Surgeons when it comes to matters of surgical training. It used to be the Joint Committee on Higher Surgical Training but its role has broadened to include core training. It is the parent body of the Intercollegiate Surgical Curriculum Programme (ISCP). Since August 2008 trainees must pay £125 per annum to the JCST. This supports the running costs of the JCST, the ISCP and the OCAP (Orthopaedic Curriculum and Assessment Project) and was introduced following the withdrawal of government funding to the royal colleges (who used to pay all of it). Core trainees, FTSTAs and specialty trainees (but not foundation doctors) must all pay it, otherwise you can't use any of the facilities such as the ISCP website and you won't be able to gain your CCT thus exiting from training.

SAC

The Specialty Advisory Committee is a subcommittee of the JCST and there is one for each of the nine surgical specialties. There are a few additional ones for so called training interface groups, which are for particular sub-subspecialties in which there is considerable crossover between main subspecialities, such as hand surgery and breast reconstruction.

Postgraduate schools of surgery

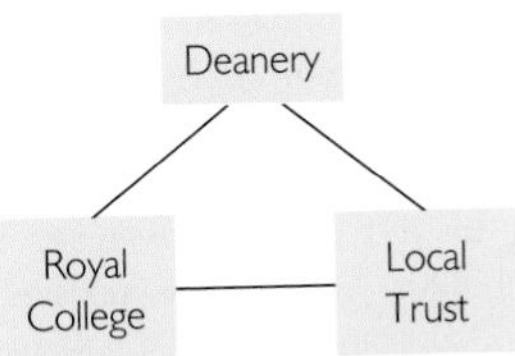

Schools of surgery have been set up in recent years to facilitate the partnership between the deaneries, the Royal College of Surgeons and the trusts. There are schools of surgery for each deanery in England, Wales and Northern Ireland (and there is equivalent of the Surgery Specialties Training Board for NHS Education in Scotland). It should oversee all aspects of training in the nine surgical specialties. Its purposes are to:

- ensure standards of education and training at programme and healthcare provider level which are commensurate with the curriculum
- meet patient needs by developing competent surgeons
- develop and nurture the trainer–trainee relationship
- champion patient needs by ensuring standards are monitored
- develop academic programmes
- provide areas of specific/speciality educational opportunities.

The school will support and integrate, at a local level, the deanery functions of:

- teaching and learning
- managing education and training programmes and posts
- faculty development
- curriculum, syllabus and content (real and virtual)
- trainee selection
- assessment of progress
- quality assurance and evaluation
- educational research
- resource management
- development of innovative education and training programmes according to service need.

(www.rcseng.ac.uk/regional/documents/college_guidance_on_schools_19feb07.pdf)

In short, from the start of core training to CCT, postgraduate schools of surgery are there to coordinate your surgical education. Each surgical school (and there are various schools across England and Wales) is accountable to the local dean but also reports to the Royal College of Surgeons and the Strategic Health Authority. Each school has a board which comprises at least: programme directors of each of the surgical specialties and the core programme director, a deanery advisor, a senior academic (usually a professor of surgery), a trainee representative (a useful role to take on if you get the chance), a college coordinator and deanery administrator.

Raven Department of Education
The Raven Department of Education is run by the Royal College of Surgeons of England and runs courses for surgeons from foundation stage to consultant. There are also education departments at the other royal colleges.

ISCP (www.iscp.ac.uk)
The Intercollegiate Surgical Curriculum Programme 'provides the framework for systematic training from completion of the foundation years to consultant level'. It is administered through the www.iscp.ac.uk under the auspices of the JCST. You pay for it, therefore, with your £125 per annum fee (to be reviewed August 2012) to the JCST. It is the central online resource for organising and recording your assessments, logbook and general career progression. It is the place to access the surgical curriculum for all nine specialties and has the following intentions.

- A common format and framework across all the specialties within surgery.
- Systematic progression from the foundation years through to the exit from surgical specialist training.
- Curriculum standards that are underpinned by robust assessment processes, both of which conform to the standards specified by PMETB.
- Regulation of progression through training by the achievement of outcomes that are specified within the specialty curricula. These outcomes are competence-based rather than time-based.
- Delivery of the curriculum by surgeons who are appropriately qualified to deliver surgical training.
- Formulation and delivery of surgical care by surgeons working in a multidisciplinary environment.
- Collaboration with those charged with delivering health services and training at all levels.

The curriculum has been mandatory since 2007 from CT1/ST1 upwards. You can obtain the full curriculum and workplace-based assessments relevant to you from the website. The initial 2007 syllabus was updated in 2010. You can download a syllabus for core surgical training, which has 10 modules. There is also a downloadable syllabus for each of the nine surgical specialties.

ASIT (www.asit.org)
The Association of Surgeons in Training, founded in 1976, is an independent body originally formed and still run by trainees for trainees. It serves both core and specialist/specialty trainees in all specialties and among other things allows a forum to air training issues. The cost is £40 per annum (£30 by direct debit).

The Silver Scalpel Award

Good trainers should be rewarded. ASIT runs an award called the Silver Scalpel Award and you can nominate a trainer who has made an outstanding contribution to your training.

BOTA (www.bota.org.uk)

The British Orthopaedic Trainee's Association, founded in 1987, has around 1,000 specialist/specialty trainees in orthopaedics on its books. It devolved from, but still works closely with, ASIT. There are three ways of joining:

1 as a stand alone member if you're a specialty registrar (StR) or specialist registrar (SpR) with a national training number (NTN) (£40 per annum)

2 as an associate member if you join the British Orthopaedic Association

3 as a junior BOTA member from FY1 upwards, and if you're more senior but without a NTN (£30 per annum).

Other specialty groups

There are a large number of other smaller groups for each of the surgical specialties and subspecialties which represent their trainees, such as the Mammary Fold for breast trainees and the Duke's Club for colorectal trainees. These are listed at the end of the relevant specialty Chapters 8–16.

Other useful sources of information

For generic information about training issues there are a number of documents in the public domain. The Gold Guide is a crucial reference document to have during specialty training. It was first published in 2007 replacing the 'Orange Book', the guide for registrars on the previous system, and has been updated annually since then. It advises on matters ranging from moving between deaneries to getting through the Annual Review of Competence Progression (ARCP) interviews.

The Gold Guide was designed to coincide with the introduction of Modernising Medical Careers (MMC) and run-through training in 2007 and thus is for trainees from ST1 upwards. It remains the guide for core trainees (the replacement of ST1 and ST2), but there is an additional supplement for those core trainees.

For foundation doctors, there is the *Foundation Programme Reference Guide*.

Recent historic changes to surgical training

It's worth knowing a little of the recent history of surgical training to give you an idea of how we are where we are today. Back in the olden days, the career structure following qualification from medical school went something like this:

- 1 year PRHO (pre-registration house officer)
- 3–6 years SHO (senior house officer)

- often a period of research to obtain an MD, MS or PhD
- approximately 3 years as a registrar
- approximately 3++ years as a senior registrar (sometimes more than 10 years).

This system was, however, highly heterogeneous; there were many different routes and rates of progression. The main criticisms of this system were its lack of a defined end-point, and the bottleneck both at registrar to senior registrar stage, and senior registrar to consultant stage. The **Calman report** in 1993 resulted, among other things, in the formalisation of the **specialist registrar (SpR)** training grade. This was termed **Calmanisation**, and from thereon appointed registrars would be called Calman SpRs and were given the holy grail of surgical training: a **national training number (NTN)** or colloquially just called – a **number**. It would see them through to appointment to consultant. It would effectively reduce the length of training in most cases, but make it a more formalised process. This remained the training pathway for the registrar years at least, until 2007.

The next main sea change was the introduction of **Modernising Medical Careers**, the first phase of which began in 2005 with the replacement of the old PRHO grade and first year SHO grade with foundation year 1 (FY1) doctor and foundation year 2 (FY2) doctor respectively.

The next phase commenced in August 2007 (in time to greet the newly graduating FY2s) when the era of basic surgical training, consisting of a number of senior house officer jobs leading to the completion of a Certificate of Completion of Basic Surgical Training (CCBST), was over. Applicants would apply directly from the end of their FY2 year to the start of run-through specialty training at ST1 stage right up to consultant. There were also other staggered entry points for the first year of its introduction because of the wide range of levels that other more senior doctors in SHO grades were at. This was a highly controversial time as it resulted in what was termed the **lost tribe** – there were too many old-style SHOs to fit into the limited number of staggered entry points into specialty training, and this affected surgical trainees particularly badly. It wasn't that there was suddenly a drop in the number of higher surgical training posts available, it was that a large number of people in a wide range of levels of seniority were suddenly forced into an all or (almost) nothing selection process. This was made worse by the deficits in the **Medical Training Application Service (MTAS)**. One of the purposes of this change, however, was to try and set an end-point for SHO training and also to improve the structuring and supervision of these posts, as the previous system was deemed to be inadequate on these fronts (Unfinished Business, Liam Donaldson, 2002). This decision was and remains controversial among surgeons.

Present day

Run-through training was not repeated in future years (except in neurosurgery across the UK and orthopaedic surgery in Scotland), therefore creating **two stages** of competitive entry: from FY2 to the newly created core trainee years, or CT1 and CT2 (which were equivalent to ST1 and ST2), and then a separate stage of competitive entry from CT2 to ST3. Successful appointment to an ST3 post proffers that 'golden ticket': a national training number.

New Deal and the European Working Time Directive

There are two aspects of legislation that govern the working hours of junior doctors:

- **New Deal Contract** (1991, implemented 1996)
- **Working Time Regulations** (the European Working Time Directive's implementation in UK law) – applies universally to all workers, juniors and consultants alike.

This has led to some significant confusion among doctors and has been a bone of great contention for the surgical specialties who believe more time is needed for training in the craft specialties than is currently allowed. Nevertheless this is currently the law of the land and it's far better to understand it and see whether you can manipulate your circumstances locally to maximise your training than just to whinge about it. Bear in mind that the EWTD didn't make the New Deal defunct – the New Deal remains in place and is the basis of our Terms and Conditions, including matters such as banding; EWTD mainly modifies the upper end of how many hours we can work.

The main points of the New Deal are:

- agreement between government, royal colleges and BMA
- response to health and safety concerns about such trifling matters as 1:2 rotas with a mere 120 hours/week
- 56 hours of actual work per week on average
- formalised full and partial shifts.

The main points of the EWTD regulations are:

- a minimum of 11 hours continuous rest in every 24-hour period
- a minimum rest break of 20 minutes after every six hours worked
- a minimum period of 24 hours continuous rest in each seven-day period (or 48 hours in a 14-day period)
- a minimum of four weeks paid annual leave
- a maximum of eight hours work in each 24 hours for night workers.

Opting out of EWTD

There is room in law to opt out of some of the EWTD regulations, but even if you do, the New Deal still prevents you working more than 56 hours a week and you cannot break the rest requirements. Opting out of the EWTD is entirely voluntary and can be cancelled if you change your mind. The main problem with opting out of the EWTD is that it won't necessarily help your training at all. Rotas will still have been arranged so that your working time is New Deal and EWTD compliant; when making the rota your hospital won't be able to rely on the off chance that all the new trainees will sign an opt out, and not later relinquish it. Trusts may also

Table 20.1 New Deal summary

	Maximum duty hours	Maximum actual weekly hours	Maximum continuous duty hours	Minimum time off between duties (h)	Minimum off duty (h)	Rest
On-call rota	72	56	32 (56 at weekend)	12	48 + 62 every 21 days	8 h/32, 5 h continuous at night
24-hour partial shift	64	56	24	8	48 + 62 every 28 days	6 h/24, 4 h continuous at night
Partial shift	64	56	16	8	48 + 62 every 28 days	4 h or ¼ of OOH period
Full shift	56	56	14	8	48 + 62 every 28 days	Only breaks

Source: www.bma.org.uk

have saved money by down banding your post and it's unlikely they'll jump at the chance to up band you just because you want to spend some more time in theatre learning how to take out a colon or put in a new hip. You would need to discuss this with your employers; it's more likely, if anything, you will be remunerated for specific hours worked at national locum rates.

Working time and medical indemnity

Sometimes the best training opportunities happen out of your allotted hours. There is understandable concern about what would happen if something involving your clinical care goes wrong when you have gone over and above your maximum hours. Will you still be covered in the unfortunate outcome of a litigious event?

The NHS Litigation Authority (NHSLA) is the body that indemnifies you as a practitioner working within the NHS when something occurs and a patient or relative attempts to sue you. In other words, providing you were working reasonably within Trust protocols and guidelines, they will take on the legal case for you. The NHSLA has previously made the statement:

> *Any activity carried out by clinicians which would be the subject of an indemnity if carried out during 'alotted' hours will be treated no differently under our schemes because that work was being done outside these hours.*

There are however, two separate scenarios this could apply to.

1 Where you have had to stay late, for instance because an operation is taking much longer to finish than anticipated.

2 Where you decide to come in on an assigned day off because there's an operation you want to do.

It would be hard to imagine the NHSLA not supporting you in the first scenario. The second is less clear-cut. As yet, further clarification through statement or case law has not been forthcoming. You should ensure you haven't volunteered for extra work when you are obviously going to be tired (at the end of a stretch of nights for instance) and that you have put the patient's needs first. It would be preferable in all circumstances to clarify this issue with your trust before any such event and ideally have something on paper.

Money

Money seems to be rarely discussed among junior doctors and doesn't feature in any books. It's surprising how often people don't know what band they're on or even what their take home pay is. But postgraduate education isn't cheap in any specialty, especially in surgery, where to remain competitive you have to go on extra courses and you're more likely to take time out to do low-paid research. So you should be aware of the financial implications of choosing surgery as a career, although it must be said that many of the costs of training will be common among all the specialties with the exception of the extra optionals such as expensive courses. When you include the costs of examinations and courses the figures really add up (see page 246) even before you add on the mandatory GMC registration and medical defence payments. Furthermore, because of the high levels of competition for surgical training, taking a course is a relatively easy, albeit expensive, way of boosting your CV points, and if everyone else is doing it you'll look worse for not doing it.

There is much debate about who should pay for training – the surgical trainee, the trust, the NHS overall, the deanery, etc. – as there are many stakeholders. Currently your pay is split equally between the employing trust and the deanery. The money from the deanery originally comes from the Department of Health via the Multi Professional Education and Training budget (MPET), who also fund study leave, postgraduate centres and the like.

In the past there has been tacit acceptance among trainees of their part in paying most of the costs of training because of a perceived eventual salary that will make it worthwhile. However, in the future this is likely to be challenged, what with increasing student loan burdens, loss of free accommodation in FY1, well below inflation pay rises, fewer band 1A/2B or even 1B jobs, career dead ends and bottlenecks, increases to pension and National Insurance contributions, probable loss of beneficial public sector pension payouts and uncertain ultimate career earnings.

Study allowances can be hard to come by and tend to be hit hard in these financially straitened times. Find out at the beginning of each job how much study allowance you are entitled to and make sure you use it. Table 20.2 gives an idea of the costs of training in 2011 money. All these costs tend to be reviewed annually. It doesn't take into account the generic costs of being a doctor, such as the annual cost of GMC registration, membership of a medical defence organisation or subscription to a union such as the British Medical Association. Neither does it include the cost of travel intrinsic to rotations where this isn't reimbursed by relocation expenses.

Pay

Pay bands

Pay bands were first introduced in 2000, becoming legally binding for the old-school PRHOs in August 2001 and for all other junior doctors in August 2003. It remains in force today. Assuming you are working full time, your basic salary is worked out based on an average working week of 40 hours between the core hours of 7am and 7pm Monday to Friday. Working more than 40 hours, or if those hours stray beyond those core times, you will get a banding supplement.

Monitoring

Your band should be worked out based on the results of monitoring exercises (diary cards), not on the theoretical band from a template rota (although the two should reflect each other). That means that if you think you are being paid unfairly, and that your rota doesn't reflect the working hours you put in, this needs to be demonstrated on the diary cards that you are asked to fill in. It is also essential that you ensure all your colleagues fill them in. Contact the BMA with issues related to banding.

Tables 20.4 and 20.5 show the gross pay depending on your stage and band.

Table 20.2 Costs of training

	Item	Cost
Mandatory	MRCS Part A	£440
	MRCS Part B	£835
	Basic Surgical Skills (BSS)	£740
	Advanced Trauma Life Support (ATLS)	£550
	Care of the Critically Ill Surgical Patient (CCrISP) (not mandatory in all subspecialties)	£550
	FRCS (specialty) Section 1	£520
	FRCS (specialty) Section 2	£1275
	Certificate of Completion of Training (to join the Specialist Register (GMC))	£500
Optional	STEP Foundation	£450
	START Surgery	£150
	STEP Core	£550
	The average specialty course over 3 days, usually at least one of these per year	Ranging from £400–£1000
	Postgraduate Masters degree part time total for 2 years	£5000
Annual recurring	ASIT or equivalent body	£40
	Royal College of Surgeons	£285
	JCST	£125

Source: www.bma.org.uk

Table 20.3 Pay bands

Band	Definition	Salary supplement as a percentage of basic salary
Band 3	For those working more than 56 hours per week on average or not achieving the required rest. Non-compliant with the New Deal, because of excessive hours or other matters, e.g. a lack of breaks during working hours or insufficient time off between shifts	100
Band 2A	For those working between 48 and 56 hours per week on average, most antisocially	80
Band 2B	For those working between 48 and 56 hours per week on average, least antisocially	50
Band 1A	For those working between 40 and 48 hours per week on average, most antisocially	50
Band 1B	For those working between 40 and 48 hours per week on average, moderately antisocially	40
Band 1C	For those working between 40 and 48 hours per week on average, least antisocially	20
No band	For those working no more than 40 hours per week on average, between 7am and 7pm	0

Source: www.bma.org.uk

A pay freeze is planned for two years from 2011. In practice, of course, the final column, Band 3, has been illegal since the New Deal came into force in 1996 and Bands 2A and 2B have been illegal since the EWTD came into force (for junior doctors) in August 2009, unless in the rare circumstance that you have opted out of the EWTD and your trust has agreed to pay you at a higher band. If you work in London this may be supplemented by London weighting of £2,162.

Relocation expenses

When you join a rotation, particularly the longer six-year higher surgical training pathway of ST3–8, you may be expected to move around hospitals in a

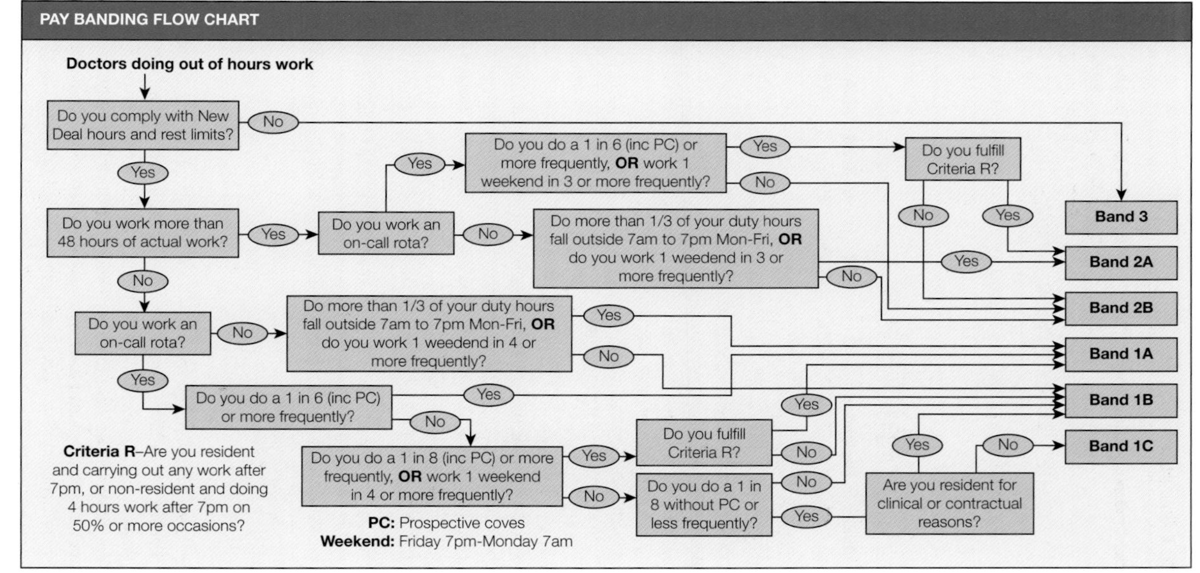
PAY BANDING FLOW CHART
Doctors doing out of hours work
Do you comply with New Deal hours and rest limits?
No
Yes
Do you work more than 48 hours of actual work?
Yes
No
Do you work an on-call rota?
Yes
No
Do you do a 1 in 6 (inc PC) or more frequently, **OR** work 1 weekend in 3 or more frequently?
Yes
No
Do you fulfill Criteria R?
No
Yes
Do more than 1/3 of your duty hours fall outside 7am to 7pm Mon-Fri, **OR** do you work 1 weedend in 3 or more frequently?
Yes
No
Do you work an on-call rota?
No
Yes
Do more than 1/3 of your duty hours fall outside 7am to 7pm Mon-Fri, **OR** do you work 1 weedend in 4 or more frequently?
Yes
No
Do you do a 1 in 6 (inc PC) or more frequently?
Yes
No
Do you do a 1 in 8 (inc PC) or more frequently, **OR** work 1 weekend in 4 or more frequently?
Yes
No
Do you fulfill Criteria R?
Yes
No
Do you do a 1 in 8 without PC or less frequently?
No
Yes
Are you resident for clinical or contractual reasons?
Yes
No
Band 3
Band 2A
Band 2B
Band 1A
Band 1B
Band 1C
Criteria R–Are you resident and carrying out any work after 7pm, or non-resident and doing 4 hours work after 7pm on 50% or more occasions?
PC: Prospective coves
Weekend: Friday 7pm-Monday 7am

Figure 20.2 Pay banding flow chart. Source: www.bma.org.uk

Table 20.4 Foundation doctor pay

Foundation year	Basic	Unbanded	1C 20%	1B 40%	1A & 2B 50%	2A 80%	3 100%
1	£22,412	£23,533	£26,895	£31,377	£33,618	£40,342	£44,824
2	£27,798	£27,798	£33,358	£38,918	£41,697	£50,037	£55,596

Table 20.5 Core and specialty doctor pay

ST point	Basic	Unbanded	1C 20%	1B 40%	1A & 2B 50%	2A 80%	3 100%
Min	£29,705	£29,705	£35,646	£41,587	£44,558	£53,469	£59,410
1	£31,523	£31,523	£37,828	£44,133	£47,285	£56,742	£63,046
2	£34,061	£34,061	£40,874	£47,686	£51,092	£61,310	£68,122
3	£35,596	£35,596	£42,716	£49,835	£53,394	£64,073	£71,192
4	£37,448	£37,448	£44,938	£52,428	£56,172	£67,407	£74,896
5	£39,300	£39,300	£47,160	£55,020	£58,950	£70,740	£78,600
6	£41,152	£41,152	£49,383	£57,613	£61,728	£74,074	£82,304
7	£43,003	£43,003	£51,604	£60,205	£64,505	£77,406	£86,006
8	£44,856	£44,856	£53,828	£62,799	£67,284	£80,741	£89,712
9	£46,708	£46,708	£56,050	£65,392	£70,062	£84,075	£93,416

NB: ST1 = CT1, ST2 = CT2.

very large area. The Kent, Surrey and Sussex deanery for instance stretches from Brighton in East Sussex to Margate in East Kent, at least a two-hour drive of more than 100 miles, including a merry jaunt in rush hour on the M25. It is written into our contracts that we should not be financially disadvantaged by having to uproot every year or travel many miles every day to our next placement (although the reality can be somewhat different). Thus you will be entitled to relocation expenses, which can be a confusing and murky world. This is mainly because there is no nationally standardised system and also the administrators of relocation expenses have in some cases changed from trusts to deaneries in recent years. NHS Employers have released guidance on relocation expenses for doctors, but even this notes the limitations of the exercise: 'The level and scope of removals expenses payable to doctors and other NHS staff are to a large extent at the discretion of the employer'. It is therefore also guidance to the administrators of relocation expenses, but how they interpret these rules differ greatly and it's important to check at the start of your rotation precisely how the rules apply in your region, and who administers them, the trust or the deanery.

In general though, you can apply for one of two things: removals expenses to help with the cost of removals or travel expenses in lieu of removals expenses if you'd prefer to commute to your next hospital instead of move.

Again, different administrators vary regarding what they'll chip in for, but as a general idea it usually covers:

- search for accommodation in the new area
- purchase and sale of property (including legal fees and stamp duty)
- removal of furniture and effects
- general/miscellaneous removal costs
- additional housing costs in the new area

Alternatively, if you are claiming travel expenses in lieu of removals, you can claim back on rail fares or petrol at a pre-agreed rate per mile. There is of course a limit to how much you can receive over the course of your training. The London Deanery for instance sets this at £8,000 from FY1 right up to CCT. Of particular note, however, the travel expenses in lieu of removals are tax deductable whereas relocation expenses are not. HMRC is now enforcing this rule, whereas in the past it has been largely overlooked. This can certainly invalidate the notion that being on rotation should not financially disadvantage you.

References

Calman Report (1993) *Hospital Doctors' Training for the Future*. The report of the Working Group on Specialist Medical Training. London: Department of Health.

College Guidance on The School of Surgery. London: The Royal College of Surgeons of England

Junior Doctors Committee (2008) *The Final Countdown. The rush to reband training posts explained*. London: British Medical Association.

Pay Circular (M&D) 1/2010 (2010). London: NHS Employers.

Royal College of Surgeons (2010) *Surgical Tutors' Handbook*. London: The Royal College of Surgeons.

www.bma.org.uk/employmentandcontracts/pay/travel_allowances/jdtravelandrelocexpenses.jsp#mileage

www.mmc.nhs.uk/colleges__deaneries/deaneries.aspx

www.nhsemployers.org/SiteCollectionDocuments/removal_guidance_doctors_training_cd_221205.pdf

Chapter 21
FELLOWSHIPS

Sofiane Rimouche

Introduction, 250
Pre-CCT fellowships, 251
Interface fellowships, 251
Post-CCT fellowships, 253
International fellowships, 253
Where to find out about fellowships, 254
Summary and general tips, 254
References, 255

Introduction

Fellowship can be described as 'additional training, beyond that available within a Certificate of Completion of Training (CCT) programme, to be undertaken as Out of Programme (OOP) experience that may or may not contribute towards CCT or CCT-holders wishing to gain additional expertise' (paraphrased from the Royal College of Surgeons [RCS]).

Fellowship opportunities have existed for many years. They can be classified into both pre- and post-CCT, as well as national and international. With ongoing changes in the NHS, the competition for consultant posts and continuing subspecialisation, it is becoming very desirable, if not essential, to undertake a fellowship. Therefore, obtaining a reputable fellowship is competitive and early planning is essential as these posts could be filled, at times, years in advance. It's essential to pick the right fellowship and one with educational value and high quality. Unfortunately there are fellowships that exist where the focus is simply on service and you will just be an extra member of staff for rota purposes. Most surgical Specialist Advisory Committees (SAC) are in the process of developing criteria that should be met in order for a fellowship to meet educational approval. According to the RCS the following are essential criteria to look for in a fellowship.

- Provides structured educational experience.
- Has an established curriculum (which includes levels of patient care, medical knowledge, practice-based learning and improvement, communication skills and professionalism).

The Hands-on Guide to Surgical Training, First Edition. Matthew Stephenson.

- Takes place in an institution that assumes ultimate responsibility for delivery of the programme of training and education.
- Providing sufficient protected time for both trainer and trainees (fellows) and necessary financial support for the programme.
- Has identified faculty that will assume educational and supervisory responsibilities throughout the programme.
- Provides opportunities for audit and research.
- Has external evaluation process.

Pre-CCT fellowships

As mentioned earlier a pre-CCT fellowship is undertaking OOP experience or training which may or may not contribute towards a CCT. It's essential that you familiarise yourself with your local deanery guidelines for OOP experience. You have to apply to the deanery for approval for OOP. You have to give notice, which is usually three to six months. OOP experience is usually for one year but could be up to two years. If you are planning to count the OOP experience towards the CCT you also have to apply prospectively to the SAC and this is referred to as OOPT (time Out of Programme for Clinical Training). If the post is currently unapproved for training or is overseas, you will require GMC approval as well. However, the GMC will recognise training in a post already approved by the statutory authority in the European Economic Area (EEA)/Switzerland and no additional approval is needed.

A list of the required documentation for SAC and GMC application for fellowship approval is available on the Joint Committee on Surgical Training (JCST) website. In order for a period of OOPT to count towards the award of CCT, on completion of the post you must apply to the SAC again to determine whether educational objectives have been met. Intercollegiate Surgical Curriculum Programme (ISCP) assessments for the entire period or a satisfactory trainer's report are required as well as an ISCP Quality Assurance survey, validated consolidation sheet of the logbook and evidence of GMC approval (for non-approved posts). Acting up as a consultant could also be classified as OOPT.

If you are planning OOP experience that you do not wish to count towards the CCT, which is referred to as time Out of Programme for Clinical Experience (OOPE) you require the agreement of the deanery. However, the SAC need not be notified.

A pre-CCT fellowship can be either a national or international one. The choice is individual and may be influenced by personal views, family and financial circumstances, the type of further experience required and where the expertise is available. The RCS is attempting to regulate and coordinate all national fellowships in terms of educational approval, workforce planning and advertising. However, this may take some time.

Interface fellowships

Special types of national fellowship that are applicable to most surgical specialties are interface fellowships. Interface fellowships are pre-CCT fellowships. They are national advanced training posts. Advanced special interest training is available through these posts. They combine curricula of at least two surgical specialties. They are recognised by the parent advisory committees. These posts are administered by the JCST through the five Training Interface Groups, which include:

- breast oncoplastic surgery: parent specialties are plastic surgery and general surgery
- cleft lip and palate surgery: parent specialties are plastic surgery, oral and maxillofacial surgery (OMFS), and otolaryngology
- cosmetic reconstructive surgery: parent specialties are plastic surgery, general surgery (breast surgery), OMFS, otolaryngology and ocular-plastic surgery (ophthalmology)
- hand surgery: parent specialties are plastic surgery, and trauma and orthopaedic surgery
- head and neck surgical oncology: parent specialties are plastic surgery, OMFS and otolaryngology.

Interface fellowships are suitable for senior trainees with a national training number (NTN) from one of the parent specialties for each programme. During the programme you have timetabled sessions with the different parent specialties. The FRCS exit exam is not essential for entry to these programmes but is highly desirable. The current interface fellowships are as follows.

- Breast oncoplastic fellowships: these are for a period of 12 months, usually advertised in the beginning of the year with start dates on the October of each year. These are open to plastic and breast surgery trainees.

- Cleft lip and palate fellowships: these are for a period of up to two years. The exit exam may be essential for these fellowships. These are open to plastic, OMFS and ENT trainees.

- Cosmetic reconstructive fellowships: these are for a period of four months and you are allowed to undertake further fellowships on top of this one. These are open to plastic, OMFS, ENT, breast and ophthalmology trainees.

- Trauma fellowships: these are administered by the Cosmetic Reconstructive Surgery Interface Group and are for a four-month period. These fellowships are based at Queen Elizabeth Hospital Birmingham in conjunction with military services. The trauma fellowships are open to most of the surgical specialities.

- Hand fellowships: these are for a 12-month period and are open to plastic and orthopaedic trainees.

- Head and neck fellowships: these are for a period of 12 months and are open to plastic, OMFS and ENT trainees.

- Lower limb trauma and reconstruction fellowship: this fellowship is not strictly speaking an interface one. It has plastic surgery SAC approval. It is based at Charing Cross Hospital and is open to plastic and orthopaedic trainees.

Interface fellowships are funded fellowships, well organised and provide excellent specialised cross-speciality training. Fellows' educational/training events (free of charge) such as a management training day are also included. The fellows get paid a decent salary. The recruitment is usually managed by the Severn Deanery. There are person specifications and standardised application forms. There is no doubt that they are becoming more competitive, and having one of these fellowships is becoming very important for certain consultant jobs. It's important to note that if you undertake one of the interface fellowships during your last year of training your CCT award date will be postponed until the end of your interface fellowship, even if you have only one day left in training. For details on the fellowships and units, visit the JCST/Interface Groups website.

Post-CCT fellowships

These fellowships are for CCT holders wishing to gain additional expertise before taking consultant posts. Post-CCT fellowships have been in existence for decades. They can be both national and international. No SAC or deanery approval is required as they are post-CCT. These fellowships may also be a way of biding your time waiting for the appropriate consultant post while gaining further expertise. Currently there are 14 national transplant surgery post-CCT fellowships administered by the RCS and centrally funded by the Department of Health (DH). Apart from the interface fellowships, which are pre-CCT, you can undertake any other fellowship as a post-CCT one. With the introduction of Modernising Medical Careers (MMC) in 2007, the RCS and specialty associations created 70 post-CCT fellowships in all surgical specialities, funded centrally by the DH. However, the funding was only for a period of a year and only the 14 transplant fellowships still exist. At the time, there was concern that this might lead to a bottleneck at the end of training and that without one of these fellowships trainees would not progress to consultant posts. However, this did not materialise. It's an individual choice to undertake a post-CCT fellowship and again the decision is multifactorial.

International fellowships

It's essential that you plan well ahead if you are considering undertaking an international fellowship, especially if it is OOPT. As with pre-CCT fellowships you need to get the required approval from the SAC and GMC for OOPT. You also need to bear in mind that whether this is an OOPT, OOPE or a post-CCT fellowship, the necessary immigration process, which if it is outside the EU may take at least six months. You need to obtain the appropriate visa for yourself and any members of the family who may be joining you on the fellowship. There is usually a significant amount of paperwork required and you may also need to have a medical assessment from a physician approved by the country where you are planning a fellowship. You need to make enquiries with the appropriate consulate or high commission. With most countries outside the EU you also need to register with the appropriate Medical Council equivalent to the GMC and to obtain the appropriate medical indemnity/insurance. For the United States you need to have passed the United States Medical Licensing Examination (USMLE) for most states (you need to check with the individual state). Australia, Canada and New Zealand seem to be the most popular destinations for an overseas fellowship. You also need to ensure that the funding, i.e. your salary, is available, as some of these fellowships may be unpaid. Most of the specialty associations and also international surgical associations and charities offer grants for unpaid fellowships. Do not underestimate the European fellowships as some of them are of high quality, require much less paperwork and are not far from home, some may even be almost commutable from the UK.

Where to find out about fellowships

Unfortunately there isn't one site or source where vacancies for fellowships are posted. Job advert websites such as BMJ Careers and NHS Jobs are a start. You can set up an email alert for jobs through NHS Careers. For the interface fellowships the JCST website is an excellent resource. The trainees' association and specialty associations both national and international are also a good source of information. However, for each specialty and subspecialty most senior trainees and consultants are aware of the most reputable national and international fellowships, so do ask around. If you were impressed by a speaker at a meeting or by a publication and you want to spend some time with that particular surgeon, do contact him or her and see if you are able to create your own fellowship – enthusiasm goes a long way. It's important to note that the RCS is in the process of trying to regulate national fellowships in terms of quality assurance, educational approval and advertising. This includes both pre- and post-CCT fellowships for all surgical specialties.

Summary and general tips

- Plan well ahead, maybe two to three years in advance.
- Ensure you are familiar with your deanery OOP regulations.
- Ensure that you meet all the SAC and GMC requirements for OOPT approval.
- Communicate with the supervisors of the fellowship you are intending to undertake well in advance: either write to them, arrange to meet them by visiting the unit or informally in meetings.
- If you are planning an international fellowship ensure you are familiar with the country's immigration regulations and allow ample time to obtain the necessary paperwork.
- For unpaid fellowships there are grants available through the national and international specialty association and charities.
- Ensure you contact previous fellows who undertook the fellowship you are aiming to get, for tips and advice.
- You need to be asking around registrars and consultant colleagues about good fellowships.

References

JCST website: www.jcst.org
Regulation for OOP: www.jcst.org/mmc_trainee_info/takingtimeout_html
Royal College of Surgeons: www.rcseng.ac.uk/
Severn Deanery: www.severndeanery.nhs.uk/
Training Interface Groups: www.jcst.org/training_interface_groups; breast: www.jcst.org/training_interface_groups/breast_surgery; cleft lip and palate: www.jcst.org/training_interface_groups/cleft_lip_and_palate; reconstructive cosmetic surgery: www.jcst.org/training_interface_groups/cosmetic_surgery; hand surgery: www.jcst.org/training_interface_groups/hand_surgery; head and neck surgical oncology: www.jcst.org/training_interface_groups/head_and_neck_surgery

Chapter 22
APPROACHING CONSULTANCY

Clare Byrne
General and colorectal consultant, Lewisham Hospital, appointed 2010

Introduction, 256
Finishing training, 256
Certificate of Completion of Training (CCT), 257
Certificate of Eligibility of Specialist Registration (CESR), 257
Making yourself competitive, 257
Deciding which consultant job to apply for, 260
Finding out which jobs are coming up, 261
The consultant application process, 261
The application form, 262
The interview, 262
Transition from trainee to consultant, 263
References, 263

Introduction

What's it all for? For most people the holy grail of surgical training is the consultant post at the end. This chapter offers advice about how to get that job. **Think early about what you want in the long term and prepare and plan for it.** By this I mean, for instance, that if you have an intercalated degree in psychology or history of medicine and you wish to become a consultant plastic surgeon in a major teaching hospital, then your BSc will be useless to you. It won't matter that you have it, but you'll have to get something else (like a PhD) as well. Your fate is not entirely determined by your early career choices, but evidence of commitment to your chosen specialty will be well received. It is important that your career progression is coherent – surgeons tend to be a very traditional bunch.

Finishing training

To be an NHS consultant you must be on the specialist register which is held by the GMC. There are two routes to finishing training and getting on to the specialist register. The first is the 'traditional' route of undergoing a formal, educationally approved higher surgical training pathway with a national training number (NTN). The second is an alternative process particularly for overseas medical graduates and those who never secured a NTN but have 'followed their own path'.

The Hands-on Guide to Surgical Training, First Edition. Matthew Stephenson.

Certificate of Completion of Training (CCT)

About six months before you are due to complete your training the college will write to you and invite you to apply for your CCT. This is done on an online form. You'll need to pay the fee upfront (£500 at the time of going to press) and then send documentation to them. There are two important pieces of paper to obtain. The first is the Record of In-Training Assessment (RITA) G form, which is given to you by the final Annual Review of Competence Progression (ARCP) panel you meet, who will sign you off as having satisfactorily completed the training programme. The second is the Royal College notification form, which must be signed by the head of the deanery. These are submitted together with photo ID, CV and your Fellowship of the Royal College of Surgeons (FRCS) exit exam certificate (see Chapter 7). As soon as you have all the paperwork you can apply.

Certificate of Eligibility of Specialist Registration (CESR)

This is another a route of entry on to the specialist register, which is open to doctors who have completed their specialist training either abroad or in any way other than completing a recognised UK specialty training programme. The application requires submission of evidence that your skills, knowledge and qualifications are equivalent to those required by your specialty as set out by the curriculum for its training programme. There is no set requirement to pass the FRCS, but evidence must be provided of an equivalent level of knowledge. Each application is treated individually. This is a long and expensive process, taking an average of six to nine months and currently costing £1,600. Success rates are low (29% for general surgery), but vary according to specialty. See Table 22.1 for details. The full list of all specialties is available at www.gmc-uk.org/doctors/eligibilitystatistics.asp.

Making yourself competitive

By the time you're a senior registrar, everyone will have a full logbook, have attended all the courses and done the exit exam. What you need is something to make your CV stand out from the crowd. You should focus on developing an area of expertise that you can bring to the department to which you are applying. Examples might include postgraduate teaching qualifications, research expertise or a highly specialised and sought after clinical skill. The directors of service on your interview panel will want to know what you can bring to the department in terms of income, innovation and prestige.

Like any other job there are person specifications to check. The following is a typical example of the kinds of things employers are looking for in a consultant colorectal surgeon.

Table 22.1 Statistics for the success of applications for CESR from September 2005–September 2010

Specialty	Success	Reject	Total	Success rate
Breast	6	1	7	86%
Cardiac surgery	3	1	4	75%
Cardiothoracic surgery	17	21	38	45%
Cosmetic surgery	0	1	1	0%
Facial plastic reconstructive surgery	0	1	1	0%
General surgery	86	210	296	29%
Thoracic surgery	1	2	3	33%
Hand surgery	1	1	2	50%
Neurosurgery	23	10	33	70%
OMFS	1	1	2	50%
Otorhinolaryngology	16	63	79	20%
Paediatric surgery	12	17	29	41%
Plastic surgery	20	39	59	34%
Transplant surgery	4	1	5	80%
Trauma and orthopaedics	86	157	243	35%
Urology	76	41	117	65%
Digestive surgery	0	1	1	0%
Vascular surgery	1	4	5	20%

NB Some of these categories have been amalgamated from the website, such as 'Thoracic surgery' and 'General thoracic surgery'
Source: www.gmc-uk.org

Table 22.2 Qualities required in a consultant in colorectal surgery

	Essential	**Desirable**
Qualifications	■ Full registration with the General Medical Council ■ On the specialist register or within six months of completion of CCT ■ Success in intercollegiate specialty examination or overseas equivalent ■ Primary medical qualification, i.e, MB BS (or equivalent)	■ Postgraduate thesis or other higher degree
Clinical experience	■ Experience and training in general and colorectal surgery ■ Ability to manage a range of emergency and elective general surgical and colorectal conditions ■ Full training in laparoscopic colorectal surgery ■ Experience of gastrointestinal endoscopy	
Management and administrative experience	■ Ability to manage and lead surgical firm ■ Ability to organise and manage outpatient priorities, surgical waiting lists and operating lists ■ Able to lead audit projects ■ Computer skills	■ Undertaken management training
Teaching experience	■ Experience of supervising foundation and core trainees ■ Ability to teach clinical and operative skills ■ Experience of teaching basic clinical skills to undergraduates	■ Experience of supervising specialty registrars ■ Formal training in teaching

(*Continued*)

Table 22.2 (*Continued*)

	Essential	**Desirable**
Research experience	■ Ability to apply current research to clinical problems ■ Publications in peer-reviewed journals	■ Ability to supervise postgraduate research
Personal attributes	■ Good interpersonal skills ■ Ability to work in a team ■ Enquiring, critical approach to work ■ Effective communication with patients, relatives, GPs, nurses and others ■ Commitment to continuing professional development	

Deciding which consultant job to apply for

There are many factors to take into account here. Geographical location is probably top of the list. You are probably going to live there for the next 30 years, so make sure that there is somewhere nearby where you actually do want to buy a house and make your home. Usually you would be expected to be able to arrive at work within 30 minutes of being called in; bear in mind that journey times may be increased at certain times of the day. The actual content in terms of subspecialty or specialist interest within your field is important too. If the entire job description is not entirely to your taste but is broadly what you are looking for then it is probably worth applying, as there may be room for manoeuvre once you're actually there. The other things to consider are whether the hospital is a district general hospital or a teaching hospital and whether you will be required to participate in a general on-call rota for your specialty or just subspecialty on calls.

Another major factor, and one that probably divides opinion, is whether it is better to try for a job in the region where you have trained or to look for somewhere new. Hospitals in your training region may know you and are probably more likely to appoint you, but the downside of working somewhere where you have been more junior is that staff there will know you as a registrar and you may find it difficult to be taken seriously as a consultant. If you are considering applying to somewhere new you do need to do your homework and find out all you can about a hospital before you apply; local reputation is important. No one wants to work somewhere that is not actually a very good hospital, so if you don't know, find out. You can get information from friends and colleagues, Doctors.net.uk (DNUK) forum, the hospital's own website and the Care Quality Commission (CQC, which is the independent regulator of health and social care in England).

Finding out which jobs are coming up

Officially, all consultant jobs must be advertised to open application. You don't want to have to scan the *BMJ* each week for anything suitable. It is important to know what is coming up where, well in advance. To do this, it's essential to keep your ear to the ground and in email contact with consultants in your specialty. You really need to plan two or three years ahead – if your almost ideal job is coming up but requires a specific skill such as renal access for a vascular surgeon then you need to give yourself time to gain competency in this. It pays to be upfront with colleagues if you work somewhere that you'd really like to come back to as a consultant. They will know if any retirements are imminent or expansion planned, it is no good holding on for your dream job at St Elsewhere's if their referrals are dwindling and they already have a plethora of young consultants. There have even been instances of jobs being created for individuals who are well known to a department and well liked and regarded. Networking at conferences and meetings is another good way to find out what jobs might be coming up and where. When you know that there is a job you would like about to be advertised then you do have to keep tabs on the *BMJ* as this is where all jobs are advertised. Applications are made directly to the hospital in question.

The consultant application process

You can apply for a job if the interview is due to be held within six months of your CCT date. Obviously, after you have your CCT certificate you are ready to go. You are exceedingly unlikely to be short-listed without the exit exam, although this is not absolutely unheard of. Most short-listing is done by means of a standardised form, although you are also likely to be required to submit your CV. I recommend getting your CV spruced up a year or so before you want to start so that as soon as a job is advertised it is ready. There is often only a week or two between advertisement and the close of applications and you need this time to complete the application form. Your CCT and FRCS, together with GMC registration, are essential criteria for short-listing. Unlike other stages in training, surgical experience is probably next most important; you really need to demonstrate that you have been fully trained in your specialty and subspecialty. A short note about 'word of mouth'; I'm sure the situation varies job to job, but it is exceedingly likely that doctors in your potential new hospital will talk to other consultants that you have encountered along your training path.

The application form

In addition to your CV you are likely to have to fill in an application form with questions similar to those you've encountered at earlier stages. The following is an example of the main questions asked in a recent application form. It doesn't matter if consultant interviews are a long way off – as explained elsewhere in this book, early preparation is key. If you're not doing audits and research in your early training years, you're no more likely to be doing them in your senior years.

- Description of your duties and responsibilities in current post (150 words).
- Describe your experience of clinical audit (150 words).
- Describe your relevant teaching experience (150 words).
- Give details of your most relevant research work and publications in peer-reviewed journals (150 words).
- Give examples of your approach to working in a team (150 words).
- Please explain your areas of clinical skill and competence relevant to the post (150 words).
- Please provide any other supporting information that you think may be helpful or that is requested in the person specification. Please ensure that this does not contain personal details or any duplicate information already provided elsewhere (500 words).

The interview

This starts with pre-interview visits, which are underestimated at your peril. I applied to a hospital in which I had been a registrar and expected these visits to be an informal chat. The director of service took me into an office and subjected me to an impromptu interview regarding the pros and cons of laparoscopic colorectal surgery in terms of operating times and costs, general and my own personal lack of experience in today's training climate, and quizzed me on my long-term career plans and private practice intentions. Be prepared. You may visit a hospital before applying but it is more usual to visit after you have been short-listed.

After you have been invited to interview you will be told the names and roles of all of those on the interview panel (officially known as the appointments advisory committee). There will be the medical director, clinical director, chief executive, lay person, college rep and if the hospital to which you have applied is linked with a university, then an academic rep. There is usually also a human resources rep to ensure fair play. In a daft game of old boys, know the system – you will be expected to contact and visit the medical and clinical directors, the chief exec and as many of your potential new colleagues as possible. However, you are not permitted to contact the college rep or the lay person as this is viewed as canvassing.

There are a number of excellent interview courses on the market. It is not the remit of this book to go through interview technique. Do a course.

The interview will have a standard structure. The chair will introduce the panel and the college representative will give you a nice easy starter for ten by asking you to summarise your training. The academic representative will go next and is likely to ask you about your research and teaching experience. Then it gets harder. You can anticipate political and financial questions from the clinical director, as well as being asked what you can bring to the trust. The medical director and the chief executive will then ask questions, and they can be on any topic. The interview concludes with an invitation for your own questions; you should not have any unanswered questions at this stage. A decision will be made and only then are references consulted.

It is perfectly acceptable to apply for a job, visit the hospital and meet the people, and then decide to withdraw. It is very bad form to withdraw after the interview itself and you could expect your referees to be contacted if you do behave badly and do this.

Transition from trainee to consultant

The most important thing about the transition from registrar to consultant is the holiday. Never again will you have the opportunity to take unpaid leave for an unlimited time, with no work pressure hanging over you, so as long as the credit card allows, make the most of it!

When you start the job, the most important thing is to be nice to everybody. It sounds obvious, but it's true. It's worth checking before your first day that you have a desk, a computer, a secretary and some passwords for PACS, etc. If an operating list has been set up for you, you must make sure that you have an opportunity to meet the patients before the day itself. Remember, you are now an independent practitioner. If something comes up that you are uncomfortable with, it's easy to postpone it to give yourself time to think and plan, and perhaps see the patient yourself in clinic beforehand. When the patient is in front of you on the day of surgery, starved and in a gown, the pressure to just get on with it will be immense.

Do not be afraid to ask for help. Colleagues will be flattered and usually only too happy to show you how they do things. If you anticipate a difficult case, try and time it so that an experienced pair of hands is at their desk waiting for your call.

You will have no admin or emails to respond to for the first few weeks. Do not worry. Play solitaire/angry birds or whatever. The paperwork and email hassle will start all too soon.

References

www. careers.bmj.com
www.gmc-uk.org/doctors/eligibilitystatistics.asp

Appendix I
PREOPERATIVE ASSESSMENT

Few things are as embarrassing as being responsible for the cancellation of a patient due to inadequate preoperative preparation, or worse, an avoidable adverse perioperative outcome. We all dread the anaesthetist turning up to see the pre-ops and finding some failure in preoperative assessment meaning that the patient's surgery is cancelled or delayed. Someone forgot to request a sickle cell test. No one ordered cross-matched blood. The INR of 5.0 went unnoticed.

Who's responsible for all this? It's usually the most junior person, the FY1, who gets blamed. But if you're reading this smugly as a senior, sorry, you also have your responsibility to oversee the process and check up on the results. Everyone is responsible, even the consultant, but try telling him that. And few things are worse than having to apologise to an anaesthetist.

Clearly there are going to be some differences in the preoperative preparation and assessment of elective cases versus emergency cases, mainly in terms of the amount of time you'll have to fully investigate a patient, but there's not much excuse for failing to fully assess elective patients.

Pre-assessing elective patients

Take a full history and thoroughly examine the patient. Concentrate first on the pathology they've come to have operated on, e.g. how long have they had their inguinal hernia? What problems is it causing them, etc? Is it possible that whoever listed that person for surgery actually got the diagnosis wrong, or that the surgery is no longer needed or desired? Next concentrate on the patient's co-morbidities and medication list. Ask specifically about the following.

1 **Cardiorespiratory disease** – Angina? MIs? COPD? Breathlessness? Cough? etc. This is probably the most crucial aspect of preoperative assessment from the anaesthetic point of view, as surgery places a strain on the physiological reserves of these organs.

2 Other **co-morbidities**, e.g. THREADS (TB, hypertension, rheumatic

The Hands-on Guide to Surgical Training, First Edition. Matthew Stephenson.

fever, epilepsy, asthma, diabetes, stroke) or renal disease.

3 What **medications** are they on, including doses and frequency? Which need to be stopped?

4 Do they **smoke**? If so it must be strongly recommended that they quit a minimum of 24 hours before anasthetic.

5 Do they drink **alcohol** and how much? Will they need detoxifying medication on admission?

6 How are they going to **manage after the surgery**? Will they have a partner at home to look after them? Will they manage the stairs?

Thoroughly examine the patient in the same order of: pathology they've come to have operated on and then signs of cardiorespiratory disease.

Then think about investigations. There is much confusion about which tests to routinely request for which patients. Generally too many tests are requested unnecessarily because we 'want to be on the safe side'. There are, however, evidence-based guidelines published by the **National Institute for Clinical Excellence** for the following investigations:

- chest X-ray
- electrocardiogram
- full blood count
- haemostasis
- renal function
- random glucose
- urinalysis
- blood gases
- lung function
- sickle cell test.

These guidelines are important reading but they are pretty complicated in their intricacies and no surgeon could be expected to memorise them all, better to consult the tables below taken directly from said guidance.

To decide which tests to perform you first need to know the grade of surgery, i.e. how invasive the surgery is.

- **Grade 1** (Minor): excision of skin lesion.
- **Grade 2** (Intermediate): inguinal hernia repair, tonsillectomy, knee arthroscopy.
- **Grade 3** (Major): endoscopic resection of prostate, lumbar discectomy, thyroidectomy.
- **Grade 4** (Major+): total joint replacement, colonic resection, neurosurgery, cardiac surgery.

Then you need to know the patient's ASA grade.

1 A **normal healthy** patient.

2 A patient with **mild systemic** disease.

3 A patient with **severe systemic** disease.

4 A patient with **severe systemic disease** that is a **constant threat** to their life.

5 A **moribund** patient, not expected to survive with or without an operation.

To be less subjective (subjectivity being a common complaint about ASA grades) about how a patient should be graded when it comes to cardiovascular, respiratory and renal disease, NICE came up with the following table.

Characterisation of 'mild' and 'severe' comorbidity, corresponding to ASA grades 2 and 3, for cardiovascular, respiratory and renal comorbidities

ASA definition	**ASA GRADE 2** **'A patient with *mild* systemic disease**	**ASA GRADE 3** **'A patient with *severe* systemic disease'**
Cardiovascular (CVD):		
Current angina	occasional use of glyceryl trinitrate (GTN) spray (two to three times per month). Dose not include patients with unstable angina who would be ASA grade 3.	regular use of GTN spray (two to three times per week) or unstable angina
Exercise tolerance	not limiting activity	limiting activity
Hypertension	well controlled using a single antihypertensive medication	not well controlled, requiring multiple antihypertensive medications
Diabetes	well controlled, no obvious diabetic complications	not well controlled, diabetic complications, eg claudication, impaired renal function

Previous coronary revascularization	not directly relevant – depends on current signs and symptoms	
Respiratory:		
COAD/COPD	productive cough, wheeze well controlled by inhalers, occasional episodes of acute chest infection	breathlessness on minimal exertion, eg stair climbing, carrying shopping, distressingly wheezy much of the time, several episodes per year of acute chest infection
Asthma	well controlled by medications/inhalers, not limiting lifestyle	poorly controlled, limiting lifestyle – on high dose of inhaler/oral steroids, frequent hospital admission on account of asthma exacerbation
Renal disease:	elevated creatinine (creatinine >100 μmol/L and <200 μmol/L), some dietary restrictions	documented poor renal function (creatinine >200 μmol/L), regular dialysis programme (peritoneal or haemodialysis)

So first you need to know the grade of the surgery (you may have to estimate it as there isn't an exhaustive list) and then you need to work out the patient's ASA grade and which system is causing them to score higher on their ASA – cardiovascular, respiratory or renal? You can then consult the following tables to work out which tests to perform. There are separate tables for neurosurgery and cardiac surgery, for paediatrics and adults. Needless to say unless you're insane, this is something to reference, not to memorise.

Of course, if you have a particular reason to get a chest X-ray, for example if you've identified something on examination, go ahead and get it regardless.

YES	Test recommended
NO	Test not recommended
Consider	The value of carrying out a preoperative test is not known, and may depend on specific patient characteristics; CONSIDER carrying out a preoperative test

6.12 Grade I surgery

ASA grade I: Children (<16 years)

Test	<6 months	6 to 12 months	1 to 5 years	5 to 12 years	12 to 16 years
Chest x-ray	No	No	No	No	No
ECG	No	No	No	No	No
Full blood count	No	No	No	No	No
Haemostasis	No	No	No	No	No
Renal function	No	No	No	No	No
Random glucose	No	No	No	No	No
Urine analysis[a]	No	No	No	No	No

[a] *Dipstick urine testing in asymptomatic individuals is not recommended (UK National Screening Committee)*

ASA grade I: Adults (≥16 years)

Test	> 16 to <40	>40 to <60	>60 to <80	>80
Chest x-ray	No	No	No	No
ECG	No			Yes
Full blood count	No	No		
Haemostasis	No	No	No	No
Renal function	No	No		
Random glucose	No	No	No	No
Urine analysis[a]				

[a] *Dipstick urine testing in asymptomatic individuals is not recommended (UK National Screening Committee)*

ASA grade 2: Adults with comorbidity from CVD

Test	> 16 to < 40	> 40 to < 60	> 60 to < 80	> 80
Chest x-ray	No			
ECG	Yes	Yes	Yes	Yes
Full blood count				
Haemostasis	No	No	No	No
Renal function				
Random glucose	No	No	No	No
Urine analysis				
Blood gases	No	No	No	No
Lung function	No	No	No	No

ASA grade 3: Adults with comorbidity from CVD

Test	> 16 to < 40	> 40 to < 60	> 60 to < 80	> 80
Chest x-ray				
ECG	Yes	Yes	Yes	Yes
Full blood count				
Haemostasis	No	No	No	No
Renal function	Yes	Yes	Yes	Yes
Random glucose	No	No	No	No
Urine analysis				
Blood gases				
Lung function	No	No	No	No

ASA grade 2: Adults with comorbidity from respiratory disease

Test	> 16 to < 40	> 40 to < 60	> 60 to < 80	> 80
Chest x-ray[b]	No			
ECG	No			
Full blood count				
Haemostasis	No	No	No	No
Renal function	No	No		
Random glucose	No	No	No	No
Urine analysis				
Blood gases				
Lung function	No	No	No	No

[b] *Chest x-rays may be considered if there has been a change in patient's symptoms or if the patient needs ventilator support*

ASA grade 3: Adults with comorbidity from respiratory disease

Test	> 16 to < 40	> 40 to < 60	> 60 to < 80	> 80
Chest x-ray				
ECG				
Full blood count				
Haemostasis	No	No	No	No
Renal function				
Random glucose	No	No	No	No
Urine analysis				
Blood gases				
Lung function	No	No	No	No

ASA grade 2: Adults with comorbidity from renal disease

Test	>16 to <40	>40 to <60	>60 to <80	>80
Chest x-ray[b]	No	No	No	
ECG	No			
Full blood count				
Haemostasis	No	No	No	No
Renal function	Yes	Yes	Yes	Yes
Random glucose	No	No	No	No
Urine analysis				
Blood gases	No	No	No	No
Lung function	No	No	No	No

[b] *Chest x-rays may be considered if there has been a change in patient's symptoms or if the patient needs ventilator support*

ASA grade 3: Adults with comorbidity from renal disease

Test	>16 to <40	>40 to <60	>60 to <80	>80
Chest x-ray	No	No		
ECG	No			
Full blood count	Yes	Yes	Yes	Yes
Haemostasis				
Renal function	Yes	Yes	Yes	Yes
Random glucose				
Urine analysis				
Blood gases				
Lung function	No	No	No	No

6.13 Grade 2 surgery

ASA grade 1: Children (<16 years)

Test	<6 months	6 to 12 months	1 to 5 years	5 to 12 years	12 to 16 years
Chest x-ray	No	No	No	No	No
ECG	No	No	No	No	No
Full blood count	No	No	No	No	No
Haemostasis	No	No	No	No	No
Renal function	No	No	No	No	No
Random glucose	No	No	No	No	No
Urine analysis[a]	No	No	No	No	No

[a] *Dipstick urine testing in asymptomatic individuals is not recommended (UK National Screening Committee)*

ASA grade 1: Adults (≥16 years)

Test	>16 to <40	>40 to <60	>60 to <80	>80
Chest x-ray	No	No	No	No
ECG	No			Yes
Full blood count	No		Yes	Yes
Haemostasis	No	No	No	No
Renal function	No	No		
Random glucose	No			
Urine analysis[a]				

[a] *Dipstick urine testing in asymptomatic individuals is not recommended (UK National Screening Committee)*

ASA grade 2: Adults with comorbidity from CVD

Test	>16 to <40	>40 to <60	>60 to <80	>80
Chest x-ray				
ECG	Yes	Yes	Yes	Yes
Full blood count				
Haemostasis	No	No	No	No
Renal function			Yes	Yes
Random glucose	No	No	No	No
Urine analysis				
Blood gases	No	No	No	No
Lung function	No	No	No	No

ASA grade 3: Adults with comorbidity from CVD

Test	>16 to <40	>40 to <60	>60 to <80	>80
Chest x-ray				
ECG	Yes	Yes	Yes	Yes
Full blood count				
Haemostasis	No	No	No	No
Renal function	Yes	Yes	Yes	Yes
Random glucose	No	No	No	No
Urine analysis				
Blood gases				
Lung function	No	No	No	No

ASA grade 2: Adults with comorbidity from respiratory disease

Test	>16 to <40	>40 to <60	>60 to <80	>80
Chest x-ray[b]				
ECG	No			
Full blood count				
Haemostasis	No	No	No	No
Renal function	No			
Random glucose	No	No	No	No
Urine analysis				
Blood gases				
Lung function	No	No	No	No

[b] *Chest x-rays may be considered if there has been a change in patient's symptoms or if the patient needs ventilator support*

ASA grade 3: Adults with comorbidity from respiratory disease

Test	>16 to <40	>40 to <60	>60 to <80	>80
Chest x-ray				
ECG			Yes	Yes
Full blood count				Yes
Haemostasis	No	No	No	No
Renal function				
Random glucose	No	No	No	No
Urine analysis				
Blood gases				
Lung function				

ASA grade 2: Adults with comorbidity from renal disease

Test	> 16 to < 40	> 40 to < 60	> 60 to < 80	> 80
Chest x-ray[b]	No	No		
ECG			Yes	Yes
Full blood count				
Haemostasis	No	No	No	No
Renal function	Yes	Yes	Yes	Yes
Random glucose	No	No	No	No
Urine analysis				
Blood gases	No	No	No	No
Lung function	No	No	No	No

[b] *Chest x-rays may be considered if there has been a change in patient's symptoms or if the patient needs ventilator support*

ASA grade 3: Adults with comorbidity from renal disease

Test	> 16 to < 40	> 40 to < 60	> 60 to < 80	> 80
Chest x-ray				
ECG			Yes	Yes
Full blood count	Yes	Yes	Yes	Yes
Haemostasis				
Renal function	Yes	Yes	Yes	Yes
Random glucose				
Urine analysis				
Blood gases				
Lung function	No	No	No	No

6.14 Grade 3 surgery

ASA grade 1: Children (<16 years)

Test	<6 months	6 to 12 months	1 to 5 years	5 to 12 years	12 to 16 years
Chest x-ray	No	No	No	No	No
ECG	No	No	No	No	No
Full blood count					
Haemostasis	No	No	No	No	No
Renal function					
Random glucose	No	No	No	No	No
Urine analysis[a]					

[a] *Dipstick urine testing in asymptomatic individuals is not recommended (UK National Screening Committee)*

ASA grade 1: Adults (≥16 years)

Test	> 16 to < 40	> 40 to < 60	> 60 to < 80	> 80
Chest x-ray	No	No		
ECG	No		Yes	Yes
Full blood count	Yes	Yes	Yes	Yes
Haemostasis	No	No	No	No
Renal function			Yes	Yes
Random glucose				
Urine analysis[a]				

[a] *Dipstick urine testing in asymptomatic individuals is not recommended (UK National Screening Committee)*

ASA grade 2: Adults with comorbidity from CVD

Test	> 16 to < 40	> 40 to < 60	> 60 to < 80	> 80
Chest x-ray				
ECG	Yes	Yes	Yes	Yes
Full blood count	Yes	Yes	Yes	Yes
Haemostasis	No	No	No	No
Renal function	Yes	Yes	Yes	Yes
Random glucose	No	No	No	No
Urine analysis				
Blood gases				
Lung function	No	No	No	No

ASA grade 3: Adults with comorbidity from CVD

Test	> 16 to < 40	> 40 to < 60	> 60 to < 80	> 80
Chest x-ray				
ECG	Yes	Yes	Yes	Yes
Full blood count	Yes	Yes	Yes	Yes
Haemostasis				
Renal function	Yes	Yes	Yes	Yes
Random glucose	No	No	No	No
Urine analysis				
Blood gases				
Lung function	No	No	No	No

ASA grade 2: Adults with comorbidity from respiratory disease

Test	> 16 to < 40	> 40 to < 60	> 60 to < 80	> 80
Chest x-ray[b]				
ECG				Yes
Full blood count	Yes	Yes	Yes	Yes
Haemostasis	No	No	No	No
Renal function			Yes	Yes
Random glucose	No	No	No	No
Urine analysis				
Blood gases				
Lung function	No			

[b] *Chest x-rays may be considered if there has been a change in patient's symptoms or if the patient needs ventilator support*

ASA grade 3: Adults with comorbidity from respiratory disease

Test	> 16 to < 40	> 40 to < 60	> 60 to < 80	> 80
Chest x-ray				
ECG			Yes	Yes
Full blood count	Yes	Yes	Yes	Yes
Haemostasis	No	No	No	No
Renal function	Yes	Yes	Yes	Yes
Random glucose				
Urine analysis				
Blood gases				
Lung function				

ASA grade 2: Adults with comorbidity from renal disease

Test	> 16 to < 40	> 40 to < 60	> 60 to < 80	> 80
Chest x-ray[b]				
ECG			Yes	Yes
Full blood count	Yes	Yes	Yes	Yes
Haemostasis				
Renal function	Yes	Yes	Yes	Yes
Random glucose				
Urine analysis				
Blood gases				
Lung function	No	No	No	No

[b] *Chest x-rays may be considered if there has been a change in patient's symptoms or if the patient needs ventilator support*

ASA grade 2: Adults with comorbidity from renal disease

Test	> 16 to < 40	> 40 to < 60	> 60 to < 80	> 80
Chest x-ray				
ECG			Yes	Yes
Full blood count	Yes	Yes	Yes	Yes
Haemostasis				
Renal function	Yes	Yes	Yes	Yes
Random glucose				
Urine analysis				
Blood gases				
Lung function	No	No	No	No

6.15 Grade 4 surgery

ASA grade 1: Children (< 16 years)

Test	< 6 months	6 to 12 months	1 to 5 years	5 to 12 years	12 to 16 years
Chest x-ray	No	No	No	No	No
ECG	No	No	No	No	No
Full blood count					
Haemostasis	No	No	No	No	No
Renal function					
Random glucose	No	No	No	No	No
Urine analysis[a]					

[a] *Dipstick urine testing in asymptomatic individuals is not recommended (UK National Screening Committee)*

ASA grade 1: Adults (≥16 years)

Test	> 16 to < 40	> 40 to < 60	> 60 to < 80	> 80
Chest x-ray	No	No		
ECG	No		Yes	Yes
Full blood count	Yes	Yes	Yes	Yes
Haemostasis				
Renal function	Yes	Yes	Yes	Yes
Random glucose				
Urine analysis[a]				

[a] *Dipstick urine testing in asymptomatic individuals is not recommended (UK National Screening Committee)*

ASA grade 2: Adults with comorbidity from CVD

Test	> 16 to < 40	> 40 to < 60	> 60 to < 80	> 80
Chest x-ray				
ECG	Yes	Yes	Yes	Yes
Full blood count	Yes	Yes	Yes	Yes
Haemostasis				
Renal function	Yes	Yes	Yes	Yes
Random glucose	No	No	No	No
Urine analysis				
Blood gases				
Lung function	No	No	No	No

ASA grade 3: Adults with comorbidity from CVD

Test	> 16 to < 40	> 40 to < 60	> 60 to < 80	> 80
Chest x-ray			Yes	Yes
ECG	Yes	Yes	Yes	Yes
Full blood count	Yes	Yes	Yes	Yes
Haemostasis				
Renal function	Yes	Yes	Yes	Yes
Random glucose	No	No	No	No
Urine analysis				
Blood gases				
Lung function	No	No	No	No

ASA grade 2: Adults with comorbidity from respiratory disease

Test	> 16 to < 40	> 40 to < 60	> 60 to < 80	> 80
Chest x-ray[b]				
ECG			Yes	Yes
Full blood count	Yes	Yes	Yes	Yes
Haemostasis				
Renal function	Yes	Yes	Yes	Yes
Random glucose	No	No	No	No
Urine analysis				
Blood gases				
Lung function				

[b] *Chest x-rays may be considered if there has been a change in patient's symptoms or if the patient needs ventilator support*

ASA grade 3: Adults with comorbidity from respiratory disease

Test	> 16 to < 40	> 40 to < 60	> 60 to < 80	> 80
Chest x-ray				
ECG		Yes	Yes	Yes
Full blood count	Yes	Yes	Yes	Yes
Haemostasis				
Renal function	Yes	Yes	Yes	Yes
Random glucose				
Urine analysis				
Blood gases				
Lung function				

ASA grade 2: Adults with comorbidity from renal disease

Test	>16 to <40	>40 to <60	>60 to <80	>80
Chest x-ray[b]				
ECG		Yes	Yes	Yes
Full blood count	Yes	Yes	Yes	Yes
Haemostasis				
Renal function	Yes	Yes	Yes	Yes
Random glucose				
Urine analysis				
Blood gases				
Lung function	No	No	No	No

[b] Chest x-rays may be considered if there has been a change in patient's symptoms or if the patient needs ventilator support

ASA grade 3: Adults with comorbidity from renal disease

Test	>16 to <40	>40 to <60	>60 to <80	>80
Chest x-ray				
ECG		Yes	Yes	Yes
Full blood count	Yes	Yes	Yes	Yes
Haemostasis				
Renal function	Yes	Yes	Yes	Yes
Random glucose				
Urine analysis				
Blood gases				
Lung function	No	No	No	No

6.16 Neurosurgery

ASA grade 1: Children (<16 years)

Test	<6 months	6 to 12 months	1 to 5 years	5 to 12 years	12 to 16 years
Chest x-ray	No	No	No	No	No
ECG	No	No	No	No	No
Full blood count					
Haemostasis					
Renal function	Yes	Yes	Yes	Yes	Yes
Random glucose	No	No	No	No	No
Urine analysis[a]					

[a] Dipstick urine testing in asymptomatic individuals is not recommended (UK National Screening Committee)

ASA grade 1: Adults (≥16 years)

Test	>16 to <40	>40 to <60	>60 to <80	>80
Chest x-ray	No	No		
ECG			Yes	es
Full blood count			Yes	Yes
Haemostasis				
Renal function	Yes	Yes	Yes	Yes
Random glucose				
Urine analysis[a]				

[a] Dipstick urine testing in asymptomatic individuals is not recommended (UK National Screening Committee)

ADA grade 1: Children (<16 years)

Test	<6 months	6 to 12 months	1 to 5 years	5 to 12 years	12 to 16 years
Chest x-ray	Yes	Yes	Yes	Yes	Yes
ECG	Yes	Yes	Yes	Yes	Yes
Full blood count	Yes	Yes	Yes	Yes	Yes
Haemostasis					
Renal function	Yes	Yes	Yes	Yes	Yes
Random glucose	No	No	No	No	No
Urine analysis[a]					

[a] *Dipstick urine testing in asymptomatic individuals is not recommended (UK National Screening Committee)*

ASA grade 1: Adults (≥16 years)

Test	>16 to <40	>40 to <60	>60 to <80	>80
Chest x-ray	Yes	Yes	Yes	Yes
ECG	Yes	Yes	Yes	Yes
Full blood count	Yes	Yes	Yes	Yes
Haemostasis				
Renal function	Yes	Yes	Yes	Yes
Random glucose				
Urine analysis[a]				

[a] *Dipstick urine testing in asymptomatic individuals is not recommended (UK National Screening Committee)*

Sickle cell

All patients fitting the ethnic criteria listed in the following table must receive sickle cell testing after giving informed consent.

Tests for the sickle cell gene in adults and children

Appropriateness of testing in patients from the following ethnic groups	
North African	Yes
West African	Yes
South/sub Saharan African	Yes
Afro Caribbean	Yes
Should informed consent be obtained?	Yes

Pregnancy

All women of reproductive age should be offered a pregnancy test after informed consent, and women should be made aware of the risks to the foetus.

Blood grouping and cross-matching

Each trust should have its own Maximum Surgical Blood Ordering Schedule (MSBOS). This idea was first developed in 1990 by the British Committee for Standards in Haematology to help guide us on when to group and save, when to cross match and when to do nothing. The following is the original 1990 version to give you an idea, but local policies vary. There hasn't been a more up-to-date national version since then.

Maximum Surgical Blood Ordering Schedule 1990	
General Surgery	
Cholecystectomy and exploration of common duct	G & S
Splenectomy	G & S
Gastrostomy, ileostomy, colostomy	G & S
Oesophageal dilation	G & S
Oesophagectomy	5
Hiatus hernia	2
Partial gastrectomy	G & S
Oesophagogastrectomy	4
Hepatectomy	4
Mastectomy (simple)	G & S
Endoerine –	
Thyroidectomy – partial/total	G & S
Parathyroidectomy	G & S
Adrenalectomy	3
Panereatectomy – partial/Whipple	4
Transplantation –	
Renal	2
Graft nephrectomy	2
Donor nephrectomy	G & S
Marrow Harvest	2
Colo-rectal Surgery	

Rectum – pouch; resection/excision etc.	2
Intra-abdominal – colectomy etc.	2
Rectopexy	G & S
Vascular Surgery	
Amputation of leg	G & S
Sympathectomy	G & S
Femoral endarterectomy	G & S
Carotid endarterectomy	G & S
Femoro-popliteal bypass	2
Axillo-femoral bypass	2
Aorto-femoral bypass	4
Bifemoral bypass	6
Aorto-iliac bypass	4
Aorto-iliac endarterectomy	4
Infra-renal aortic aneurysm	6
Thoracic or thoraco-abdominal aneurysm	10
Ruptured aneurysms	10
Cardio-thoracic surgery	
Angioplasty	G & S
Open heart operations – CAVBG, MVR, AVR, (redo*)	4 (8*)
Bronchoscopy	G & S
Open pleural/lung biopsy	G & S
Lobectomy/pneumonectomy	2

(Continued)

Sternal refashioning	G & S
Ureterolithotomy and Cystotomy	G & S
Reimplantation of Ureter	G & S
Urethroplasty	2
Head and neck	
Major H-N procedures – Laryngectomy etc, Major plastic reconstructions (see Plastic Surgery)	2
Other H-N procedures	G & S
Plastic Surgery	
Abdominoplasty	G & S
Mammoplasty	G & S
Head and neck reconstructions	2
Laparotomy – planned exploration	G & S
Liver biopsy	G & S
Vagotomy +/– drainage	G & S
Neurosurgery	
Head injury, extradural haematoma	2
Craniotomy, craniectomy	G & S
Meningioma	4
Vascular surgery (aneurysms, A-V malformations)	3
Shunt procedures	G & S
Cranioplasty	G & S
Trans-sphenoidal hypophysectomy	G & S

Vascular transformations, posterior fossa exploration	2
Disc surgery	G & S
Laminectomy	G & S
Spinal decompression for tumours	2
Peripheral nerve surgery	G & S
Orthopaedics	
Removal hip pin or femoral nail	G & S
Ostectomy/bone biopsy (except upper femur*)	G & S (2*)
Removal cervical rib	G & S
Bone graft from iliac crest – 1 side (both sides *)	G & S (2*)
Nailing fractured neck of femur	G & S
Spinal fusion	2
Laminectomy	G & S
Internal fixation of femur	2
Internal fixation – fibia or ankle	G & S
Arthroplasty – total knee or shoulder	2
– total hip	2
– total elbow	2
Changing hip prosthesis	4
Dynamic hip screw	G & S
Urology	
Cystectomy	6
Cystectomy and Urethrectomy	8

(Continued)

Nephrectomy	2
Nephrectomy and Exploration of vena cava	6
Open Nephrolithotomy	2
Open Prostatectomy (RPP)	2
TURP	G & S
TUR Bladder Tumour (large tumour)	G & S
Percutaneous Nephrolithotomy	G & S
Ureterolithotomy	G & S
Cystotomy	G & S
Obstetrics and Gynaecology	
LSCS	2
ERPC/D & C	G & S
Hydatidiform mole	2
Placenta praevia/retained placenta	2
APH/PPH	2 (variable)
Hysterectomy: abdominal or vaginal – simple	G & S
– extended	2
Wertheim's operation	4
Pelvic exenteration	6
Vulvectomy (radical)	4
Myomectomy	2
Oophorectomy (radical)	4
Termination of pregnancy	G & S

Other preparatory measures

In addition to these investigations you will want to write the patient's **drug chart** in advance of their admission and include:

1 their regular medications

2 any perioperative antibiotics you envisage they will have (for example in orthopaedic joint surgery)

3 DVT prophylaxis – TEDS and low molecular weight heparin

4 analgesia

5 antiemetics

6 preoperative intravenous fluids where appropriate

7 bowel preparation if indicated (very much depends on individual consultant preferences but is commonly favoured for left colonic resections (not right)).

Make sure all of the relevant **imaging** is available on PACS. If the patient had their CT at St Elsewhere's it may not be available and will need to be found before surgery.

In an ideal world, the patient should be **consented** well before the day of their surgery and the pre-assessment clinic is an ideal time to do this. If you aren't capable of consenting them, try and arrange for someone who is to see the patient too.

On admission

- The **side** of surgery (where appropriate) needs to be marked.
- The **consent form** must be re-checked and confirmed.
- The **drug chart** must be re-checked.
- The **imaging** must be checked.
- The **results** of any outstanding investigations must be checked and made readily available in the notes

The perioperative management of specific conditions/ medications

Diabetic patients

Usual medications are taken up to and including the day before surgery by all diabetics, although some advocate reducing the evening dose the night before going nil by mouth. Insulin-dependent diabetics should be started on an insulin sliding scale either from the night before or the morning of surgery depending on the time of surgery and when they are admitted. The sliding scale continues throughout surgery and is stopped only when the patient is eating and drinking again, when their usual regimen can be restarted.

Non-insulin-dependent diabetics should not take their antidiabetic medications on the day of surgery. Secretagogues like sulphonylureas can cause hypoglycemia and metformin can cause lactic acidosis. So these patients may require the same treatment as insulin-dependent diabetics depending on the severity of their disease. This should be checked by regular BM measurements. If the BMs are high on the day of surgery because of omission of antidiabetic medications start a sliding scale and restart the oral medications postoperatively only when they are eating and drinking again.

Remember, diabetic patients are at higher risk of a variety of complications, not least infections – always consider the use of antibiotics. Try to always put diabetic patients first on the list.

Patients on steroids

Surgery is a physiological insult resulting in release of endogenous steroids from the adrenal gland. Patients taking long-term steroids will have adrenal gland suppression and won't be able to rise to the occasion, particularly if their oral prednisolone is withheld. Give intravenous hydrocortisone or similar instead to avoid an Addisonian crisis. A dose of 5 mg of oral prednisolone is equivalent to 20 mg of hydrocortisone. Continue the intravenous doeses until the patient is able to take their oral prednisolone again.

Patients who are anticoagulated

Warfarin should be stopped five days before surgery in order to achieve an INR < 1.5. If their indication for taking warfarin is only relative, such as uncomplicated atrial fibrillation, they need no other substitute. If, however, they have had multiple pulmonary emboli, or most significantly have a metallic heart valve, they must be admitted to the hospital during this time to receive replacement anticoagulation in the form of an intravenous heparin infusion that can be switched off just four hours prior to surgery and switched back on again afterwards, thus minimising the time their blood isn't anticoagulated. In some hospitals, rather than a heparin infusion, treatment dose low molecular weight heparins such as dalteparin are preferred, with the advantage of a once daily injection and not having to measure the APTT (which is the measure of the effect of heparin).

Patients on antiplatelets

If there is no absolute indication for taking aspirin it should be stopped seven days before surgery. There is no point stopping it on the day of surgery, it will take another seven days before platelet function normalises, i.e., new platelets have been made. Clopidogrel should ideally be stopped for two weeks before. The main absolute indication for keeping antiplatelets going is the presence of coronary drug eluting stents, which usually absolutely need to continue for one year post insertion. For less absolute indications weigh up the pros and cons of a higher risk of bleeding and bruising versus a lowered risk of thromboembolic events, or whatever the patient is taking it for. This comes down to individual surgical preference. In general most surgeons will be happy to operate if the patient is taking one of these pair, but aspirin *and* clopidogrel can cause considerable difficulty with haemostasis. In emergencies, a bag of intraoperative platelets may be necessary.

Patients with sickle cell disease

These patients need maximum oxygenation, hydration and warming to prevent sickle cell crises. Their haemoglobin should be checked as they run a chronic anaemia, so blood should be available where necessary.

References

National Institute for Clinical Excellence (2003) *Preoperative Tests. The use of routine preoperative tests for elective surgery*. London: NICE.

Voak D, Napier JAF, Boulton FE *et al*. (1990) Guidelines for implementation of a maximum surgical blood order schedule. *Clinical and Laboratory Haematology* 12: 321–7.

Appendix 2
CONSENT

It is well established that, as a general rule, the performance of a medical operation upon a person without his or her consent is unlawful, as constituting both the crime of battery and the tort of trespass to the person.

Lord Goff 1990

Introduction

Consenting the patient means that irritating step of getting them to sign that yellow form before the porters take them down to theatre, doesn't it? Well unfortunately that's how it's often interpreted, and practised. Consent, to many, may sound like a boring, dry subject, but if you want to be a surgeon you'd better get interested in it, and fully understand it. If you don't, a career's worth of disgruntled patients, lawsuits and even (theoretically) a spell in one of Her Majesty's prisons awaits you. This will by no means be a comprehensive review of consent – it would take up several tomes – rather it is a brief whistle stop tour.

Issues of consent for surgical procedures fall into two broad categories: those patients who **can consent for themselves**, and **those who can't**. In most of your practice, unless you're destined to be a neonatal paediatric surgeon, it's likely that the majority of your patients fall into the former group, and the distinguishing feature of the two groups is whether the patient has the mental capacity to make a decision.

Assessment of capacity

To decide which group your patient falls into, you need to decide if they have capacity to make decisions about their treatment. The first principle is that you **assume all patients over the age of 16 to have the required capacity** unless shown otherwise.

According to the **Mental Capacity Act (MCA) 2005**, a patient will not have capacity if they are unable to do one or more of the following:

1 **understand** the information relevant to the decision

2 **retain** that information

3 **weigh up** the **pros and cons** related to the decision

4 **communicate** the decision

The Hands-on Guide to Surgical Training, First Edition. Matthew Stephenson.

Often, the above is not completely clear-cut and everyone, including the courts, accepts this. What is important is that you make reasonable decisions and **document clearly** in the notes anything that may seem contentious and how you've come to your conclusion. Furthermore, a patient may have the capacity to make decisions about one thing, but not another, or this may vary over time.

Patients with capacity

Assessment of capacity is just the first step for this group, there are two other vital ingredients to obtaining consent. The three components are:

1 the patient has **capacity** (see above)

2 the patient is **fully informed** about the procedure

3 the consent is **voluntary**

In other words, it's no good getting a perfectly competent intelligent patient to consent to a procedure unless you have fully informed them of the nature of the procedure, the pros and cons, and the alternatives. Equally, consent isn't valid if you've twisted their arm because you really wanted to do their operation, or you misrepresent the value of an alternative option, or the patient is being bullied into it by a caring relative.

This second point is a bit sticky – just how much do you tell the patient about the risks of a procedure? For this we must look to some **English case law**. You may have heard of the **Bolam (and Bolitho) tests**. As Mr Justice McNair put it in Bolam in 1957:

> *I myself would prefer to put it this way, that he is not guilty of negligence if he has acted in accordance with a practice accepted as proper by a responsible body of medical men skilled in that particular art. I do not think there is much difference in sense. It is just a different way of expressing the same thought. Putting it the other way round, a man is not negligent, if he is acting in accordance with such a practice, merely because there is a body of opinion who would take a contrary view. At the same time, that does not mean that a medical man can obstinately and pig-headedly carry on with some old technique if it has been proved to be contrary to what is really substantially the whole of informed medical opinion. Otherwise you might get men today saying: 'I do not believe in anaesthetics. I do not believe in antiseptics. I am going to continue to do my surgery in the way it was done in the eighteenth century.' That clearly would be wrong.*

This applied to consent in that a doctor would be expected to tell their patient about whatever risks a responsible body of doctors would tell their patients in the same circumstances.

In other words, if Doctor X never warned his hernia repair patients about the risk of chronic groin pain and a patient sues Doctor X because he didn't warn him, Dr X could get away with it if he could find a group of his mates who wouldn't have warned the patient in those circumstances either, *providing* that those mates held a view that was capable of withstanding logical analysis; a decision which would ultimately fall to be made by the court.

This dominated the legal scene for a long time – and amounted to telling the patient about all of the common potential risks – but the crucial factor has been: how common does a risk have to be to tell the patient? In the case of **Sidaway v Bethlem Royal Hospital** (1985), the claimant failed in her lawsuit against her neurosurgeon for not telling her about the 1% risk of paraplegia (which she unfortunately developed) during a cervical cord decompression. The court felt that the surgeon was not under a duty to warn the patient about remote side effects, they felt a risk of 10% was a reasonable cut off. In the case of **Pearce v United Bristol** (1999), the pregnant defendant was overdue by about two weeks and requested an induction or Caesarean section. She was advised by her consultant to proceed with a natural delivery but this resulted in a stillbirth. She lost her case because the risk of proceeding with a natural birth was only in the order of 0.1–0.2%, but the court did contend that doctors should **err on the side of generosity** in giving information to their patients.

Importantly in the Pearce case, the court found that if there was a significant risk that would affect the judgement of **a reasonable patient**, then in the normal course* (*only if the doctor believes that the disclosure of such information would not cause the patient significant harm or distress – the 'therapeutic privilege') it is the responsibility of a doctor to inform the patient of that significant risk so that the patient can determine for themself as to what course they should adopt.

The next big case to challenge the received wisdom of risk was **Chester v Afshar** (2004). Mrs Chester suffered neurological injury following neurosurgical intervention for her lower back and claimed to have never been warned about it, the risk being in the order of 1–2%. She won. A precedent had been set in which serious complications, even if they were unlikely, should be raised with the patient.

As if that didn't make it complicated enough, there was then the case of **Birch v UCL Hospital** (2008). Mrs Birch was admitted with a third nerve palsy and underwent a diagnostic angiogram to look for a cerebral aneurysm. She was appropriately counselled about the risks of the angiogram. She suffered a stroke, sued the hospital, and won – why? Because she wasn't told about the **alternatives**, and the pros and cons of the alternatives (and in particular an MRI which would not have had the risk of a stroke) so she was found to have been denied an opportunity to properly weigh the comparative risks and benefits of competing procedures.

So there has been a paradigm shift away from warning patients about risks that seem **reasonable to the doctor** (or body of doctors), to warning the patient about risks that would seem **reasonable to the patient**. In other words, a 0.5% risk of causing ischaemic orchitis following a primary inguinal hernia repair may not seem too troubling to you as the surgeon, but if you were the patient, you may have wanted to know. What's more – have you told your patient that while you can offer an open inguinal hernia repair, Mr X down the road could do it laparoscopically (and all that that might entail)?

In short, consent, even for a patient with capacity, can be very, very thorny.

But in general you are far safer by telling the patient more, rather than less, even if the risk is small. And by the way, what if you don't actually write down on the consent form or in the notes that you've warned the patient that the varicose veins might come back? Who do you think the civil courts are going to believe – you or the patient? Sorry, but it will be the patient almost all of the time. Remember civil courts need only prove, on the 'balance of probabilities' (not 'beyond all reasonable doubt' as in criminal courts) and who will the court consider is more likely to remember what you said on that day three years ago when you saw the patient in day surgery? The patient who's only had one operation in her life and for whom it was a major event, or you, who's done hundreds of operations since then and can't even remember her name?

So essentially, it's not about getting that patient to scribble a mark on a yellow form – it's a matter of confirming they have capacity to make that decision, ensuring they are fully informed of the procedure and all it entails, including the alternatives, and finally letting them think and cogitate on it. Therefore it is best not left until the day of surgery, unless in emergency situations – it's far better done in the outpatient clinic. The scribbling on the 'form' is merely evidence that you said what you did, when you did – it is not 'consent'.

Patients without capacity

But what about patients who you think don't have capacity to make decisions? The **Mental Capacity Act (MCA) 2005**, which came into force in October 2007 pulled together much of the ad-hoc case law that had accumulated over the years. It was designed to codify the underlying principles to protect patients who lack capacity. Let's say for instance a man with Down syndrome with associated severe learning disabilities comes to see you in clinic – he has an inguinal hernia (this isn't an emergency). The patient has no living relatives and no other legally recognised directive. In the past, if the doctor felt it was in the best interests of the patient to have his hernia repaired, he would proceed.

So what should you do now? First, is it possible that the patient **may regain his capacity** and you must consider if the decision for treatment is **delayable** until then? If so, you should wait, but this usually isn't the case. Second, you must **enable the patient** as much as possible in taking part in the decision-making process – even if you can't get a full and clear idea of what they would want, the little information you can still glean is useful. Third, you must consider any **premorbid wishes expressed** – either verbally or written, for instance an an **advance directive** (a legally recognised statement made by the patient when they have capacity, to be invoked if they lose capacity) or if the patient has appointed a **lasting power of attorney** (someone who the patient appointed when they had capacity to take on such decisions in the event that they lose capacity, it replaced the **enduring power of attorney**). Fourth, you must take the views of those closest to the **patient** (even if not appointed as lasting powers of attorney) – usually the family, but also healthcare professionals. Normally this is sufficient to form a decision, but that decision to treat must be a reasonable one and made only after, and on the basis of, this holistic assessment of the patient's interests. It must be written in the notes in full, with a thorough explanation of why and how the decision was reached. There is usually a special form in your hospital to fill in too. This should be enough to make a safe, considered decision in the best interests of the patient and keep you out of trouble.

But what happens if the patient has no family? They live in a nursing home and all their friends and family are dead. They have no advance directive and there's no lasting power of attorney. They are unbefriended. Meet the **Independent Mental Capacity Advocate (IMCA)**. These are non-medical individuals who you must get in contact with in these circumstances; your hospital will have a local IMCA service. They will arrange to meet with you to discuss the best interests of the patient, the IMCA representing what one would hope to be the best interests of the patient. In other words, the paternalism of days gone has vanished – doctor does not necessarily know best. Ignoring this would be extremely unwise.

Special circumstances

Emergencies

In the emergency situation where the patient has capacity to make decisions, you can obviously proceed as you normally would, although the steps are bound to be quicker and you, the patient and the court would accept that their time for cogitation would be limited. Worrying about being sued over this must not delay a vital operation. In emergencies, what needs to be done gets done. For the patient without capacity to make decisions, which may be an unconscious patient or one with long-term lack of capacity, you must act in the patient's best interests and provide only that treatment which is necessary (until capacity can be re-established) – in true traditional paternalist style – and without further ado.

Paediatrics

In the 16- to 18-year-old category, patients can consent for procedures, but strictly they can't refuse them against medical advice if this would not be in their best interests. Such rare situations require great tact and care. In the rarest of situations, an application to court may be necessary. In the under-16 category, in general, patients are deemed to be children and their parents must consent for them and act in the child's best interests. However, the case of **Gillick v West Norfolk** (1985) in which a child was prescribed contraception without the knowledge of her mother set a precedent. If the minor is able to understand the information, in much the same way as an adult – they are deemed '**Gillick competent'** – i.e. they are treated as an adult and can consent as such. The decision is reached on a case-by-case basis and will require you to consider the mental, emotional and chronological age of the child, their ability to understand

and their ability to appreciate the consequences of their decision.

Summary

- **All patients over the age of 16 have the capacity** to make decisions unless shown otherwise.
- A patient must be able to **understand**, **retain** and **weigh up** the information and be able to **communicate** it.
- In a patient with capacity, consent must be **fully informed** and **voluntary** to be legally recognised.
- Inform patients of all the **common risks** and any **potentially serious risks**, even if the chances are small. Err on the side of more, rather than less.
- The **Mental Capacity Act 2005** changed the management of patients without capacity.
- **Advance Directives** and **Lasting Power of Attorney** need to be considered in decision making in those without capacity
- If in doubt, appoint an **Independent Mental Capacity Advocate** (IMCA).
- In **emergencies**, if in doubt, act in what you see as the **best interests** of the patient
- Patients aged **16–18 can consent** to treatment but **can't refuse** it.
- Patients **under 16 can consent** to treatment if they are **Gillick competent**.

Appendix 3
LOCAL ANAESTHETICS

You need to know how much of which local anaesthetic drug to give, not only for procedures done purely under local anaesthetic but also as an adjunct during a general anaesthetic (if you numb the surgical field before cutting, you reduce the amount of systemic analgesia the anaesthetist has to give, and the patient wakes up in less pain).

Don't forget, local anaesthetics don't work well in inflamed, infected areas as these are acidotic. Local anaesthetics are weak alkalis and only diffuse through the cell membrane in their unionised (unprotonated) form. If there's a bunch of protons hanging around, as obviously there are in acidic environments, the local becomes ionised and can't cross the membrane. Also, the higher tissue vascularity carries the injected local away quicker.

Local anaesthetics are divided into **esters** and **amides**, examples of the former being benzocaine and cocaine, which are infrequently used. Amides are far commoner, the commonest being **lignocaine** and **bupivocaine**, with or without added adrenaline. The adrenaline locally vasoconstricts and stops the local getting away so quickly, so you can use more of it and its effects last longer. Bear in mind that these amide local anaesthetics are metabolised by the liver so their half-lives may be far longer in someone with liver failure; you may want to be sparing with it. Lignocaine's onset of action is quicker and will last one to two hours, whereas bupivocaine will last three to four hours.

Quite frustratingly, if you want to look up how much local you can safely give you'll find many sources giving different concentrations per kilogram (body weight). The following is a safe guideline:

Lignocaine	4 mg/kg
Lignocaine with adrenaline	7 mg/kg
Bupivocaine	2 mg/kg
Bupivocaine with adrenaline	3 mg/kg

Now some maths for surgeons.

- In *1 ml* of *0.5%* local anaesthetic there is *5 mg* of local anaesthetic.
- In *1 ml* of *1%* local anaesthetic there is *10 mg* of local anaesthetic.
- In *1 ml* of 2% local anaesthetic there is *20 mg* of local anaesthetic etc

Example 1

You want to use some 1% concentration plain lignocaine on a 70 kg patient.

- Maximum allowed = 70 (kg) × 4 (mg/kg) = 280 mg.

The Hands-on Guide to Surgical Training, First Edition. Matthew Stephenson.

- Total volume allowed = 280/10 = 28 ml of 1% lignocaine.

Example 2

You want to use some 0.5% concentration plain bupivocaine on a 50 kg patient.

- Maximum allowed = 50 (kg) × 2 (mg/kg) = 100 mg.
- Total volume allowed = 100/5 = 20 ml of 0.5% bupivocaine.

Don't give too much! Do this calculation for each patient before you start drawing anything up. Bupivocaine is particularly cardiotoxic with a narrower therapeutic window. The first warning signs are circumoral tingling or numbness, lightheadedness and tinnitus. This can then progress on to tonic-clonic convulsions, coma, respiratory arrest or cardiac arrest, and that would be pretty terrifying if someone's come in for excision of their mole.

The antidote

If you're using local anaesthetics you must know what to do if you inadvertently give too much and cause cardiac dysrhythmias or worse, a cardiac arrest. Aside from the obvious: stop injecting it and attending to the basic ABCs of resuscitation, the magic drug you must demand is Intralipid. Give 1,000 ml of 20% Intralipid IV in incremental amounts while resuscitating the patient.

Reference

The Association of Anaesthetists of Great Britain and Ireland (2007) *Guidelines for the Management of Severe Local Anaesthetic Toxicity*. London: AAGBI.

Index

ABCDE (primary survey) 68, 84–6
abdominal drains 54–5, 75
abdominal incisions 26, 30
abdominal wound dehiscence 64
abscesses 55
absolute risk reduction (ARR) 229
academic surgery 225–32
  clinical fellowships 106–7, 231
  foundation programmes 93
  getting published 188–9, 230
  higher degrees 138, 151, 196, 231–2
  questions likely to come up in interviews 225–30
  see *also* research
admissions 283
  take handovers 51–3
adrenaline 292
advance directives 289
Advanced Trauma Life Support (ATLS) 83–8, 118
airway management in the primary survey 68, 84–5
alcohol consumption
  alcoholic patients 83
  dehydration caused by 80
  preoperative assessment 265
Allis forceps 4
anaesthesia
  epidural 56, 62
  local 16, 292–3
anal/anorectal conditions 74–5
anal/anorectal investigations and procedures 73
analgesia 50, 62, 82
anaphylaxis 62
anastomoses, dehiscence 65–6
angiography 76
ankle-brachial pressure index (ABPI) 76
Annual Review of Competence Progression (ARCP) 120–1, 137–8, 257
antibiotics
  patients admitted on-call 82–3
  postoperative 62–3
  preoperative 20
  ward round review 50
anticoagulants 50, 284
antiplatelet agents 284
antispasmodic agents 82
aortograms 76
appendicectomy 26–31
application process 201–2
  academic training 93, 106–7
  consultant posts 261–3
  core training 101–6
  CVs 206, 208–9, 261
  failure in 115–16, 217–18
  forms 90–1, 102, 209–10, 262
  foundation training 90–3
  interviews 102–5, 210–17, 225–30
  portfolios 105, 202–8
  specialty training 127–36
  see *also* recruitment
ARCP (Annual Review of Competence Progression) 120–1, 137–8, 257
arterial investigations/procedures 76
artery forceps (haemostatic clips) 3–4
arthroplasty 38, 44, 187
ASA grades 265–7
ASIT (Association of Surgeons in Training) 238–9
aspirin 284
assigned educational supervisors 236
atelectasis 60
ATLS (Advanced Trauma Life Support) 83–8, 118
audits 94, 108, 150, 207, 216
AVPU scale 68

Babcock forceps 4, 28
Bailey bone cutters 8

The Hands-on Guide to Surgical Training, First Edition. Matthew Stephenson.

banding (of pay) 244–8
banding (of piles) 74–5
Bard–Parker handles 7, 8
barium swallows 75
Barry, Dr James 221
Basic Surgical Skills (BSS) course 117–18
bile duct, drainage using a T-tube 54, 75
biopsy procedures 75, 77
Birch v UCL Hospital (2008) 288
bleeps 15
blood loss
  haemostatic equipment 3–4, 6, 7
  perioperative 18–19
  postoperative 62, 64–5, 68
  transfusions 81, 85, 277–84
  in trauma 85
blood pressure, low 62
body language during interviews 211
Bolam test 287
bone spikes 7, 8
BOTA (British Orthopaedic Trainees Association) 239
bowel clamps 7
bowel surgery
  appendicectomy 26–31
  postoperative complications 65–6
breast surgery 141
  courses 145
  investigations and procedures 76–7
  oncoplastic surgery/fellowships 252
breathing in the primary survey 68, 85
Bristow periosteal elevators 9
British Orthopaedic Trainees Association (BOTA) 239
BSS (Basic Surgical Skills) course 117–18
bupivocaine 292, 293
buscopan 82

Calman report (1993) 240
capacity 286–90
cardiothoracic surgery xiv, 156–9
  MSBOS 279–80
  preoperative investigations 277
cardiovascular system
  postoperative complications 49, 61, 62
  preoperative assessment and investigations 264, 266, 269, 271, 273, 275
Care of the Critically Ill Surgical Patient (CrISP) course 119
career advice 217
career breaks 137, 220–1
career path
  as it is now xvi, 100–1, 111, 122–7, 240–1
  as it was in the past vii, 239–40
  cardiothoracic surgery 156
  ENT surgery 167
  general surgery 142
  interview questions about 214
  neurosurgery 180
  OFMS 161
  orthopaedic surgery 187–8
  paediatric surgery 172
  in the person specification 131, 132
  plastic surgery 194
  urology 148–9
case-based discussion (CBD) 98, 109
catheters, urinary 56, 86
CCT (Certificate of Completion of Training) 257
cellulitis 62–3
central lines 56
Centre for Workforce Intelligence (CfWI) 122
certificates 206–7
  CCT 257
  CESR 257, 258
cervical rib 76
CESR (Certificate of Eligibility of Specialist Registration) 257, 258
chest drains 54
Chester v Afshar (2004) 288
circulation in the primary survey 68, 85
cleft lip and palate surgery/fellowships 252
Clinical Anatomy of Practical Procedures course 96
clinical evaluation exercises (Mini-CEX) 98, 109
clinical fellowships 106–7, 231
clinical governance 216
clinical lectureships 231
Clinical Skills in Examining Orthopaedic Patients course 97
clinical skills (item in the person specification) 133
  see also competence (clinical)
clinical supervisors 236
clinical trials 225–30
clinics 71–7
clopidogrel 284

colleagues, behaviour towards
360 degree assessments 109, 203
at referral 73, 79–80
interview questions about 215
as a new consultant 263
in theatre 12–17
colonography 74
colonoscopy 73
colorectal surgery 141
appendicectomy 26–31
courses 145
investigations and procedures 73–5
MSBOS 279
qualities needed in consultants 259–60
communication
handover procedures 50–3, 84
interview questions about 214–15
language skills 131
in theatre 14, 15, 19
see *also* documentation
comorbidities in elective patients 264–5, 266–7
competence (clinical)
ARCP 120–1, 137–8, 257
in the core training years 107, 109, 110, 120–1
ENT surgery 169
in the foundation years 94, 98–9
neurosurgery 182–3
paediatric surgery 174–5
urology 151, 152–3
competence (to give consent) 286–91
complications, postoperative 60–6
computed tomography (CT) 74, 76
conferences 207
confidence interval (CI) 229
confidentiality 51
consent 283, 286–91
consultants
cardiothoracic surgery 159
ENT surgery 170
female 221–2
general surgery 146
getting a post 257–63
neurosurgery 184–5
OFMS 164–5
orthopaedic surgery 190–2
paediatric surgery 177
plastic surgery 198–9
qualifying for the post 256–7
in training roles 236
urology 154–5
consultations with patients 71–2
core biopsy 77
core training 100–21
cardiothoracic surgery 156–7
ENT surgery 167–8
general surgery 142–3
OFMS 161–3
orthopaedic surgery 188
paediatric surgery 172
plastic surgery 194–5, 197
recruitment 101–6
syllabus 110–11, 238
urology 150–1
cosmetic reconstructive surgery/fellowships 252
costs
CCT 257
CESR 257
courses 95, 96, 118, 119, 120
FRCS exam 139
Masters degrees 138
MRCS exam 114
overall costs of training 243–4, 245
courses
cardiothoracic surgery 158
in the core training years 108–9, 117–20, 150, 172, 197
ENT surgery 169
in the foundation years 95–7
general surgery 144–5
on interview technique 213
neurosurgery 181, 184
OFMS 164
orthopaedic surgery 189, 191
paediatric surgery 172, 175–6
plastic surgery 197–8
urology 150, 154
Covidien sutures 13
CrISP course (Care of the Critically Ill Surgical Patient) 119
critically ill patients
admitted on-call 80–8
courses on management of 96, 119
postoperative 66–70
cross-match guidelines 277–83
curriculum vitae (CV) 206, 208–9, 261
cysts, breast 77
Czerny retractors 5

deaneries 234, 235, 237
Deaver retractors 5
decision-making skills xii, 48, 134
deep venous thrombosis, prophylaxis 20, 50

dehiscence
bowel anastomoses 65–6
wound 64
dehydration 62, 80–1
dental syringes 9
dentistry 161, 164, 222
diabetic patients 284
diathermy equipment 6, 7
Diploma in Otolaryngology (DOHNS) 167
direct observation of procedural skills (DOPS) 99, 109
disability in the primary survey 68, 86, 87
discharge letters 24
disclosure of risk 287–8
diuretics, and blood transfusions 81
DNAR orders 69
Doctorate degrees 232
documentation
consent 287, 289, 290
handovers 52–3
operation notes 22–5
patient lists 51
preoperative 283
referral letters 72–3
of training see portfolios
ward rounds 46, 50
WHO surgical checklist 18–21
Doppler ultrasound 76
DOPS (direct observation of procedural skills) 99, 109
drains and tubes 53–6, 75, 86
dress codes
during ward rounds 45–6
in interviews 211
in OSCEs 116
in theatre 14–15
dressings 58–60
drug charts 24, 50, 283
dying patients 69–70
dynamic hip screw insertion 37–44

e-learning modules 98, 196–7
ear, nose and throat (ENT) surgery xv, 166–70, 252
equipment 9
electrolytes 81–2
eligibility
for foundation training 90
for MRCS exams 113
for specialty training 130
email addresses on application forms 202
emergency surgery 23
consent for 290
see also on call work
end of life care 69–70
endocrine surgery 142
endoscopic retrograde cholangiopancreato-graphy (ERCP) 75
ENT surgery xv, 166–70, 252
equipment 9
epidurals 56, 62
equipment
needed for ward rounds 46
surgical instruments 1–9
ethical issues 69, 216–17
Ethicon sutures 13
European Working Time Directive (EWTD) 153, 164, 241–3
evidence levels 228
examination under anaesthetic (EUA) 74
examinations (professional)
FRCS see exit exams
MRCS 98, 111–17, 167
exit exams 138–9
cardiothoracic surgery 159
ENT surgery 169–70
general surgery 146
neurosurgery 184
OFMS 164
orthopaedic surgery 190
paediatric surgery 176–7
plastic surgery 198
urology 153, 154
exposure in the primary survey 68, 86

failure, coping with 115–16, 217–18
family life, part-time working 219–20, 222
Fellowship of the Royal College of Surgeons (FRCS) see exit exams
fellowships 106–7, 158, 197, 231, 250–5
femoral neck fractures 37–44
fever 61–2
financial issues 243–9
see also costs
fine needle aspiration (FNA) 77
fistulograms 76
flail chest 85
flatus tubes 55–6
flexible training 219–22
fluid balance 50, 62, 80–1
follow-up procedures 72, 73
foot and ankle surgery 187
foot ulcers 57
forceps 2, 7
artery forceps 3–4
for ENT surgery 9
tissue-holding 4, 28

foundation training 8
9–99
urology 149–50
FRCS (Fellowship of the Royal College of Surgeons) see exit exams

gallbladder, investigations 75
Garden classification (femoral neck fractures) 37–8, 39
gastrointestinal assessment 49
gastrointestinal surgery 141
appendicectomy 26–31
investigations and procedures 73–5
General Medical Council (GMC) 233–4, 236, 251
general surgery xiv–xv, 140–7
appendicectomy 26–31
inguinal hernia repair 31–6, 75–6
MSBOS 278–9
Gillick competence 290–1
Gillies forceps 2
Gillies skin hooks 5, 6
Glasgow Coma Scale 87
GMC (General Medical Council) 233–4, 236, 251
Gold Guide 124, 239
Good Medical Practice 203–4
GPs 73, 79–80
grading
ASA 265–7
invasiveness of surgery 265
granulation tissue 57
groin, hernia repair 31–6, 75–6
group and save guidelines 277–82
haematoma 64
haematuria clinics 152
haemoglobin 81
haemorrhage see blood loss
haemorrhoids 74–5
haemostasis
diathermy equipment 6, 7
haemostatic clips 3–4
haemothorax 85
hair removal 20
hand surgery/fellowships 252
handover procedures 50–3, 84
hangovers, as example of dehydration 80
Hartmann's solution 81
head and neck surgery 252, 280
see also ear, nose and throat surgery; oral and maxillofacial surgery
heads of school 236
healing of wounds 56–8
health declaration 206
heart failure 61
heparin 50, 284
hepatopancreaticobiliary surgery 142
hernias, inguinal 31–6, 75–6
herniography 75
hierarchy of evidence 228
hip fractures 37–44
hip replacements 38, 44, 187
history of surgery vii, 220
recent changes to career path 239–41
hospital trusts 236
Howarth elevators 7, 8
hydrocortisone 284
hypotension 62
hypothermia 86
hypoxia 60–1

ilioinguinal nerve injections 75–6
image intensifiers (II) 40
impact factor (journals) 226
incapacity 289–90
incisions
abdominal 26, 30
for hip repair 40–1
for inguinal hernia repair 32
Independent Mental Capacity Advocate (IMCA) 290
infected wounds 57, 62–3
prevention 20
inguinal hernias 31–6, 75–6
inguinoscrotal hernias 36
insulin 283
insurance 243
Intercollegiate Surgical Curriculum Programme (ISCP) 107, 204, 238
interface fellowships 251–3
international fellowships 253–4
interviews 210–17
for consultant posts 262–3
for core training 102–5
questions likely to be asked 213–17, 225–30
for specialty training 128–9, 143, 157–8, 163, 189, 195
Intralipid 293
intravenous lines 56
investigations
preoperative 14, 265–77
specialty-specific 73–7

ISCP (Intercollegiate Surgical Curriculum Programme) 107, 204, 238

Joint Committee on Surgical Training (JCST) 236–7, 238

Killian nasal speculums 9
Kocher forceps 7

Lahey artery forceps 3, 4
Lanes forceps 2, 3
Lanes tissue-holding forceps 4
Langenbeck retractors 5
language skills 131
Lanz incision 26
laparotomy drains 55
larval therapy 58–60
left ventricular failure 61
legal issues
  consent 286–91
  working hours 241–3
less than full-time training (LTFT) 219–20
lignocaine 292–3
Liverpool Care Pathway 69–70
local anaesthesia 16, 292–3
location, location, location 91–2, 129, 260–1
locum appointments for service (LAS) 124, 218
locum appointments for training (LAT) 124
logbooks 94, 98–9, 109, 207–8
lower limb trauma and reconstruction fellowship 252
lower respiratory tract infections 61

maggots 58–60
magnetic resonance imaging (MRI) 74, 76
mallets, orthopaedic 8
mammography 76
management issues, at interview 216
marking of patients 18
Masters degrees 138, 151, 196, 197, 232
maternity leave 220–1
Maximum Surgical Blood Ordering Schedule (MSBOS) 277–82
Mayo scissors 3
McBurney's point 26
McDonald dissectors 7, 8
McIndoe double-prong skin hooks 5, 6
McIndoe forceps 2
McIndoe scissors 3
mean 228
median 228
medical indemnity 243
Membership of the Royal College of Surgeons (MRCS) 98, 111–17, 167
Mental Capacity Act (2005) 286, 289
meta-analysis 230
metabolic assessment 49
mini-CEX (clinical evaluation exercises) 98, 109
mini-PAT (peer assessment tool) 109
minors, consent 290–1
Modernising Medical Careers (MMC) 240–1
money 243–9
Morris retractors 5
motherhood
  delaying 222
  maternity leave 220–1
MRCS (Membership of the Royal College of Surgeons) 98, 111–17, 167
MRI (magnetic resonance imaging) 74, 76
MSBOS (Maximum Surgical Blood Ordering Schedule) 277–82
multiple-choice questions (MCQs) 114, 115
muscle-splitting techniques 27, 32

nasal surgery, equipment 9
nasogastric drains/tubes 55
nasojejunal tubes 55
National Patient Safety Agency (NPSA) 17
national training numbers (NTN) 123, 173, 220, 240
necrotic tissue 57, 58–60
needle holders 4–5
needles 11–12
negative pressure wound therapy 58
neonatal critical care 173
neurological assessment 49, 87
neurosurgery xv, 179–85
  MSBOS 280–1
  preoperative investigations 276
New Deal Contract 241, 242
non-steroidal anti-inflammatory drugs (NSAIDs) 82
non-take handovers 53
Norfolk and Norwich retractors 5, 6
Northern Ireland 129, 136
Northfield bone nibblers 8

NTN (national training numbers) 123, 173, 220, 240
null hypothesis 229
number needed to treat (NNT) 229
nurses, being polite to 14
nutrition 49
nylon sutures 12

obese patients 30
Objective Structured Clinical Examinations (OSCE) 114–15, 116–17
observational studies 229–30
obstetrics and gynaecology 282
odds ratio 229
oesophagogastroduodenoscopy 75
OFMS (oral and maxillofacial surgery) xv, 160–5, 252
on call work 78–80
  ENT surgery 167–8, 169
  during flexible training 220
  general surgery 143
  New Deal requirements 242
  OFMS 164
  orthopaedic surgery 189–90
  paediatric surgery 175, 177
  plastic surgery 196, 199
  urology 153
OOP see Out of Programme years
operation notes 22–5
opioids 62, 82
oral and maxillofacial surgery (OFMS) xv, 160–5, 252
orthopaedic surgery xv, 129, 186–92, 252
  BOTA 239
  courses 97, 191
  dynamic hip screw insertion 37–44
  instruments 7–9
  MSBOS 281
OSCE (Objective Structured Clinical Examinations) 114–15, 116–17
otorhinolaryngology see ENT surgery
Out of Programme years (OOP) 136–7, 174
  fellowships 250–1, 253–4
  maternity leave 220–1
overseas doctors 113, 131, 257
overseas fellowships 253–4
oxygen therapy 60, 82

P value 229
paediatric surgery xv, 171–8, 187
  consent for 290–1
  preoperative investigations 268, 270, 272, 274, 276, 277
pain relief 50, 62, 82
palliative care 69–70
pancreatic drains 55
paracetamol 82
paralytic ileus 66
part-time training 219–20
patient lists 51
patients
  behaviour towards 16, 17, 47, 215
  confirming identity preoperatively 18, 19
  feedback from 203
  safety of 17–22
  see also critically ill patients
pay 244–8
PBA (procedure-based assessment) 109
Pearce v United Bristol (1999) 288
peer assessment tool (mini-PAT) 109
percutaneous endoscopic gastrostomy (PEG) 55
peripheral lines 56
peritoneum, opening 27–8
person specifications 127, 130–5, 136, 157, 209–10
  consultants in colorectal surgery 259–60
personal questions asked at interview 214
personal skills (item in the person specification) 134–5
piles (haemorrhoids) 74–5
plastic surgery xv, 193–200, 252
  MSBOS 280
pledgets 7
PMETB (now part of the GMC) 233–4
pneumothorax 62, 85
Polysorb sutures 12
Pooles suckers 6
portfolios 202–9
  core training years 105, 107–8, 109
  foundation years 94–5, 98–9
  interview questions about 213–14
  presentation 151, 202
postgraduate degrees 138, 151, 196, 197, 231–2

postgraduate schools of surgery 237–8
potassium 82
power of attorney 289
prednisolone 284
pregnancy tests, preoperative 277
preoperative assessment 264–5
 admission checks 283
 ASA grade 265–7
 consent 283, 286–91
 grade of surgery 265
 investigations 14, 265, 268–77
 MSBOS 277–82
 WHO safety checklist 18–20
presentations 150, 207
pressure sores 49, 57
primary survey 67–8, 84–6
private practice 146, 165, 199
prizes 150, 207
probity declaration 205
procedure-based assessment (PBA) 109
proctoscopy 74
professional bodies 113, 233–9
professional integrity (item in the person specification) 135
Prolene sutures 12
psychological assessment (of a patient) 50
publications 108, 150, 188–9, 207, 209, 230
 how to critically review a paper 225–7
pulmonary embolus (PE) 60–1
punch biopsy 75
pus 57
pyrexia 61–2
quality of training, regulation of 233–4
questions asked in interviews 213–17

Rampley sponge holders 2
Ramsey forceps 2, 3
randomised controlled trials (RCTs) 226–7, 229
Raven Department of Education 238
RCS (Royal College of Surgeons) 113, 234–6
recruitment
 academic training 93, 106–7
 application process 201–18
 cardiothoracics 157–8
 consultants 257–63
 core training 101–6
 ENT 168
 foundation training 90–3
 general surgery 143
 interface fellowships 253
 neurosurgery 180–1
 OFMS 163
 orthopaedics 188–9
 paediatrics 172–3
 plastic surgery 195–6
 regional variations 103–4, 126, 129
 specialty training in general 124–36
 urology 151
referees 209
referrals
 to clinics 71–3
 when on-call 79–80
reflective practice 208
registrars 123, 240
 see *also* specialty training
relative risk (RR) 228, 229
relocation expenses 246–9
renal function 49, 56
 preoperative investigations and 267, 270, 272, 274, 276
research 225–32
 academic training 93, 106–7, 231–2
 during core and specialty training 108, 150, 188–9, 196, 231
 getting published 188–9, 230
 higher degrees 138, 151, 196, 231–2
 how to critically review a paper 225–7
 interview questions about 215, 225–30
 OOP 137
 recorded in the portfolio 207, 209
research skills (item in the person specification) 133
respiratory system
 postoperative complications 49, 60–1
 preoperative assessment and investigations 264, 267, 269, 271, 273, 275
 in the primary survey 68, 85
resuscitation
 patients admitted whilst on-call 80–8
 patients on a ward 67–8
retractors 5
revision 14, 112–13
ring handled spikes 7, 8

Royal College of Surgeons (RCS) 113, 234–6

SAC (Specialty Advisory Committee) 237
salaries 244–8
scalpel handles 7, 8
schools of surgery 237–8
scissors 2–3
Scotland 113, 129, 234
scrubbing up 15
secondary survey 86–8
sensitivity (statistics) 228
sick patients
  admitted on-call 80–8
  courses on
    management of 96, 119
  postoperative 66–70
sickle cell disease/trait 277, 284
Sidaway v Bethlem Royal Hospital (1985) 288
sigmoidoscopy
  flexible 73
  rigid 74
silk sutures 12
Silver Scalpel Award 239
skill sets needed by good surgeons xii
smoking 265
So You Want to be an Orthopaedic Surgeon? course 97
specialist registrars (SpR) 123, 240
Specialty Advisory Committee (SAC) 237
specialty registrars (StR) 123
specialty training 122–39
  academic training within 137, 231–2
  cardiothoracic surgery 157–9
  ENT surgery 168–70
  general surgery 143–6
  neurosurgery 180–5
  OFMS 163–4
  orthopaedic surgery 188–90
  paediatric surgery 172–7
  plastic surgery 195–8
  urology 151–4
specificity 228
spinal boards 88
spinal surgery 187
ST3 posts see specialty training
standard deviation 228
START Surgery course 96
statement of health and probity 205–6
statistics 227, 228–9
STEP (Surgeons in Training Education Programme) courses 95, 119–20
steroids 284
students xiii–xiv
suckers 5–6
surgical instruments 1–9
surgical site infection bundle 20
surgical tutors 236
Surgipro sutures 12
sutures 10–12, 13
swab-on-a-stick 2
syllabus for core surgical training 110–11, 238

T-tubes 54, 75
TAB (team assessment of behaviour) 98
tachycardia 62
take handovers 51–3
teaching
  interview questions about 216
  in the portfolio 95, 99, 108, 208
  on ward rounds 47
team assessment of behaviour (TAB) 98
teamwork
  interview questions about 215
  on-call 78–9, 84
  in theatre 14, 15
  during ward rounds 47
terminal patients 69–70
thank-you letters 208
theatre etiquette 12–17
  patient safety 17–22
thromboprophylaxis 20, 50
Tilley–Henkel forceps 9
toffee hammers 9
training programme directors (TPDs) 236
transfusions 68, 80–1
transplant fellowships 253
transplant surgery 142, 159
trauma fellowships 252
trauma surgery xv, 187, 189–90
  courses 118, 146
  emergency admissions 83–8
travel expenses 249
Travers retractors 5, 6
tubes 53–6, 75, 86
type I/II errors 227

ulcers, foot 57
United States of America 254
upper limb surgery 187
urinary catheters 56, 86
urological assessment 49, 56
  preoperative investigations and 267, 270, 272, 274, 276
urology xvi, 148–55
  MSBOS 281
  paediatric 177

VAC dressings 58
vascular surgery 141–2, 145
  investigations and procedures 76
  MSBOS 279
venous duplex 76
venous thromboembolism, prophylaxis 20, 50
Vicryl sutures 12
Volkmann spoons 7, 8

Wales 129
ward rounds 45–50
warfarin 50, 284
West retractors 5
withholding of consent by minors 290
withholding treatment in terminal cases 69
women in surgery 221–4
  part-time training 219–21
work-based assessments 98–9, 109, 121, 174, 207
working hours 153, 241–3
World Health Organization (WHO) safety checklist 18–22
wounds
  closure methods 10–12, 29, 35, 44
  complications 57, 62–4
  drains 55
  dressings 58–60
  healing 56–7

Yankauer suckers 6